THE VARIETIES OF
PSYCHEDELIC EXPERIENCE

THE CLASSIC GUIDE TO THE EFFECTS OF LSD ON THE HUMAN PSYCHE

ROBERT MASTERS, Ph.D.
and JEAN HOUSTON, Ph.D.

Park Street Press
Rochester, Vermont

For Our Parents

Katherine Masters	Mary Houston
Col. Robert Masters	Jack Houston

Park Street Press
One Park Street
Rochester, Vermont 05767
www.InnerTraditions.com

Park Street Press is a division of Inner Traditions International

Library of Congress Cataloging-in-Publication Data

Masters, Robert E. L.
    The varieties of psychedelic experience : the classic guide to the effects of LSD on the human psyche / by Robert Masters and Jean Houston.
        p. cm.
    ISBN 0-89281-897-2 (alk. paper)
    1. LSD (Drug) I. Houston, Jean. II. Title.

BF209.L9 .M3 2000
154.4—dc21

00-026625

Printed and bound in Canada

10 9 8 7 6 5 4 3 2

Contents

Preface

Almost thirty-five years have passed since *The Varieties of Psychedelic Experience* was first published. Jean and I wrote it together during the months just after we were married and, unlike a great many book collaborations, we were almost completely in agreement about what we would say and how we wanted to say it. The collaboration was further enhanced by a tiny and immensely devoted Siamese cat named Psychedelic who sat on my right shoulder while I was typing and seemed to purr and occasionally to tread when I was making my best points.

We had each been involved in research with psychedelics for quite a few years before writing the book—my work beginning in 1954—at first working independently, then working together as a research team. It was of great interest to discover that many of the observations each of us had made working independently were very similar or even identical.

The so-called Drug War was unheard of in those days and there was great excitement and often enthusiasm surrounding the work with psychedelics, especially LSD-25. Thousands of papers had been published in scientific journals describing psychotherapeutic and other work with LSD. Although Timothy Leary and a few other self-anointed messiahs were already generating some opposition, in general the public mind at least remained open concerning the value of psychedelic research. The Drug War would all but destroy that open-mindedness, and even criminalize work with psychedelics, but it had not yet done so and many agreed with us that LSD and some similar substances provided unparalleled access to a great variety of mental processes and to the personal unconscious with its rich images and many other treasures. Some agreed that this included openings also into the collective unconscious and into dimensions where access usually is given only to those who achieve it by means of deep, intense, and prolonged psychophysical and psychospiritual disciplines.

Shortly after *Varieties* was published we picked up a copy of the Sunday *New York Times* and found to our delight that we had been given the front page of the *New York Times Book Review*—something that almost guaranteed many other book reviews and a substantial audience for the book. The review was written by a psychiatrist not altogether friendly to LSD research and he described the book as "offering a whole new system of psychopathology." He mostly praised the book as a serious and important study but generally hewed to the line that the psychedelic experience was pathological. That view, which has been espoused by most psychiatrists who first worked with LSD, had been abandoned by many at the time. The label "psychotomimetic (mimicking a psychosis) had already largely been replaced by the term "psychedelic" (mind-manifesting), which was proposed by the distinguished British psychiatrist Humphry Osmond after he collaborated with Aldous Huxley on a term that could gain widespread acceptance while escaping negative meanings.

The *Varieties of Psychedelic Experience* was in fact very widely and favorably reviewed in many different kinds of publications, including scientific ones, and in many countries. Besides making the book well-known, these reviews had the effect of bringing to the door of our New York City apartment quite a large number of interesting and diverse visitors. They included a spectrum of psychotherapists, scientists of various sorts, philosophers, theologians, psychiatrists, other physicians and psychologists, swamis of yoga and Tibetan lamas, Zen Buddhists and Sufis, anthropologists, authors and artists, and even an occasional offer of funding for new research. Clearly the interest in psychedelics was worldwide and included a host of exceptionally intelligent and learned people from many different occupations and areas of interest. In the case of the artists, a movement of sorts was being born and we eventually described it in another book, *Psychedelic Art*.

SOME CONCLUSIONS AND RECOMMENDATIONS

It has been said of the ancient Persians that when they had some matter of real importance to consider they went over it once while sober and a second time while in an intoxicated state. Then they made their decision based on the best thinking and understandings gleaned from the two approaches. If a matter was important, they felt, it should not be examined solely by means of *ordinary* states of consciousness.

Herodotus, who speaks of this, does not say just what kind of intoxicant was used. It could have been alcohol, since there are many ways of using that substance which are little if at all known to people at present. The ancient religious uses, for example, call attention once again to the extreme importance of set and setting. But the Persians might have used some other substance to achieve their altered or intoxicated states of consciousness.

In *The Varieties of Psychedelic Experience* we wrote that psychedelics such as LSD "afford the best access yet to the contents and processes of the human mind." Removed now from that conclusion by more than three decades, I find no reason to alter it. And I would add that there is an *enormous* range of valuable applications of psychedelics which has not been explored because of our society's failure to recognize the constructive possibilities. As matters stand, it well may occur that all of those persons who became experienced in the very complicated work with psychedelics will die of old age before our society gains enough maturity and wisdom to let the work proceed. Alas, very few understand the magnitude of that loss.

When it finally happens that psychedelic research—left sufficiently free to realize the potentials—is permitted, then that freedom must include an agreement that *under no circumstances must it be monopolized by psychiatrists.* Psychologists, philosophers, theologians, anthropologists, artists, scientists, engineers—those from many different disciplines and fields—must be allowed to contribute to the body of knowledge that will be generated. Given the range and diversity of the psychedelic experience—and truly nothing human is alien to it—*investigation must be multidisciplinary if it is not to be warped and stunted.* And we must understand and agree that some of this work will be *exploration,* not subject to the kinds of constraints imposed if it were to be more narrowly defined.

I will mention just a few areas where work with psychedelics seems to me to be most promising. These include research into the levels and dimensions of consciousness; psychotherapy; creative process and problem-solving; neural and sensory reeducation; nature and regulation of pain; enhancement of pleasure, including sexual pleasure; expanded awareness of self and world, including aesthetic appreciation; paranormal capacities; exploration of the worlds of myth and religion; and the pursuit of self-knowledge and personal growth, including perhaps some sanctioned "rites of passage."

Psychotherapy. Few people now remember that by 1965 there had appeared in scientific journals well over two thousand papers describing treatment of thirty to forty thousand patients with psychedelics. There were additional reports from hundreds of psychotherapists working in many of the countries and cultures of the world, and therapy with psychedelics continued to proliferate on into the 1970s, up to the time when prohibited. Many different kinds of patients were successfully treated, often in just a few sessions, including—ironically—alcohol and other drug addicts, along with habitual criminals, sexual deviates, violence-prone individuals, and people suffering from chronic anxiety states, depression, and many other disorders of the kinds with which therapists frequently must deal.

In more recent years other kinds of mind-altering substances have been employed, including, notably for its therapeutic potentials, the "empathogen" MDMA (or "Ecstasy"). MDMA, before being banned by a drug prohibition reflex, proved itself to be the most effective tool ever available for "couples therapy." It is now possible to develop other substances which might be highly specific for various kinds of problems, but in the present climate those too would be prohibited—"criminalized."

As one experienced in both psychotherapy and work with psychedelics, I am unequivocally certain that the success rates in therapy could be increased, and treatments shortened, by means of substances such as LSD and MDMA. I also have no doubt that such work would stimulate new and more effective therapeutic methods.

Consciousness Research. Under this heading I would include explorations of different states of consciousness and their characteristic phenomena, along with most of the territories usually assigned to psychology and related disciplines. This includes perception and mind-body relationships, but it also includes a great deal of experience which psychologists rarely attempt to examine—religious and spiritual dimensions, for example.

The use of psychedelics to investigate "mind" has frequently been likened to the use of a telescope in astronomy and a microscope in medicine. One often is able to focus on particular psychodynamic phenomena and observe them in a kind of isolated and naked state that has proved extremely useful. Mind-body interactions are often very easy to demonstrate—particularly because of the unwavering intensity with which consciousness may be focused on images of (or symbolizing) body parts and functions. Consciousness Research is a field of inquiry so vast that its limits must be arbitrarily imposed, if there are to be any limits.

Problem-solving and Creative Process. Psychedelics offer a means of gaining new creative insights into almost any kind of problem and there is considerable evidence that psychedelic experience also stimulates the creative process in many people. The problem-solving and/or new insight possibilities of psychedelics are such that they could probably increase the creativity and productivity of any culture or smaller unit in which their skilled use was encouraged.

Much more could be said, but let us go back to the Persians and share their insightful recognition that important matters should never be left just to ordinary states of consciousness and their belief- and habit-limited mental and perceptual processes. We are at a time when existing as well as new and unexplored psychedelics could be providing important understandings and knowledge so urgently needed by our people and our planet. Given the multitude of our problems, how foolish and how tragic it is to deny ourselves such treasures of experience and such vehicles of multifaceted empowerment. And, of course, psychedelics offer experiences of such wonder and beauty that no wise and benevolent society should fail to find ways to make them accessible.

Robert Masters, Ph.D.

The Varieties of
Psychedelic Experience

One:
Some Varieties of the
Psychedelic Experience

The once impenetrable mysteries of matter have begun to unfold and to point to consequences still incomprehensible to thought and beyond the farthest reaches of vision. Unlocked by such keys as the work of Einstein and Heisenberg the gates of the physical universe open upon possibilities that already have resulted in the drastic transformation of man's position not only with respect to his own planet, but also to the measureless vastness around it.

Now, as research advances, the psychedelic (mind-manifesting) drugs give promise of providing access to another of the great and hitherto largely impenetrable realms—the vast, intricate, and awesome regions we call *mind*. Our own research, which will be described here, like all other research in this area, can be no more than an early, tentative exploration. Even so, we hope to make entirely credible our belief that the psychedelic drugs afford the best access yet to the contents and processes of the human mind.

Much already has been written about the psychedelic drugs as they have been used in the treatment of severely disturbed individuals. The present volume, however, is principally concerned with the psychedelic drug-state as it is experienced by the comparatively normal individual—

3

the "average person" rather than the psychotherapist's patient. It is, then, the remarkable range and richness of the inner life of normal individuals, as revealed in purposeful, controlled drug sessions, that will be described. And the effort will be made to detail means by which the average person may pass through new dimensions of awareness and self-knowledge to a "transforming experience" resulting in actualization of latent capacities, philosophical reorientation, emotional and sensory at-homeness in the world, and still other changes beneficial to the person. We also will try to make unmistakably clear the enormous potential importance of psychedelic research for many scholarly and scientific disciplines. And, while our major concern has not been with exploring the many implications for therapy, we believe so abundant and novel a detailing of the contents and processes of mind cannot fail to interest those whose business is the mind in its various conditions of distress. Especially, this may be the case since the data so strongly suggest a tendency or impetus towards self-actualization, that can be set into motion and then may carry the person to a high degree of self-fulfill-ment in the psychedelic drug experience.

The dimensions of human fantasy life revealed here should, we think, have a liberating effect upon many persons who may find a greater degree of self-acceptance once they have understood what a complicated being is man and how many and varied are his ideas, imaginings and tendencies, in health as well as in sickness. We hope that equally beneficial will be this first detailed presentation of a Western-oriented, non-mystical phenomenology and approach to the direction of the psychedelic session.

That there are dangers in the use of these drugs is something we very well appreciate and many of those dangers will be pointed out and described. However, where we think alleged dangers have been exag-gerated or otherwise misrepresented, that aspect, too, will be discussed. Here, we will remark that we emphatically do not agree with those who would make these drugs available to everyone, or almost everyone, to use under any conditions at all. The psychedelic experience is one that has to be responsibly directed if it is to be of maximum benefit to the drug subject. The same responsible direction should eliminate the dan-ger of psychological damage to the subject and should minimize the frequency as well as the intensity of some painful experiences always possible in the drug-state and which we will discuss along with the other phenomena.

To be hopeful and optimistic about the psychedelic drugs and their potential is one thing; to be messianic is another. Both the present and the future of psychedelic research already have been grievously injured by a messianism that is as unwarranted as it has proved undesirable. The present work, then, should be understood as hopeful and optimistic, but realistic.

The materials here presented are based upon first-hand observation of 206 drug sessions and upon interviews with another 214 persons who have been volunteer subjects, psychotherapy patients, or who have obtained and taken the drugs on their own. Our own work, covering a combined total of more than fifteen years, has been very largely with two of the psychedelic drugs: LSD-25 and peyote.[1] The former is a synthetic chemical substance more lengthily known as d-lysergic acid diethylamide. The latter is a cactus plant (*Lophophora williamsii*) found in the American Southwest and contains a number of alkaloids, the best known and most important of these being mescaline.

LSD and peyote are potent psycho-chemicals that alter and expand the human consciousness. Even the briefest summation of the psychological effects of these drugs would have to include the following: Changes in visual, auditory, tactile, olfactory, gustatory, and kinesthetic perception; changes in experiencing time and space; changes in the rate and content of thought; body image changes; hallucinations; vivid images—eidetic images—seen with the eyes closed; greatly heightened awareness of color; abrupt and frequent mood and affect changes; heightened suggestibility; enhanced recall or memory; depersonalization and ego dissolution; dual, multiple, and fragmentized consciousness; seeming awareness of internal organs and processes of the body; upsurge of unconscious materials; enhanced awareness of linguistic nuances; increased sensitivity to nonverbal cues; sense of capacity to communicate much better by nonverbal means, sometimes including the telepathic; feelings of empathy; regression and "primitivization"; apparently heightened capacity for concentration; magnification of character traits and psychodynamic processes; an apparent nakedness of psychodynamic processes that makes evident the interaction of ideation, emotion, and perception with one another and with inferred unconscious processes; concern with philosophical, cosmological, and religious questions; and, in general, apprehension of a world that has slipped the chains of normal categorical ordering, leading to an intensified interest in self and world and also to a range of responses moving from extremes of anxiety to extremes of pleasure. These are not the only effects of the psychedelic drugs, but the listing should suffice to convey some idea of the potency of the drugs and the range of the experiences they afford.

Concerning our use of the term "psychedelic," meaning mind-manifesting, first proposed in this connection by Humphry Osmond, we have used it in preference to such other current terms as "hallucinogenic" and "psychotomimetic" (mimicking a psychosis) because it is both more accurate and less pejorative than those others. And while it may be vague, "psychedelic" does have the merit of being comprehensive. We will make occasional use, when appropriate, of the terms "hallucinogenic" and "psychotomimetic," since it is true that hallucinatory and psychosis-like phenomena do emerge in some of the drug sessions. But the main interest of the authors should be understood to lie in exploring the full range of the consciousness-*changing* aspects of the psychedelic experience and in recording the phenomenology of that experience.

Turning now to the forthcoming examples of psychedelic drug experiences, it is not possible to say that they are "typical." Every such experience is in many significant ways very *individual* and depends for its structure and content upon what the subject brings to the session in the way of personal history and frame of reference—"who he is" at that time. The other principal determinants of the experience will be the physical environment and the other person or persons present, most notably the *guide* conducting the session. The drug itself makes certain experiences possible; but rarely would it be accurate to say that the drug in any other sense determined a particular experience.

Finally, before passing on to the examples, something should be said about the remarkably high quality of the writing of those drug subjects who have given us first-person accounts of their psychedelic experiences. In many cases, the style is worthy of a professional author and the idea content is almost equally impressive. As others before us have noted, this surprising display of literary talent is not at all uncommon among former psychedelic subjects writing accounts of their experiences, and we think the reasons for it are clear. First of all, the subject has had what he regards as an enormously impressive and important experience and this valuation of the experience provides a very high degree of motivation to describe the session well and to try to convey to others the details, flavor, and impact of what occurred. Also, the psychedelic experience almost always is so unusual and richly various that all the materials are at hand for a vivid prose statement that requires no imagination to construct while, at the same time, the contents seem to the writer to rival the creative productions of even the most imaginative authors. In the case of our own subjects, it is relevant, too, that many were persons of superior intelligence and considerable education. Moreover, many were educators, clergymen, attorneys, and other such persons whose day-to-day work demands a fairly high degree of verbal facility.

Example No. 1. This contains no especially unusual elements but does describe a good many of the more common components of the psychedelic experience. Of particular interest is the summation by the subject (S), at the end of his account, of the reasons why he considers the term "consciousness-expanding" to be warranted.

S, a thirty-six-year-old assistant professor of English literature, had his peyote session in the company of the guide and S's wife, neither of whom took the drug. Several pre-session interviews and some correspondence and other reading had prepared S for his experience and eliminated misconceptions and most of the anxiety concerning it. S's own account follows:

"My peyote experience began in a house on a farm in the rugged hill country of Northwest Arkansas. A kind of tea had been brewed from the green 'buttons' or tops of the cactus plants and I had no trouble consuming an amount the guide told me was sufficient. The Dramamine I took ahead of time apparently was instrumental in keeping the hour or so of nausea within manageable proportions.

"Apart from this nausea and some feelings of being alternately too hot and too cold, no effects of the drug were noticeable for about one and one-half hours from the time of consumption. Then I suddenly became extremely aware of the croaking of frogs and then of the chirping of crickets. The former came from a stream about a block or so away from the house but sounded very close and I fancied that the frogs had come down to stand before the door and serenade me.

"Darkness had come on almost unnoticed and my attention was first called to the dimness of the light when my wife got up to turn on a small lamp that was standing on a table in one corner of the room. Very shortly after this I saw moving toward me across the room a ball of red fire about the size of a golf ball. It drifted, swaying a little from side to side, while moving toward me at about the level of my shoulders as I was seated in a chair. I felt no uneasiness, only interest, and when the ball of fire had come close enough I poked at its center with my finger. It then exploded, a lavish shower of multicolored sparks cascading and dropping on the rug at my feet. I smiled happily at the others and remarked: 'It has started. Now let's see what kind of traveler I am going to make.'

"Ever since I first had heard of the peyote I had wanted to observe the effects of such a drug on myself. I sought no particular experience but I expected to have a happy and interesting time and also possibly to learn a good bit about my own psychology. The beautiful images some writers have described were something I hoped would be a part of my experience. While outside the house were lovely natural surroundings that later I planned to explore.

"To see if the images would come I closed my eyes and perceived at first a succession of geometric forms, mostly circles and triangles. The colors were soft pastels and aroused in me a kind of emotional warmth that encompassed my wife, the guide and all of my surroundings and remained with me throughout most of the session. This warmth was accompanied by a sensation of relaxing muscles, although the mind kept very much alert and alive. Then began the images I had wanted to see, brilliantly colored and drenched in white and golden light. Also, objects in the images seemed to generate a light of their own and cast off glowing and pulsating or rippling waves of color. The first image I remember was of an Egyptian tomb made of granite, alabaster and marble. Behind it great golden sculptures of pharaohs rose to awesome heights and there was the fragrance of eucalyptus burning in brass bowls mounted upon tripods of iron that had the feet of falcons. Priests in ornate headdress ringed the tomb and raised their arms to greet a procession of many brightly robed figures bearing torches and with faces obscured by masks resembling the heads of various beasts. Funerary orations seemed to blend into marriage ceremonies where fruit and great platters of meat, even the forbidden pig, were served up by fierce glistening black slaves. The platters were placed upon massive stone steps leading to a dais upon which were seated royal figures in carved black chairs whose arms were the heads of solemn cats.

"From a distance, after that, I saw pyramids and knew that in one of these the ceremony just observed was unfolding. But the pyramids were transformed into haystacks, golden under a huge red sun, and then these became dunes in a great desert. Here, tents were clustered half-buried by swirling stinging sands. Inside one of these, in appropriate garb, my wife and I were seated on pillows of camel's hair. Girls in filmy garments were dancing, their dark eyes flashing above gleaming white teeth. There were tambourines, a drum, and strange stringed instruments, playing a music I could hear and that seemed intended to lay bare and set quivering the elemental passions of the listeners. Swarthy, scowling, bearded men were ranged near the tent's entrance. They had black, glaring eyes, wore daggers, and some held naked swords in lean weather-beaten hands.

"In many of the images that came to me I saw myself, sometimes with my wife, more often alone. I was a fur-capped Mongol huntsman, cold-eyed and cruel, bow in hand, striking down a running rabbit from the back of a racing, gaunt half-wild stallion. I was a stark black-robed figure, protected by an amulet suspended from a heavy gold chain that was worn about my neck, somberly wandering, lost in bitter ascetic reflection, among the crumbling walls of old temples overgrown by thick, twisted and gnarled vines. At other times there were legions of warriors, darkening deserts or in ranks that extended across immense bone-littered plains. There were brown-cowled monks, pacing cloisters in silent, shared but unadmitted desperation. Image after image after image, flowing in succession more rapid than I would have wished, but all exquisitely detailed and with colors richer and more brilliant than those either nature or the artist has yet managed to create.

"Again and again I returned to the images, so numerous I could not begin to recount them, but in between times many other curious phenomena came to my attention. So extended was time that once it seemed to me I lighted a cigarette, smoked it for hours, looked down and noticed that the cigarette still had its first ash. A few moments were hours, possibly longer, and any one event seemed to take almost no time at all. I remarked to my wife that 'We are out of time, but that is not to say that time has run out.' What I meant was that, in the moment when I spoke, time's fingers had ceased their nervous, incessant strumming upon the space that contained us. But that space was—how can one put it?—*irregular*. A space that expanded and contracted and imposed upon us (actually, of course, upon *me*) the arbitrary quickening rhythms of its pulsations. For, as I remarked, this timeless space was a bubble, and would burst. Then I experienced a dull sort of sadness, since I wanted to remain forever out of time. Or, if not that, then in a world of moments which, like those I was experiencing, were enormously extended. I wanted to know that those moments would not, in some instant to be dreaded, snap back like an elastic drawn out for a while but then released as if God were punishing some pleasure so great as to be an unforgivable transgression.

"I believe it was simultaneous with this that I became aware of the body that encased me as being very heavy and amorphous. Inside it, everything was stirring and seemed to be drawing me inward. I felt that I could count the beats, the throbbing of my heart, feel the blood moving through my veins, feel the passage of the breath as it entered and left the body, the nerves as they hummed with their myriad messages. Above all, I was conscious of my brain as teemingly alive, cells incredibly active, and my mental processes as possessing the unity of perfect precision. Yet this last, I suspected, was not really true and instead my mind, 'drunk on its own ideas,' was boastfully over-estimating its prowess.

"Sensations were acute. I heard, saw, felt, smelled and tasted more fully than ever before (or since). A peanut butter sandwich was a delicacy not even a god could deserve. Yet, I took only a few bites and was too full to eat more. To touch a fabric with one's fingertip was to simultaneously know more about both one's fingertip and the fabric than one had ever known about either. It was also to experience intense touch-pleasure and this was accentuated even further when, at the guide's suggestion, I 'localized consciousness' in the fingertip with the consequence that all phenomena at that point were greatly enhanced.

"I took my wife's hand and it seemed to me a great force of love flowed through my hand into hers, and also from her hand into mine, and that then this love was diffused throughout our bodies. Her smile, her whole face was beautiful beyond description, and I wondered if I would be able to see her like this when the drug experience had ended.

"Together we walked to one end of the room, where a large reproduction of Rousseau's *Sleeping Gypsy* was hanging on the wall. Try as I might I could not at that time decide if the Gyspy was a man or a woman, but my wife said 'A man,' and I accepted her judgment. Studying the bulging-eyed beast in that painting, I saw that its mane is all dendrites and energy pulses through each branch and is transmitted to the brain of the sleeping Gypsy. The beast seemed to be sniffing, while the moon shimmered and winked and smiled, and the strings of the instrument that lay upon the ground were plucked by an invisible hand. I saw that in the painting gray-green waters never stir to wash upon brown sands. The sleep of the Gypsy was endless. The beast hovered, rooted forever in its place, and the life that I now breathed into that scene gave new life to me but not to those figures transfixed in captive immortality projected by a brain long since gone to its rest and returned to the dust. Better, I said, to be a live beholder than to be a great artist in his grave. Better life, than to be an immortal but immobile Gypsy or moon or sea or beast. My life suddenly seemed to me infinitely precious and I cried out with joy at the thought that I was now living so much in so short a span of time.

"Later, we walked in the woods and by the river and it seemed that my love was so great it evoked a response from animals, birds and plants, and even from inanimate things. On the river bank, as the sky began to brighten, I threw my arms around my wife and at once the birds broke into a song that bespoke a universal harmony always existing but requiring that one approach it in a certain way before it can reveal itself. The silver-surfaced river, bathed in fresh dawnlight, reflected trees reaching down as if yearning toward the heart of the earth. The leaves of the trees were as intricately patterned as great snowflakes and at other times resembled webs spun by God-inspired spiders of a thread of unraveled emeralds. The beauty of nature was such that I cannot describe it, although I have managed to retain some measure of the *feeling* it awakened in me.

"Along with all this there were torrents of ideas, some amplifications of my own past thinking, but others that were strange and entered my mind as if from without. At the house, when we returned and the effects were much less, it seemed to me that what I had experienced was essentially, and with few exceptions, the usual content of experience but that, of everything, there was MORE. This MORE is what I think must be meant by the 'expansion of consciousness' and I jotted down at that time something of this MORE I had experienced.

"The consciousness-expanding drugs, I wrote then, enable one to sense, think and feel MORE.

"Looking at a thing one sees MORE of its color, MORE of its detail, MORE of its form.

"Touching a thing, one touches MORE. Hearing a sound, one hears MORE. Tasting, one tastes MORE. Moving, one is MORE aware of movement. Smelling, one smells MORE.

"The mind is able to contain, at any given moment, MORE. Within consciousness, MORE simultaneous mental processes operate without any one of them interfering with the awareness of the others. Awareness has MORE levels, is many-dimensioned. Awareness is of MORE shades of meaning contained in words and ideas.

"One feels, or responds emotionally with MORE intensity, MORE depth, MORE comprehensiveness.

"There is MORE of time, or within any clock-measured unit of time, vastly MORE occurs than can under normal conditions.

"There is MORE empathy, MORE unity with people and things.

"There is MORE insight into oneself, MORE self-knowledge.

"There are MORE alternatives when a particular problem is considered, MORE choices available when a particular decision is to be made. There are MORE ways of 'looking at' a thing, an idea or a person . . ."

In an appraisal of the effects of his session, made about five months later, S said that his view of the psychedelic experience as "essentially a MORE" still seemed to him to be valid. What he had "carried away from" his session was "above all a feeling of very great enrichment." He retained "a more acute awareness of color, a much increased appreciation of the great beauty of my wife, and a wonderful awareness of the almost infinite detail that objects will yield up if only one will give them one's attention."

Most important of all, S thought, was "the knowledge and certainty I now have that it is truly possible to attain to a sense of harmony with all creatures and things." He felt that this sense of harmony as he had experienced it during his session provides the person with "a strength, serenity and capacity for loving not possible when the experience of harmony is wanting." S was having some success at "re-invoking" the harmonious state and making it a part of his everyday life. He felt that this must be done without the "invaluable help of peyote which shows one the way but then, quite properly, leaves one to follow that way through one's own efforts. This has to be so, since the way pointed out has its application in this world, not in the peyote wonder-world." S added that his experiencing of the "universal harmony and what it confers was the richest single event of my session and probably, also, of my life."[2]

In evaluating the session just described, we regarded it as being a very positive and pleasant one for the subject. However, it was not one of those more profound experiences met with in the drug-state in which the subject confronts himself on the deepest levels of his being, receives some basic insight or understanding, and emerges transformed in some fundamental way.

Possibly these deeper levels were not reached because the subject had no *need* to reach them. His adjustment already was superior and this is reflected in the thoroughly wholesome or healthy-minded character of his session. Few psychedelic experiences are so free of "negative" elements as this one, although *all* of our subjects had to meet such basic requirements as: 1) successful present functioning; 2) absence of detectable signs of psychosis or serious neurosis; 3) absence of past history of major mental illness; and 4) adequate preparation for and positive expectations concerning the drug experience.

We would add that when these and a few other preconditions are met and when the session is adequately managed, the chances of any subject's "getting into trouble" are reduced to very slight proportions.

Example No. 2. The second example to be presented is of an unguided "session." The "subject" was, of course, not observed during his experience, but he was interviewed subsequently on several occasions and at length. He also submitted a written report of his experience.

We present an example of an unguided drug experience both so that it may be compared in certain respects with the examples of guided ones and because it illustrates some of the more common painful and delusive varieties of ideation and perception met with in the sessions. Most of these negative aspects will not be found in the other examples given in this chapter, but will be further exemplified and discussed later on. In general, the negative aspects of the experience occur less often and in much milder form in the properly guided session than in the unguided or mismanaged one.

In this case, S, a male university student, age twenty-two, obtained a supply of LSD by "borrowing" it from his older brother, a physician. He took a very strong dose of the drug (estimated afterwards to have been 400 to 500 micrograms) and experienced what he believes was a "transient psychosis." The following is a condensed account by S of his experience:

"I had been thinking for some time about having some LSD. I finally made a decision and at about nine o'clock in the morning I went to the refrigerator where my brother kept a supply and took what I thought would be a sufficient amount. The amount, as I soon discovered, was more than sufficient! For the next ten hours I moved through a world that sometimes was beautiful and intensely interesting, but more often resembled a nightmare. For four of those hours I seem to have an almost complete amnesia. The experience as a whole I regard as a temporary psychotic distortion of consciousness.

"The experience did not begin badly. At first there was a very strange sense that all perception and abstract cognition had become kinesthetic—that these were no more than extensions of one's neuromuscular being. Then came a profound sense of the tragic and comical aspects of life, with a sense of walking around inside of my own brain.

"I closed my eyes and at once there appeared to me a great variety of Egyptian motifs, statues and *bas relief* forms with a rigorous symmetry. Everything was very precise and geometrical. When I opened my eyes and looked at the objects around me, it was as if they were made of tallow and were melting. There was a drippiness of colors, and it also seemed that these things might be made of waxen candy. It occurred to me that this was probably due not only to my heightened awareness of objects, but also to the liquid in my eyes that now imparted to everything a liquid coating. Along with these perceptions there was the sense of the intense sensuality of oneself, an extremely luxurious sensuality.

"I had several hallucinations that I recognized as such. At one point elves appeared and accepted me as a jolly fellow spirit. They spoke to me in verse and wanted to guide me to magical places—to castles and mythological realms. Many different personalities, all of them part of oneself, became autonomous and spoke of various things. There was a great concern with personal destiny and a sense that the total attention and concern of the universe was focused upon me. I thought that I was participating in a test, was being observed, and that the observing forces were benevolent. All people seemed to me to be no more than simply different forms of oneself, different masks of oneself. They were all of the different lives that one has, or that one is to live. And there was the sense that the world has no greater claim to substance than does a dream; that all authority, all validity rests with oneself and the world is entirely one's possession. Later, when I went out, this resulted in a total unconcern for social forms, such as not sitting down on the sidewalk or in the street; for now one knew that the sidewalk was a part of one's brain and one could do with it what one liked.

"My solipsism was accompanied by delusions of grandeur not logically consistent with it, yet reconcilable for the reason that they had a logic of their own. Although I was the All, I participated in the test of living that somehow was connected with the training of the future God. I was awed by the stereoscopic solidity of reality, the sheer substantiality of it all. Yet reality was my own thought and I was struck with wonder that one's thoughts could suddenly become so substantive and stereoscopic. I congratulated myself upon being able to create reality so well. I felt that others should be grateful to me for supporting their existence. I was holding them up, containing them, giving them air. I was benevolent, and did not kick them.

"I went out and walked through the streets where people were experienced as epiphenomena of oneself. They were also waxen mechanical toys, part of a mechanical toy process and were made out of candy. (This may have been because they were seen as having the bright colors of those little candies that are sometimes made in images of persons.) People were an utter absurdity as they went about their rituals, which I contained completely and knew to be absurd in their circularity, unconstructiveness and superstitiousness. But they went about their rituals with a sense of absolute self-righteousness, hilarious zombies who failed to recognize me as the one who beneficently supported their existence. I forgave them for failing to recognize me, knowing them to be as ignorant as children or animals. I took in the world as my private menagerie, a banquet I have provided for myself. It occurred to me to give them commands, but I knew it was better that I respect their ignorance; at the same time I was telling myself: 'You are under drugs and in a psychotic state and had better be as withdrawn and restrained as possible in a world that is liable to blow up if you make the wrong move.'

"The streets bounce, of course. The world is experienced as a physical extension of oneself, of one's own nervous system. Consequently I felt the blows of pick axes wielded by construction men tearing up the street. One possessed a kinesthetic identity with the street, and yet the blows did not hurt. For the street knows in its own being that it is being broken up and yet does not experience the judgment of pleasure or pain. Related to this was an acute awareness of energy in the world. One felt one's body to be supercharged with 'energy,' a word that was variously associated with 'nervous' and 'spirit.' Or it could be associated with tension of the spirit. The other, when it is person, is supercharged with energy like neonized electric generators, sizzling firecrackers as distinguished from the other when it is object and is perceived as static electricity. Only water fountains, among things, have energy. Other objects are frozen.

"The persona of people, I thought, are not to be respected. With this thought, they became the absence of materiality—smiling ghosts. However, they are similar to oneself and therefore are no more to be respected than oneself, or feared or approved of. All of my ideas about politics, religion, state and race were, at this point, embellished. I thought about all of the perversions of myself, by which I meant the rest of humanity. These perversions were not to be hated, just to be pitied and forgotten. They are the dead-end of evolution.

"I noticed that events in the world occurred or started just where one's own thought left off. One could think 'It's getting warm,' and then naturally someone just behind you would say 'It's getting warm.' One always anticipates—no, *knows*—the next stage, the next link in the process, or something in the world may take up at the point anticipated by one's thought. For example, I created a symphonic structure that reached a peak calling for a solo instrument, but there I broke off and at once was answered by an event in the world that was the objective resolution in the world of my subjective harmonies. This event was a man who came up to me and asked 'Are you all right, buddy?' This was the completion of the symphony, and I had anticipated his words and even his very tone of voice.

"A phenomenon of importance under the drug is the non-connective tactile awareness of things that consists of an extension of visual awareness to incorporate tactile awareness into its scope. The substance of a thing was both seen and felt through the visual perception. And along with this there was the sense that one must speak to beauty and commune with beauty in all of its forms, including persons. This included not just pretty girls, but also trees. A major revelation was that of the spiritual nature of trees: the obedient benevolence of trees. One was obliged to commune with them, and with statues. This imperative was part of a larger imperative that seemed to stand out absolutely from all other thought as the one overriding imperative statement: That one must seek God. The beautiful is a part of the imperative that one must approach the Godhead. This was the ultimate procedural prescription. All of the rest of thought was dispensable and this prescription alone could guide one. Related to this was the falling away of all the normal power and authority sanctions and seeming rightness of familiar social and prescriptive forms of behavior and purpose and attitude. These melted away with awareness of what was truly important, valid and authoritative. Since there was no reason not to, I sat down in the middle of a busy sidewalk and let people pass around me. I noticed that mannikins in windows were smiling and Elizabeth Taylor from an enormous poster advertising the film *Cleopatra* several times gestured for me to come to her.

"I got onto the subway thinking that I would ride it to the end of the line. At once these words, 'end of the line,' assumed awesome and multiple proportions. I felt drawn and impelled toward this 'end of the line' where Some Thing was waiting, and beckoning. I felt that I might find there fulfillment or destruction, or both. I recognized now that always at the core of the experience there had been this nightmarish rhythm of acceleration toward some impending unknown. Even so, there was some part of oneself that held to one's sense of mature sobriety.

"I remembered a patient described by my brother. He was schizophrenic, oblivious to circumstances and to his orientation in the world, and concerned himself only with considering what was going on in his head—a 'buzzing' in his head, as if it contained a nest of hornets. Now, with all of the stimuli from the environment swarming in upon me, I also felt my internal state to be one of a vast and buzzing colony of bees. Tingling, vibratory feelings overwhelmed my nervous system and I felt myself lifted upwards toward some unknown bliss or terror.

"I left the subway and lay down on a bench in a park and it was there that I lost my four hours. I had long nightmare dreams that came to me in a state that was different from sleeping but still somehow resembled it. These dreams, I think I have forgotten in self-defense against their horror. Yet I recall that they were just as vivid and real as conscious experience, but had gross although somehow symmetrical distortions as one would go through the same motions countless times. One would walk through the same door again and again, endlessly passing out through the door. There was a sense of the normal world having run riot and that it was now transformed into its antithesis. At other times, I 'awakened' into increasingly incredible and terrifying worlds. It seems to me that giant elevator shafts extended down into the infinite and insane-looking men kept passing into the elevators and coming out again—the same men, over and over. I sensed that I was moving toward some final undefined cataclysm of total damnation, but then awakened into what I supposed was another of the nightmare worlds and discovered that instead it was the 'real world.' The vividness and verisimilitude of the dream world is demonstrated by the length of time it took me to realize that now I was back in the 'real world.' From this point on, the drug intoxication diminished steadily and I made my way back home. Afterwards I felt that I had been in a feverish, drunken state that had left me with a head tied in knots and a feeling of shellshock, or possibly a feeling like that of one who is undergoing withdrawal from a schizophrenic state.

"I felt also that things might have been much worse: That in the drug intoxication one might lose one's sense of balance and be in utter terror and helplessness before the nature of the universe—just as, for instance, should one lose one's sense of gravitational balance, of upness and downness, one would find oneself in terrified estrangement from the normally beneficent, supporting terrestrial environment."

Several things need to be said about S's account of an experience that contained psychosis-like elements if it was not, as he believes, an actual temporary psychosis. First of all, while the drug experience was definitely a very bad one, it also contained (as interviews brought out) a good many positive elements that S has played down in his account and which suggest that the "psychosis" may have been sporadic and intermittent, rather than continuous. It is characteristic of those persons who have painful experiences with psychedelic drugs that they attack the experience with great vehemence. Thus S, in his summation, insists that the "cosmic and mystical unions some drug subjects claim to experience in the drug-state are *always* [our italics] mere chemically imbalanced, epileptic-type states." And that all of the drug-state insights "are the insights of madness, which may or may not be valid but whose validity only can be determined by one in a normal state of consciousness."

The unfortunate experience of this subject almost certainly resulted in the main from several crucial factors. First of all, S would not have been accepted by a responsible researcher as a volunteer subject. Although a very brilliant young man, he has a history of *petit mal* seizures and this alone would have been a basis for disqualification. Secondly, he took the drug with the expectation of experiencing a "model psychosis"; and this expectation, as the scientific literature makes painfully evident, is frequently fulfilled. Third, not only did he have no supportive and directional guidance, but he exposed himself to a variety of stress situations that generated anxiety and accentuated his pathological ideation.

In the following example we offer a first-person account of an LSD experience that was thoroughly pleasurable to the subject, but comparatively innocuous. The drug was administered by a guide who was on hand for the session, but whose role was only to provide support and to deal with difficulties should any arise (as they did not). S, apart from the few tests she was given was allowed complete free rein to experience what she would and her session, although she termed it rewarding, was relatively shallow and in that sense typical of sessions where the guide does no real guiding, only observes and, by his presence, enables the subject to feel more secure than she might feel otherwise.

Example No. 3. S, a twenty-four-year-old university instructor, was given 225 micrograms of LSD. (She had had one previous LSD experience with a 100-microgram dose.) Her account is as follows:

"The experience began in my fourth floor walk-up in Greenwich Village. After the initial physical sensations (a very mild nausea and stiffness of the neck) had passed, I began to notice that the wooden floor had started to ripple. I walked across the floor, climbing up its steep waves and sliding down its inclines. Occasionally, I would catch one of its oaken crests and ride it to the wall in much the same way that a surf rider travels on the waves.

"I looked first at the guide, whose appearance was unchanged, and then at my co-subject R, who was sitting in the lotus position. His well-fringed face was alternately shifting from Christ to satyr, then back to Christ again, and he opened his eyes and came out of his private Nirvana for a moment to say to me: 'Well, this is ιτ! What more is there to say?'

"I directed my attention towards the room and suddenly everything was holy. The stove, and the pottery and the chairs and the record player and the soup ladles and the old bottles—all were touched with sacrality, and I bowed to each of them in turn and worshiped. One pot in particular was so well endowed with divinity I dared not come closer to it than four or five feet lest I be burned to ashes for my unclean lips and impure heart. But a godly peach proved friendlier and accepted my adoration with kindly beneficence, radiating on me the preternatural light of its numinous fuzz. I bowed my gratitude and moved on, transfigured by the deity of things.

"I remember looking at a finely detailed photograph of the Swiss Alps. I had admired this photograph before, in my pre-LSD days an hour or an aeon ago, but now its precision became reality and the temperature plunged and fine crystals of snow whipped across my face and I circled like an eagle above the crags and snowy summits of the mountain top. An expedition of climbers waved up at me and I lifted one talon to wave back.

"I was called back to Greenwich Village by obscenity. A sound, a chant, lascivious and brutal, a whining pornography assaulted my ears and left me furious with moral indignation. "How dare you say things like that to me!" said I to the disembodied chant. It suddenly ended, as quickly as it had begun, and I saw R removing a record which he explained to me was a recording of fertility mantras directed to the goddess Kali. A Bach toccata then was put on the phonograph and the music of the spheres left their archetypal abode and took up residence in the walk-up on——Street.

"It was at this time that I closed my eyes and experienced a vision of the future that unfolded in vivid colors before my closed eyes and was accompanied by voices that were audible, however, only inside my head. I found myself and the rest of mankind standing together on the foothills of the earth, being addressed by two splendid and luminous figures many hundreds of miles high. They could be seen plainly in spite of their height and they told us that they were the elders of this particular part of the cosmos and had lost their patience with the human creatures of this earth. The recalcitrance of greedy, warring, barbarous mankind had overexceeded itself and now that nuclear power had been discovered the outrageous breed evolved on our planet might yet attempt to subvert the whole cosmos. And so it had been decided in the Council of Elders that unless mankind could find something in its creations with which to justify itself, it would have to be destroyed.

"Having heard this message, we earthlings scattered and searched our libraries, museums, histories and parliaments for some achievement that might be seen as a justification for our being. We brought forth our greatest art objects, our Leonardos, Michelangelos, Praxiteles—But the elders only shook their heads and said solemnly: 'It is not sufficient.' We brought forth our great masterpieces of literature, the works of Shakespeare, Milton, Goethe, Dante. But these also were deemed insufficient. We searched in our religious literature and offered the figures of the religious geniuses—Jesus, Buddha, Moses, St. Francis, but the elders only laughed and said: 'Not sufficient.'

"It was then, when destruction seemed imminent and all had given themselves up to their fate, that I came forward and offered to the elders the music of Johann Sebastian Bach. They listened to the entire corpus and great silver tears of incredible brilliance shimmered and trickled down the length of their luminous bodies, after which they were silent. On and on this silence extended, until they broke it to say only: 'It is sufficient. You of the Earth are justified.' And then they went away.

"For a period of time I had neither capacity nor wish to measure, I pondered this vision. Then, when the music had ended, I lay on my back and looked up at the ceiling where a kaleidoscope of images from ancient civilizations flickered rapidly before my eyes. Egypt and Greece, Assyria and old China sped across the ceiling. Flickering pharaohs, fluttering parthenons and a palpitating Nebuchadnezzar—all contributed to this panoramic, historical agitation.

"And suddenly—destruction! The air was thick with the ammonia smell of death. Noxious vapors stung the eyes and choked the throat. The stench of the Apocalypse rose up with the opening of the graves of the new and old dead. It was the nostrils' view of the *Night on Bald Mountain*, an olfactory *Walpurgisnacht* rite. The world had become a reeking decay. Then I heard R rebuking someone with the words: 'Christ, Timmy, couldn't you have used your sandbox?' Timmy was the cat and the apocalyptic smell had issued from a single turd he had deposited in the middle of the floor.

"I turned my attention from Timmy's tangible residues to Timmy himself. He stretched himself with infinite grace and arched his back to begin—*The Ballet*. Leaping through time and space, he hung like Nijinsky—suspended in the air for a millennium, and then, drifting languidly down to the ground, he pirouetted to a paw-licking standstill. He then stretched out one paw in a tentative movement and propelled himself into a mighty spiral, whirling into cosmic dust, then up on his toes for a bow to his creation.

"He was a cat no longer—but Indra, the primeval God dancing the cosmic dance in that time before time, setting up a rhythmic flux in non-being until it at last had attained to Life. The animating waves of the Dance of Creation pulsed all around me and I could no longer refuse to join in the dance. I arose to perform a *pas de deux* with the cat-Indra, but before I could allow myself more than a cursory leap into the cosmic fray a great flame erupted somewhere in the vicinity of my left elbow and I felt obliged to give it my attention. The guide had started a fire burning in the hearth and it commanded I concentrate upon it to the exclusion of all else.

"It was a lovely fire. Mandalas played in it and so did gods, and so did many hundreds of beings, known and unknown, rising in El Greco attenuations for one brilliant moment, only to lapse again into nothing. I fell into musing and after aeons had gone by and worlds within worlds within worlds had been explored, I looked up and said something to R. It was an attempt to define our relationship at that precise moment, and I said: 'You and I, we are ships that sometimes pass one another on the seas but never meet.' 'Bull——!' said R—and my vast, rippling reflections were shattered.

" 'Let's get out of here!' I said. 'Where to?' he asked, and seemed to find his question very funny. 'Where to?' he asked again, convulsed with laughter, and managed to add: 'as if there were any other "where" or "to." ' 'Where to, Bruté?' he howled, and along with our guide we headed for the second-floor apartment of a friend whose roomful of Buddhas I had planned to inspect.

"We began to descend the two flights of stairs and they never ended.

Down, down, down, down, down, down, down—into the bowels of some ultimate cavern—into the center of the earth, no doubt—or perhaps into nowhere—to descend the stairs, forever and ever. 'Will they never end?' I asked, starting to panic. 'Only one more flight,' I was assured. And then, an infinity of stairsteps later, we arrived and entered the roomful of Buddhas and everything brightened.

"The room was a cacophony of Buddhas! Screaming gold Gautamas seared the eye from their sun-spot Satoris. Seething stone saviors revealed a Buddha-to-come in each of their granular particles. Wooden hermaphrodite Lords-of-the-East reconciled all opposites, all dualities, all dialectics. 'Yin, Yang, Jung!' I cried, and dragged R toward another room with a balcony just over the street. But the journey was long, and I felt like Alice when she had to go twice as fast in order just to stay in the same place.

"From the balcony the crowded street leaped up to greet us and it seemed we had only to reach out to touch the passersby. A painted elf skipped past us and I looked after him in astonishment. 'Just a fairy,' R explained. 'I thought it was an elf,' said I—for all double meanings were lost on me. A decrepit old gargoyle tottered by. 'Poor old gargoyle,' said I. 'He can't find his chapel.' And suddenly I felt very sad, for the whole of life became explainable in terms of men losing their potentialities by default and decaying into gargoyles which could yet be happy if only they could find their proper niche—their own flying buttress, overlooking eternity.

"Continuing to observe the scene below from the balcony, it seemed that my consciousness was projected downward, and with it my perceptions, so that I saw the passersby as if I were standing on the sidewalk and confronting them. From this perspective, they became an animated waxworks, escapees from Madame Tussaud, who bit their wax nails, clutched their wax newspapers, and knit their wax brows as they thought waxen thoughts. I kept wondering how long they could keep up this charade before they melted down into puddles and oozed away along the pavement.

"One strange creature approached us slowly, then yawned to reveal little stalagmite clay teeth set in a grotto of red dust. Suddenly, as if just making his decision, he turned and climbed onto a bus. I then noticed that people got on and got off of this bus. On and off. On and off. On and off. The eternal return. Primitive yet Christian. Circular but linear. And the bus plunged ahead along the route of its manifest destiny, then stopped a short distance down the street, while people kept climbing aboard at intervals to catch its life force, but only to be deposited unceremoniously along the byways of their partial, all-too-partial life segments. But where was the bus going? Toward what ultimate destination? Heaven? Fort Tryon Park? Utopia? Perhaps it was a million years away.

"It seemed that a horde of people came bearing down upon us— tides of gray automata threatening to engulf us. 'Don't worry,' I counseled R. 'I shall be Moses.' And, raising my arm, the crowd parted and we were free to enter the Promised Land.

"People continued to stream towards us and past us. I focused on an old lady in her late seventies, a dowdy pathetic creature dressed in shabby black and carrying impossibly huge shopping bags. As she made her way heavily towards us I saw, no longer much to my astonishment, that she began to lose years. I saw her as an Italian matriarch in her sixties, then in her fifties. As she continued to bloom backwards in time, she entered her portly forties and, after that, her housewifely thirties. Her face softened, her body grew more shapely, and still the years kept on dropping away. In her twenties she was carrying a child, and then she was a bride and carried orange blossoms. A moment later and she was a child who, in turn, shrank into a newborn baby carried by a midwife. The baby's umbilical cord was still intact and it let out a howl of awakening life. But then the process was reversed and the baby grew back into childhood, became again a bride, passed through her thirties, forties, fifties, sixties, and was the old lady in her seventies I had seen at the beginning. The old woman blinked, her eyes closed for a fraction of a second, and in that instant I clearly saw her death mask. She passed us by and had moved a little down the street when I heard from the direction she had come a baby's howl of awakening life. I turned my head, expecting to perceive afresh Our Lady of the Eternal Return, but saw instead the vortex of a crowd.

"The vortex was streaming into the giant doorway of a giant building. It atomized into points of energy, radial lights and shimmering vortices converging into a single solar concentration that seethed in thermal fury to explode at last into a kaleidoscopic burst of falling jewels. Some sound had evidently come to my attention and a golden shovel crunched into a mound of opals near which was a sign that bore the incomprehensible words: DIG WE MUST FOR A GROWING NEW YORK. An iron-clad tympany bruised the ears with a raucous counterpoint of digging. Construction, destruction or something was in process and two protean tractors loomed before us, large and living. In their cabs these vital creatures bore little robot mannikins—absurd toy trinkets which undoubtedly they wound up every morning to mimic the motions of life. How proper it all seemed—the Man-machine playing at *noblesse oblige* with the machine—man. But between themselves, the living tractors maintained an uneasy truce. A crystal shelf shattered under the collective impact of their heavy, separate blows. Its sonic vibration stung the nervous system and prepared one for war. The tractors made ready for mutual assault, swinging their shovel-antennae high in the air and bellowing metallic curses at one another. Dive and attack! Attack and dive! But then their clanging vituperations acquired a primeval resonance. Voices were screaming from out of an early swamp. And I saw that the warring tractors were warring dinosaurs, their long necks diving and attacking in sinuous combat. 'Too much!' I thought, and with what seemed a great effort of will I returned through the centuries to—— Street.

"We continued our vigil from the terrace, but now I looked down on the scene below as if from a very high place. I chanced to observe a particularly rough square of pavement and what I saw there caused me to cry out to R to come over and share in this latest wonder. For there below us in that square of pavement lay all of Manhattan—its canyons, and skyscrapers and parks and people—laid out beneath us in miniature. The proportions, the infinite detail were perfect. We could have been in an airplane flying low over the city. But here it was in a common block of pavement—the city within the city. We could have swooped down like gods and lifted up the Empire State Building if we had so wished. But our ethics precluded that, and we left the little microcosm as it was.

"And so it went—a ten thousand years'-long adventure condensed somehow into a few brief hours. It all ended very suddenly for me, when a parking meter I was watching abruptly flipped its red Time Expired flag. And I knew it was over."

The account just concluded describes quite a few of the usual phenomena of the psychedelic drug experience. The altered awareness of time is frequently mentioned and is well exemplified in the subject's description of the interminable descent down the stairs. Mood changes abruptly, often in response to awareness of some perceptual stimulus. A great many altered perceptions—visual, auditory, and olfactory—are mentioned. There are vivid eyes-closed images, the empathic experiencing of a picture and the "projection" of consciousness to a point some distance from the body with visual perception appearing to be from that point and not from the actual physical location of the organs of sight.

Making some order out of and deriving something of value from these curious experiences and others like them will be a main concern of this book.

Necessarily, the subject describing a psychedelic experience is able to mention only a very few items selected from the wealth of events that make up the total experience. Usually the subject writes down what seems most important, unusual, or entertaining to her, or what she thinks will be of most value to the guide. In practice, these accounts by the subject are supplemental to the extensive notes made by the guide in the course of the session—notes recording both what the subject has said, and what the guide is able to observe apart from what is said.

In the following, fourth example we offer some excerpts from a guide's report on several hours of one session. In a few instances, and where so noted, the subject's post-session write-up has been drawn upon to amplify the guide's in-session observations.

Example No. 4.   S, a forty-year-old editor and former medical student, was given 125 micrograms of LSD at 11:00 A.M. and a similar dose at noon. About fifteen minutes later he complained about nausea and said that he was feeling quite depressed. He explained that although he "knew better," he was being influenced by papers he had read describing the LSD experience as a psychotomimetic one. He proceeded to enumerate his symptoms and listed them as "irrational ideas, a slight paranoia, and a fear of being unable to distinguish the unreal from the real," along with a generalized anxiety. He felt "like the fellow who was cast adrift in a lifeboat with nothing to read but a medical textbook and developed every single symptom except a broken leg." He noted a speed-up in his mental processes and felt this was a "flight of ideas" while "flight of ideas = mania = maniac."

S was temporarily distracted from this unpleasant trend when the guide encouraged him to examine his associational processes, about which he had commented. He distinguished "two radically different processes, one continuous and associational, the other marked by discontinuity and sharp breaks." He remarked that so long as his thoughts continued unbroken the ideas were associational, each flowing out of the preceding, along a line, as: A - B - C - D - E - F and so on.

However, the line might be "broken," or so it seemed, and S would "stop thinking." For example, the line A to F might be broken off at that point and S would then take up at some new and seemingly unrelated place and begin a new chain of associations, as: A - B - C - D - E - F /break-off point/ new A - B - C - D, and so on.

When this occurs, S wondered, "what is the cause of the new A —the new idea apparently unrelated to what has preceded it? How is the sequence able to come to a halt and how, the flow of ideas being halted, is it able to start up again?" He became very interested in this problem and also in the fact that he seemed to be able to follow the chain of his associations "back over at least forty associations, possibly more." He declared his nausea almost gone and his depression lifted.

12:30 P.M.: S decides to observe his eyes-closed imagery and soon declares himself once again quite depressed. He has been imaging material from his days as a medical student: surgical procedures, gaping and infected wounds, "all terribly ugly," and this is the cause of his depression.

At this point the guide does not haphazardly attempt to change the subject's ideation or imagery. Instead, as experience has proved to be effective, the guide suggests a new image *but retains the formal structure of the old one.* Thus, the guide speaks to S about (wound-like) caverns and molten lava flowing through the center of the earth (like S's "red, oozing gashes"). It is suggested to S that he descend into the center of the earth and report on what he finds there. Attempting this, he soon found himself able to divert his imagery into a more positive setting and described his consciousness as being localized in his "legs, stomach, the room, and also down there in the center of the earth" (this putting a final end to his depression).

The "world at the center of the earth," which S is imaging, he describes as cavernous and having "a thick atmosphere of air that appears to be divided in the manner of a honeycomb or cluster of fish eggs. The inhabitants are fishlike creatures who seem to swim or float through this atmosphere, although it is not watery." The inhabitants are aware of S's presence in their world, but ignore him and seem to be pretending he does not exist. Finally, however, one of the creatures communicates with him telepathically and agrees to be his guide. The creature is then immediately ostracized by his own people, who regard him as a traitor.

In the very remote past, S is told, the sun once reached this world when some great fissure opened in the earth. The fissure has long since closed, but around their glimpse of the sun the members of this society have constructed an elaborate religion, mythology, etcetera. The religion has its priests and among the "people" there are visionaries who claim to be able to see the sun while in their mystic states. But there is some debate as to whether these visionaries are charlatans, or possibly experience hallucinations.

The creatures of this world at the center of the earth have fishlike faces with long snouts and porcupine-like hairs extending outward from their cheeks. Their form suggests that originally they moved by spiraling through the earth or a much more solid substance than is now the case. And now, with a "softer atmosphere" to move in, their bodies, too, have become soft. S adds that they resemble "fishes with faces like possums, only their noses are still more pointed. Their shape is cylindrical and their skins silvery and shining. There is kind of light although no source of light can be detected."

12:40 P.M.: S opens his eyes and looks at some Bird of Paradise flowers in a vase. He describes them as unbelievably beautiful and says that they resemble great fiery serpents with flicking tongues of flame. The room is "enormous, like an airplane hangar or huge factory building" and two briefcases sitting at the end of the room about 20 feet away appear to him to be "two suitcases that seem so small because they are so terribly far away." (Here one notes that S is simultaneously aware that, in fact, he is seeing briefcases and that the distortions he is seeing are only that.) Asked about the time, he can only estimate that "many hours" have passed. In fact, the drug effects began to be noticed by him less than half an hour ago.

S is told to look at the flowered fabric of the couch on which he is sitting and to relate what he sees there. He perceives a great number of faces and scenes, each of them belonging to a different environment and to a variety of times: some to the American Gay Nineties, some to the nineteen twenties, some later. There are Toulouse Lautrec café figures, Berlin nightlife scenes and German art from the late twenties and mid-thirties. Here and there, a "Black Art" appears and he recognizes the work of Felicien Rops and drawings like those of the artist who has illustrated Michelet's *Satanism and Witchcraft*. There are various Modigliani figures, a woman carrying a harpoon, and persons such as appear in the classical Spanish art of the seventeenth century. Most interesting to him are "paintings" like those of Hieronymus Bosch, and he describes a great complex of sprawling yet minutely detailed figures which combine to make up a larger complex of a mountain scene of trees and snow. In another variation, this same complex consists of "a great face with the trunk of an elephant that is blowing liquid on the face of a demon whose body has been trampled into the ground. The elephant is blowing liquid on the face of the demon either in an attempt to revive him or as a gesture of contempt. A herculean male figure rises next to the elephantine face. He is trapped to the waist in stone and this marbled stone looks like sea foam, it is so delicate and lacy. Everything blends into everything else. The herculean figure is also the ear of a face and the elephant-like trunk is the bridge of the nose of another larger, still more complicated figure.

The guide asks a question and S responds that it is very difficult to give an answer entirely his own because it is almost impossible to eliminate the implied, suggested answer from a question. When he attempts to answer he finds that, simultaneously his mind "goes out" to find what the guide is asking for; he feels "closing in" on his mind and influencing him what he feels would be the guide's answer to the question; and "irrational impulses and instincts" come up "out of nowhere" to influence his answer and also in revolt against his feeling that an answer is being imposed from some external source. S remarks that these processes probably go on under nondrug conditions, but one is unaware of them. Concerning his own ideas he observes that "It is odd that what one thinks at some given moment should seem so important when one knows that one will be thinking something entirely different a few moments later." He further remarks that he is conscious of a different physiological reaction to the emergence from within or the imposition from without of each different idea. This physiological reaction to ideas, images, and perceptions was referred to repeatedly during S's session. The reaction was felt particularly plainly in his "nervous system." At this point S was also conscious of his mind as "a big, involved computer."

Closing his eyes, S images mind in terms of a great domed interior supported by the steel frames of a giant Erector set. He thinks about "a mind with a screw loose" and images an exquisitely jeweled screw that has come loose and is banging around inside this interior. "It is all presented like a television commercial, but in very vivid colors." He laughs at some length and when asked the cause for his merriment reports another image: He has been "seeing the human brain as a behind that gets more sore and unwholesome-looking as the years go by." After this S attempts to image the brain of Bertrand Russell and reports that Russell's brain "at this stage of the game looks like an old pair of patched trousers with the stitches coming loose around the patches."

Following this "low level cartoon production," S reports a "magnificent, staggeringly beautiful" sequence of images. He is seeing immense zodiacal figures laid out in jeweled definition with blue and gold stones against the heavens that glow with a black interior light. Then vast ships drift through the heavens "on a grand cosmic scale." S speculates that the zodiacal signs that man has "imposed upon the stars" derive from corresponding physical structures in the brain. He "feels" in his brain the patterns that man once employed in creating the zodiacal patterns. He remarks that the physiological pleasure responses experienced by his brain in comtemplating the imagery reinforces the images so that those images eliciting the most pleasurable reponses are the ones that persist for the longest periods of time.

1:00 P.M.: S images a number of additional cartoon sequences including a rather lengthy one set in Harlem that has to do with "a Negro making a cartoon about how a Negro would make a cartoon about a Negro making a cartoon about Negroes." Asked why he thinks the mind produces so many cartoons and caricatures while a person is in the drug-state, S replies that a kind of partial mental economy is involved. The brain "rests" when it produces these images requiring a minimum expenditure of psychic energy, in order that it should be able to "afford" the other fantastic and lavish things with which it provides itself. He makes the analogy of a French laborer who six days out of the week endures an impoverished existence in the provinces in order that on the seventh day he will be able to deck himself out like a prince and enjoy a free-spending "hell of a good time" in Paris.

S lies unmoving on a couch and reports that "nothing much" is going on his body and any activity is limited to the "central communication box." Apart from relaying routine messages, his body feels to him like that of a big lazy alligator lying on a beach: an extremely sensual feeling. He has experienced this serpent-like identification previously but did not mention it. Always, it "gives great pleasure of a very sensual type."

S speaks at some length but in half-sentences and verbally incomplete statements about the "traditional spirit vs appetite struggle that ever rages in man." He says that since appetite can be weaned away from the body or pulled in various directions so easily, it has set up a "great competition" between persons and groups. Man is very much a creature of appetites for all his pretensions. He is able to "put down" other creatures, but—and here S is convulsed with laughter. He has closed his eyes and at once has seen an image that anticipates his thinking. He is imaging man as "a god-damned little mangy, scurvy ape that is sitting on top of an ant hill scratching his head and thinking that his is the top brain in the universe." This image "is of mankind generally, and also of specific individuals who think they are sitting on the apex of everything."

1:20 P.M.: S amuses himself for some time by "playing a lot of psychedelic games." In his report on this "game-playing" he writes (we have condensed his material) as follows:

"I found that I could flatten out the room, including myself, and make of it a painting—some part of my awareness then standing away from the result and looking at this painting in which I lay upon a couch in a room completely flattened and projected on a screen-like surface by an effort of my imagination.

"Then, I created a world in which the imaginary was the real and the real the imaginary. My mind was a stocking, its outside the real, its inside the imaginary. Reaching down, I turned the stocking inside out, making the imaginary real, the real imaginary. When I tired of this, I just turned the stocking inside out again, restoring my world to what it had been before.

"I imagined myself a character in a novel, and had some bad moments when I seemed to be imprisoned on a printed page from which I could not escape. I wondered if all fictional characters were not thus alive and imprisoned between a book's covers, or on the pages where they appear?

"I did a great many things like this and except for those moments when I seemed to be trapped as words on the pages of a book, none of these odd mental events and gymnastics aroused in me the slightest anxiety or even any very great astonishment. I seemed always to have known that the mind is capable of these things and did them instinctively."

2:18 P.M.: S enters into the most important phase of his session. He speaks of experiencing a "powerful sense of the whole evolutionary process." This process is symbolized by an incredibly long snake that extends back through time from the present to the beginnings of all life. The snake is seen as an image but S also *feels* himself, his body, to *be* what he is imaging. The feeling of snakeness he has may be a kind of "evolutionary consciousness, an awakening of a consciousness traces of which are always present in the nervous system, but ordinarily dormant." The seen-felt snake image is retained but along with it, and sometimes superimposed upon it, S sees-feels the "primordial evolutionary beginnings. From minute independent organisms tiny lines extend out, touch, intermingle, and unite to form the nucleus of new organisms that continue to organize themselves in various kinds of life." Most of these primordial life forms perish, but a few survive and new forms continue to emerge. "All of this is felt in the deepest roots of one's body. One descends into these roots and relives the prehistoric process."

Suddenly, as he describes his ascent up the evolutionary process, S becomes extremely excited. His whole demeanor changes from that of curious observer to the manner of one experiencing an important revelation. Slamming his fist against his palm he reports with mounting excitement that "Something cuts across the Evolutionary process at this point! Something blasts into it! Cuts it clean in two! Changes its course!" The severed chain snaps back together quickly, but although the evolutionary process is deflected only slightly, the consequences are enormous. "Had this not happened man would have evolved into just another kind of animal!"

S now is experiencing his vision in terms of immense, panoramic and detailed imagery, brilliantly illumined. But, "when something is not quite clear," he also receives illustrative animated cartoons and diagrams "that make everything understandable." As he finds himself increasingly able to feel the evolutionary chain in his body and especially in his nervous system, he seems to understand that "If each nerve were allowed to dance its own dance, then all would be confusion. Some music, some form simply must be imposed upon the dancing. This imposition of form and pattern on Being is one of the survival functions of the brain." Asked by the guide: "What is music?" S responds that music is a derivative product of a mathematical function that the brain was forced to develop in order that the organism might survive and progress. "That is why music is never as great as philosophy. Music has to be derived from ecstatic impulses of the body filtered through the mathematical ordering screen of the brain and is shaped by the structure of the brain. But philosophy is a pure emanation from the brain and owes nothing to the lower bodily processes." S emphasizes that his "understanding is all experienced as simultaneous visual and felt thinking."

Returning to his main vision, S declares that if one is not to see man as only a machine then one must recognize that alien force has blasted into the evolutionary sequence at a certain point and altered its course in the direction of a higher, more sophisticated process. But can one be certain that this alien force is something *other* instead of just a better disguised mechanism? S here experienced briefly another cartoon image that provoked much laughter: that of "a fellow who keeps looking up into the sky for something good, but always gets clobbered by falling vultures."

S continues that man possesses two distinct varieties of consciousness. One is the higher consciousness that came into being at the time when the alien blast cut through evolution. The other, primitive consciousness had its origins much earlier and is capable only of feeling and a very low order of intellection. The alien blast into matter initiated a process whereby the higher consciousness evolved along with but did not extinguish the lower, primitive consciousness. The force that struck into the pre-established evolutionary animal pattern was God or Spirit. This Higher Force burst in like a bullet. It imposed itself upon the creation of the "other, earlier God-Force" that had conceived of and created the material world. The subject later reported himself amazed at this gnostic ideation; in fact, amazed at "the whole religious content" of his experience. He described himself as profoundly antagonistic to "religion" and said that these ideas were previously certainly not his and quite foreign to his "usual way of thinking."

S reports a series of images showing "how it would have been" without "the infusion of spirit into matter." Consciousness would have developed along continuous evolutionary lines, would have been "entirely animal in nature," and man would have been a creature entirely ruled by his appetites. S sees these "degenerate beings" and their world of "low waterfront cafés." Man "as he might have been" is seen by S as a creature who rather resembles himself. But, unlike himself, this might-have-been man is about three feet high, thick, squat, and coarse, with a head hunched over to one side and with frog's weblike protuberances growing out from the sides of the head. The legs are thick and gnarled and the feet are rooted in some "slimy stuff." One effect of the infusion of spirit, then, may be physically observed in the refinement of man's body—his angularity and attenuation. Did the blast, S muses, serve to diminish the effect of the "gravitational squash?"

Both seeing and feeling the images, S continues to experience "the accident of this thing exploding into this planet and sending out its rays and particles through the faults of the earth and the organismic structure it had penetrated. The blast touches off a profound reaction in matter and in the animal consciousness. These are infused by the *other*, but not wholly conquered by it. "Between the lines of silver that surge through the body of matter the chunks of meat remain." S is able to move up and down the evolutionary chain and to pass back beyond the point when the higher consciousness evolved. He descends down his physiological past to a level that seems to be of feeling alone and remarks that "the older consciousness is still there in our bodies. The new consciousness is spirit and must be of a different order since it has cut into the evolutionary process and redirected it from outside of the process."

S continued this discussion for some time, elaborating further upon the basic "revelation." He concluded this phase of his experience by saying that the original creation might be understood as "the Self" while the source of the second creation or infusion of spirit might be understood as "the Other." The self, so long as it exists by itself, can only develop in its own terms. If it is to transcend itself, to become something more than itself, it must receive its impetus from something other than itself. This led into a discussion of the interpersonal psychology of Sartre which S summed up as "a Darwinian snarl."

For the many hours remaining in his session, S experienced a wealth of ideas, images, and a wide range of other psychedelic phenomena. But he returned repeatedly to the "infusion of spirit into evolutionary process" and felt that in some as-yet-undetermined way this idea-complex must be of some importance to him. He regarded this phase of his experience as being "not a religious one in any conventional sense, or any kind of revelation from God, but a message probably from the unconscious" to the effect that he had been suppressing a "real interest in fundamental questions that now I propose to go into seriously and in depth." S was particularly impressed with his "new and firm conviction" that "otherness is an essential condition for growth [and that he must] open myself to an 'infusion' of otherness in order to escape the narrowness of my self-limiting self-concern. Whether the impulsion to this actually comes from the unconscious or not is unimportant. It's still a good idea." Subsequently, S embarked on an extensive program of readings in philosophy and also scientific material dealing with evolution—this last "on the off chance that somewhere along the evolutionary line there is actually a discernible point of disruption or deflection that might give credence to the LSD notions."

Every reader of the popular literature concerning the psychedelic drugs knows by now that some persons are drastically changed by what occurs during their sessions. A great mass of evidence has piled up and apparently demonstrates that chronic alcoholics may stop drinking, "hardened" criminals may be rehabilitated, and other equally important and beneficial results may come out of a psychedelic session. These transformations, often involving a major reorientation of values, have resulted even from psychedelic experiences where the aim was not "therapeutic" and none of the technical procedures of therapy was employed. The drug experiences have also, although far less often, resulted in a *dis*orientation of the subject and some other harmful effects. Most subjects, however (and we here make no comment on treatment of *patients*), seem not to be significantly changed in any way that would alter the overt patterns of behavior. Positive behavioral changes may ensue in time; but this usually requires that the subject keep working with the data of his session to further break down conditioned responses and preserve his ability to be open to, and accepting of, external stimuli and his own positive ideas and feelings.

The subject whose case has just been discussed was not dramatically transformed by his LSD experience; and we have refrained from introducing at this point any instances of what we will term the "transforming experience." The subject did have what he regarded as an intensely interesting and rewarding session—"probably the most interesting ten hours" of his life. He enjoyed several days of "unusual calm" just after the session; and he regarded his new philosophical and scholarly pursuits as constructive and personally fruitful. He felt, moreover, that his insight into the "fructifying nature of otherness" was helpful to him in his interpersonal relations and would be still more helpful in time to come. Whether this long range benefit in fact was forthcoming, we are unable to say. The last possible follow-up on the subject, who as previously planned departed for Europe and new employment, was only six weeks after his session and therefore no assessment of any long-term effects could be made.

In presenting these four examples of the psychedelic drug experience we have not attempted to "glamorize" the experience. Nor will we glamorize it elsewhere. We believe the experience to be of enormous potential value, both to subject and researcher; but it also has negative elements that not all who have written about the drugs have felt it essential or desirable to mention. This needs to be remedied, but by means of objective data rather than a collection of horrendous "scare stories." It is equally necessary to place in proper perspective the numerous ill-informed and hostile reports concerning the drug experience and its aftermath.

Even the materials already presented should suggest that the psychedelic drugs have legitimate uses beyond the strictly medical, or still more limited experimental psychiatric and psychotherapeutic, ones to which some persons would restrict them. Support for a wider use has come from prominent individuals in a variety of fields who believe that psychedelic research will be of great value in such diverse areas as philosophy, parapsychology and the creative arts, and in the study of literature, mythology, anthropology, comparative religion, and still other fields. The possibility of such applications was remarked at the turn of the century by the German toxicologist Louis Lewin, sometimes described as the founder of psychopharmacology. His view has been often reiterated since and its accuracy proved by accomplished work. Even so, the effort to close off non-medical research has been very largely successful.

Obviously we, as the authors of this book, do not agree that psychedelic drug research should be confined to medical and psychotherapeutic areas of use. And it is toward a much wider horizon of productive exploration and application that we intend our book to point.

Two:
History and Controversy

There exists an abundance of evidence to indicate that mind-changing drugs have been used since remotest antiquity by many of the peoples of the earth, and have importantly affected the course of human history. The plant sources of these drugs—the visionary vegetables—have been worshiped as gods in many times and places, and the persons employing the drugs as a means of acquiring "super-natural powers" have been the priests, prophets, visionaries, and other leaders of their respective societies. East and West, civilized and primitive, religious thought and all that flows from it almost certainly has been importantly influenced by the psychedelic drugs, a point we examine in some detail in our chapter on drug-induced religious experience. Some magical and occult uses are mentioned in a subsequent discussion of extrasensory perception; and here we will only very briefly suggest something of the temporal, geographic, and functional range of the drugs before focusing upon LSD and peyote; the substances with which we are principally concerned.

Three millennia ago, the East already had its legendary *soma*, reputedly involved in the origins of yoga, and the West had its *nepenthe*, immortalized by Homer. What these substances were is unknown, but descriptions of their effects suggest that nepenthe probably was opium, while soma was probably a substance more closely resembling the "con-sciousness-expanders" well-known to us today.

Possibly still more ancient in its usage is the hemp plant (*Cannabis indica* or *Cannabis sativa*), mentioned at a date often given as 2737 B.C. by the Chinese emperor Shen Neng. A hemp derivative—such as hashish, marijuana, bhang or gangha—appears to have been known to the Assyrians eight centuries before Christ, and to the Scythians not later than the fifth century B.C. In India, various types of hemp deriva-tives, yielding visions, heightened concentration, and other psychedelic effects, have been in use for hundreds and possibly thousands of years as aids to spiritual development and as sources of occult power. Pres-ently, an estimated ninety per cent of the Indian holy men use hemp, often along with other drugs; and the not-so-holy men of India and other countries of the East employ the same substances in a frank search for "kicks" and to escape a sometimes barely tolerable reality. This escapist motive also underlies the widespread use of hashish in the Moslem countries, where alcoholic beverages are prohibited to the faithful. Hashish, habitually used, appears to produce a gradual deteri-oration in the Eastern user. It accounts for a high percentage of Arab worker absenteeism and for a large percentage of the mental illness, especially in Egypt. (However, the common practice of mixing hashish with Datura seeds and opium may have to be considered in assessing these ill effects.) Thus, in both the Indian and Moslem cultures, the social impact of hemp has been enormous, and rarely favorable. The impact of hemp use has been great, too, in many African Negro cul-tures, where the plant is worshiped and its use bestows supernormal powers on witch doctors and produces in the native masses effects that range from sodden intoxication to orgiastic frenzy and a homicidal ferocity such as that displayed by Lumumba and his hemp-intoxicated followers in the Congo. In our own country, the use of marijuana was until a few years ago largely limited to members of various subcultures, often of the outcast variety. Presently, its widespread use among uni-versity students is creating something of a national furor. Although physiologically nonaddictive, and possibly less harmful than alcoholic beverages, marijuana use can hardly be justified on the basis that it makes a major and positive contribution to society. Certainly, as com-pared to LSD, peyote, and other powerful psychedelic drugs, its value as a consciousness-expanding agent, vehicle of self-transcendence, or source of visions, is not very great. On the other hand, it is sheer nonsense to lump marijuana together in punitive legislation with heroin, morphine, or even cocaine.

In pre-Columbian Mexico and at the time of the Spanish Conquest a number of plants containing psychoactive agents were in use, including the peyote. Unfortunately, the Aztec records were destroyed upon the orders of Cortez, so that what we know of the native drug use has come down to us mainly in the form of pious attacks upon pagan practices made by the Spanish clergy or those under their influence. We do know that the Aztec priests used the plants to commune with their gods and to induce visions, and that the plants were more widely employed for purposes of sorcery and healing. One of the drugs described as being in use at the time of the Spanish Conquest was *ololiuqui*, long thought to be a species of *Datura*. However, it now has been established that ololiuqui is the white-flowered morning-glory, *Rivea corymbosa*, whose effects resemble those of LSD. (That certain morning-glory seeds selling on the American market yield psychedelic effects not long ago came to the attention of scientists, Beatniks, the public, and finally the U.S. Congress, where it was seriously proposed that morning-glorys be eliminated—raising the specter of policemen or government agents armed with plant poisons colliding with little old ladies defending their flower-covered trellises. Apparently, no action was taken on the measure.)

The Aztecs also had a sacred mushroom, *teonanacatl* ("flesh of god"), which they used in rites that bore a strong resemblance to the Christian sacrament and so were especially detestable to the Spaniards. This particular mushroom, *Psilocybe mexicana*, still is in use in parts of Mexico today and is dispensed by local *curanderas* (witch women) and *curanderos* (witch doctors), some of whom conduct their rituals in the curious tonal language of the Mazatecs. The chant of the *curandera* includes many references to Christ and the saints, but still more references to the reputation and prowess of the witch herself, who speaks directly to Jesus when in the drug-state. The Mazatecs believe that Christ gave them the drug—as certain Indians believe the peyote to be a gift of God. In recent years, a number of the *Psilocybe* mushrooms were obtained by mycologist R. Gordon Wasson, who several times participated in the rites, and Roger Heim, director of the National Museum of Natural History in Paris. Heim and the famed Swiss chemist A. Hofmann discovered the psychoactive alkaloid, *psilocybin*, which Hofmann synthesized in 1958. Hofmann is well-known as the discoverer of the similar mind-changing effects of LSD-25. Psilocybin has been one of the most widely used of the various synthetic psychedelic drugs.

Another mushroom productive of curious mental effects is the fly agaric (*Amanita muscaria*). The plant is extremely poisonous, but the toxicity is reduced by removing the skin and through other preparations. It has been used for centuries in the dismal regions of Northeast Asia, mostly as an inebriant but also by shamans to induce visionary states, out-of-the-body experiences, and other typical drug phenomena. In Scandinavia, as well, the use of this mushroom has a long history and attempts have been made to link it to the legendary ferocity of the Norwegian Berserkers. In fact, the effects of the drug—depending upon quantity taken and use context—may range from dullness or mild euphoria through delightful visions and communion with deity to delirium and murderous frenzy.

Also dangerously toxic and of considerably more importance to history, are the *Solanaceae* family of drugs—the plants Thorn Apple (*Datura stramonium*), belladonna, mandragora, and the henbanes. They contain the alkaloids atropine, hyoscyamine and scopolamine, among others. These plants or their relatives are found almost everywhere in the world and for countless centuries have served as poisons, intoxicants, love potions, sources of dreams and visions, and for a host of magical purposes. Datura and the henbanes were known to the ancient Greeks and the former possibly was the drug used by the oracle at Delphi as a means of inducing possession by the god. But the greatest claim to fame (or infamy) of the *Solanaceae*, is as drugs employed by the European witches; and it has frequently been argued that the Witch Mania would never have occurred had it not been for these drugs.[1]

Under the influence of Datura, henbane, or belladonna, or some mixtures of these, the witches of the fifteenth to seventeenth centuries experienced dreams and visions of flying to the Witches' Sabbats, where they participated in orgies and blasphemous rites with the Devil and demons. By the same means, they were visited at night by demon lovers (incubi and succubi). Often these experiences were so vivid that the individuals later believed them actually to have occurred—so confessing to the Inquisitors only what they thought to be a fact.

The witches prepared *Solanaceae* potions, which they drank; and also an ointment, which was rubbed over all the body or upon especially sensitive areas, such as the armpits, the palms of the hands, or the vaginal walls. That the witches' ointment already was known in the fifteenth century, and that it was thought to produce dreams or illusions of flying and attendance at the Sabbat, is clear from a case cited at the time. A Dominican had watched a woman rub herself with the ointment and fall into a "trance." When she awakened, she claimed to have been transported to the Sabbat and to have joined in the revels there. The witches' ointment was actually analyzed in the sixteenth century by Andreas de Laguna, physician to Pope Julius III. Of a tube taken from a witch, Laguna reported that the ointment was green in color and contained hemlock, salanum, mandragora, and henbane.

More recently, the *Solanaceae* "Devil Drugs" have been put to other malign purposes. In less than fatal doses they still may produce extreme confusion and the appearance of psychosis, so that individuals have been drugged with the substances as a preliminary to obtaining from some unsuspecting physician an order committing the victim to a mental hospital. Similarly, the confused drug-state has been used to facilitate robbery and the commission of still other crimes against drugged individuals.

In addition to the few mentioned, we find throughout most or all of the world a great many other mind-changing plants, varying widely in the range of mental phenomena produced, and in importance for the cultures in which they exist. But to further explore this array of psycho-chemicals is impossible here, and we now will limit ourselves to a brief historical discussion of peyote and LSD-25.

The first of these, peyote (*Lophophora williamsii*),[2] is a small cactus with a spineless gray-green top or "button" and a brown carrot-shaped root. Found in the southwestern United States and in Mexico, its use for religious and magical purposes has been traced back as far as 300 B.C.

The peyote cactus contains a combination of apparently interactive alkaloids which together constitute the psycho-chemical also known as peyote (or, sometimes, pan-peyotl). These nine alkaloids are Anhaline, Anhalamine, Anhalonidine, Anhalonine, Anhalinine, Anhalidine, Lophophorine, Pellotine, and Mescaline. Mescaline is the principal psychoactive alkaloid and is responsible for the vivid imagery always emphasized whenever peyote is discussed, but the combination of alkaloids yields the peyote effects which differ from those of mescaline alone.

Peyote alkaloids are contained in the "button," which is tufted with clumps of white "hair" or "fuzz"—explaining the botanical name *Lophophora*, or "crest-bearer." This button may be eaten, or a "tea" may be made from it, or it may be dried and then powdered and put into gelatin capsules. Since the methods of preparation are crude, and since the strength of the alkaloids varies from plant to plant, no exact measurement of dosage is possible when the drug is so consumed. The person preparing the drug learns to produce an effective concoction of approximately the strength desired. Although toxic elements are present, the margin of safety is very great and serious poisoning is virtually unheard of.

The psychological effects of peyote are usually experienced within one to two hours from the time of ingestion and after some preliminary physical discomfort, most notably nausea. The effects then persist for from ten to twelve hours, on the average. They may include any of the psychedelic phenomena mentioned in the previous chapter.

Peyote first was described as a narcotic in 1560 by the Spanish historian Sahagún and a botanical description was provided by Francisco Herandez, a naturalist, in 1638. The Spaniards, first encountering this plant, which had been sacramentally ingested since pre-Columbian times by the Aztecs and the Huichols, denounced it as a diabolical root and in 1620 a law was passed by the heresy-hunting conquistadors that tells us something of the uses to which peyote then was being put:

"We, the Inquisitors against heretical perversity and apostasy, by virtue of apostolic authority declare, inasmuch as the herb or root called peyote has been introduced into these provinces for the purposes of detecting thefts, of divining other happenings and of foretelling future events, it is an act of superstition, condemned—as opposed to the purity and integrity of our Holy Catholic faith. The fantasies suggest intervention of the Devil, the real authority of this vice."

Gradually, under the pressure of continuous suppression, the use of peyote largely died out among the Indians of central and southern Mexico but continued to survive among various tribes of northern Mexico. During the second half of the nineteenth century Indian tribes from the United States appropriated the ritual use of peyote as a result of their raids on the territories to the south. The years 1870 to 1890 witnessed a remarkable proliferation of the peyote religion as it spread by way of the southwestern Apaches and Texan Tonkawas to the Comanche and Kiowa of the southern Great Plains. It now has spread to tribes throughout the United States and has reached as far north as the Canadian province of Saskatchewan. Presently, peyotism can be considered the native religion of more than fifty American tribes including the Cheyenne, Arapaho, Chippewa, Blackfoot, Crow, Delaware, Shawnee, Pawnee, and Sioux.[3]

By 1922, the peyote communicants numbered some 13,300 persons, their rites being a combination of Christian and aboriginal elements serving as the mythic structure for the sacramental eating of the peyote. In order to protect themselves against various attacks from religious and political antagonists, participants in the peyote worship joined together to have themselves legally incorporated as the Native American Church. According to their charter, "The purpose for which this corporation is formed is to foster and promote religious believers in Almighty God and the customs of the several tribes of Indians throughout the United States in the worship of a Heavenly Father and to promote morality, sobriety, industry, charity and right living and culti-vate a spirit of self-respect, brotherly love and union among the mem-bers of the several tribes of Indians throughout the United States and through the sacramental use of peyote." The pan-tribal membership of the Native American Church now is said to number some 225,000 Indians. This extraordinary growth of the peyote religion among the American Indians merits some further consideration.

The beginnings of this growth are to be found in the late nineteenth century when, as a result of the Indian's unsuccessful resistance to the territorial and cultural encroachments of the white man, he was placed within the restrictive reservation system. On these reservations tribal disintegration and demoralization took a heavy toll of the Indian cul-ture. As well as destroying established economic and political struc-tures, the system served to ethnically, psychologically, and spiritually de-mythologize the Indian, stripping him of his heritage, his hope, and his spiritual identity. It would seem to be for this reason, then, that the past eighty years have yielded so great an expansion of the peyote religion. The cactus serves as a re-mythologizing agent for the Indians' exhausted mystique. It awakens the knowledge that the spirit of God has come to strengthen and comfort the red man. The humbled pride of hunter and warrior finds solace in the feeling of universal fellowship and empathic communion encountered in the peyote rites.

The frequency with which the peyote rites are held may vary ac-cording to circumstances, and tribal and local custom. In general, when meetings may be easily arranged, the rites are held weekly and last from Saturday evening to Sunday morning. Special ceremonial occasions, such as New Year observances, add to the total, as do rites held when some person is sick or for a variety of other reasons. The Indians begin their long peyote ceremonies early in the evening. The participants enter a tipi and sit around a fire in front of which has been placed a crescent moon altar of earth adorned with a single peyote button (or, sometimes, two buttons: one "male," one "female"). The Road Chief (one of the terms for the leader), representing the Great Spirit, sings a traditional opening song, calls upon God to share in the rite, and cautions the communicants to prepare their hearts for the sacred ceremony. The peyote songs are often very simple and short. For example, an opening song of the Winnebago goes:

> God's Son says: "Get up and follow Me."
> Jesus said: "You shall enter into the kingdom of God."

Repetition lengthens the songs, as in another Winnebago example collected by the ethnologist Frances Densmore:

> We are living humbly on this earth,
> We are living humbly on this earth,
> We are living humbly on this earth,
> We are living humbly on this earth,
> We are living humbly on this earth,
>
> Our Heavenly Father,
> We want everlasting life through Jesus Christ.
> We are living humbly on this earth.

To the right of the Road Chief sits the Drum Chief who, in Christianized rites, represents Jesus Christ and who sets the percussive rhythms for the ceremonial. The Cedar Chief, representing the Holy Ghost, attends to the use of incense and after the opening prayers throws cedar chips into the fire and censes the communicants. In addition to these three peyote priests, there is a Fire Chief who takes care of the fire, guards the door, tends to the sick, and is representative of the angelic host.

Following the "smoking [with special tobacco] of a prayer," the peyote buttons are distributed and slowly eaten. All-night singing is begun and instruments are played. The participants sing hymns together and take turns at singing alone. This singing moves clockwise, each singer when his turn comes holding a holy staff and a gourd rattle and singing four peyote songs of his own choosing. Each man drums for the singer at his left as the songs go around the circle. The songs consist of rhythmic chants and tend to be of three kinds: the Opening and three other ritual songs, which may be sung in an ancient and now undecipherable tongue of probable Mexican origin; songs in the singers' tribal language; and Christianized songs in which the person of Jesus figures very prominently. In the Christian peyote rites the songs are believed to have come from Christ and the singing is regarded as a way to communicate with the divine.

The singing continues all night, interrupted briefly at midnight when the Road Chief sings the Midnight Song, walks around the outside of the tipi, and blows an eagle wingbone whistle to the four corners of the earth. As a participant describes this moment, "The sound shrilled through aeons of space and corridors of time. It echoed to eternity. When he came back to us he (the Road Chief) prayed, 'That the Universe may prevail.' "[4]

The subtly changing rhythms of drum, rattle, and voice continue until dawn, bringing communion and revelation, dissolving the self into "life universal," and accompanying the emergence of visions both dreadful and glorious. In the Christian rites the flesh of the peyote is considered to be the flesh of Christ, and the subsequent visionary and other experiences may unfold in Christian archetypes. At dawn the Morning Song is sung and Peyote Woman, usually the Road Chief's wife, enters the tent and is greeted with songs of thanksgiving. She brings with her food and drink which she deposits before the altar. The worshipers then approach the altar, pray, and partake of the refreshments she has brought.

This, in brief, is a fairly typical peyote ceremonial, to which some tribes have added public confession, expression of remorse over sins, and other public declarations. The major ceremonies of life also may be celebrated during the peyote rites, the sacrality of the occasion lending its providence to the healing of the sick, the joining of couples in marriage, and the laying of the dead to rest.

Such use of the non-addictive and otherwise harmless peyote has been of very great value to the Indians. Spiritual sustenance apart, peyote has been conspicuously instrumental in effecting rehabilitation of countless Indian alcoholics; and the use of the substance should be credited, too, with preventing much additional destructive use of alcoholic beverages. Yet, so dangerous and wicked have the peyote rites seemed to a good many churchmen and politicians, that the peyote religion and its members have been the target of repeated attacks, and punitive legislation has been proposed and sometimes passed by various state law-making bodies. This sometimes has meant the classification of peyote as a dangerous narcotic, use of which is to be regarded as equivalent to the use of, say, morphine or heroin.[5] These attempts to legally ban peyote, begun in the last century and continuing up to the present time, have been vigorously opposed by an array of distinguished anthropologists and other experts who have made first-hand studies of the uses and effects of the drugs among the Indians. Sometimes these experts have carried the day, but on other occasions the courts and lawmakers have proved opaque to all authoritative evidence; and the future of the peyote religion remains uncertain at the time of this writing—the question of the new psychedelic drugs, especially LSD and other synthetics, having arisen to complicate the issue. That peyote, for many sound reasons, should not be considered along with the synthetic psycho-chemicals, is evident to any careful student; but that this fact also will be evident to legislators and government agencies may be too much to hope for.

Modern scientific study of peyote began in the 1880's both in the United States and abroad. In this country, although long marketed by Parke, Davis & Co., the drug created only slight interest. It fared much better in Europe, mainly owing to the efforts of Louis Lewin, a German toxicologist often referred to as the founder of psychopharmacology.

Lewin, who first obtained peyote in 1886, published a number of articles and books in which he described in a highly provocative way the psychological and other effects of the drug and also outlined most of the more promising areas of psychedelic drug research. For example, in a preface to his much-acclaimed volume, *Phantastica*, a study of psychedelic and other drugs, Lewin declared:

"Not only are these (mind-changing) drugs of general interest to mankind as a whole, but they possess a high degree of scientific interest for the medical man, especially the psychologist and the alienist [psychiatrist], as well as for the jurist and ethnologist."[6]

The ethnologist, Lewin thought, would find psychedelic drugs especially valuable in the area of comparative religion where the researcher might find a key to the understanding of the genesis of religious experiences. For the psychiatrist, he proposed the psychotomimetic hypothesis, suggesting that some of the drug effects resembled, if they were not identical with, the mental states of psychotics and so might cast light upon the psychotic process and its etiology. This lead was followed by a colleague of Lewin's, K. Beringer, who subsequently published a monograph entitled *Experimentelle Psychoses durch Mescalin*. Lewin further suggested inquiries into possibilities of psychotherapeutic use, along with studies of creativity, perception, and the emotions.

While Lewin regarded the images produced by peyote as less important than some of the other drug-state phenomena, it was just this vivid and seemingly exotic eidetic imagery that impressed some other influential authors including S. Weir Mitchell and Havelock Ellis. Mitchell and Ellis, by giving the impression that the drug experience was primarily an aesthetic one, probably—however inadvertently—did much to discourage scientific psychedelic research for at least half a century in English-speaking countries.

For example, Mitchell, a physician, described the eidetic imagery of his peyote experience so vividly that parts of his account repeatedly have been republished, creating a widespread impression that the images constitute almost the whole of the experience. To select some quotations:

"The display which for an enchanted two hours [after entering a darkened room] followed was such as I find it hopeless to describe in language which shall convey to others the beauty and splendor of what I saw. Stars, delicate floating films of color, then an abrupt rush of countless points of white light swept across the field of view, as if the unseen millions of the Milky Way were to flow in a sparkling river before my eyes. . .

"A white spear of gray stone grew up to huge height, and became a tall, richly furnished Gothic tower of very elaborate and definite design, with many rather worn statues standing in the doorways or on stone brackets. As I gazed, every projecting angle, cornice and even the face of the stones at their jointings were by degrees covered or hung with clusters of what seemed to be huge precious stones, but uncut, some being more like masses of transparent fruit. These were green, purple, red, and orange, never clear yellow and never blue. All seemed to possess an interior light, and to give the faintest idea of the perfectly satisfying intensity and purity of these gorgeous color fruits is quite beyond my power. All the colors I have ever beheld are dull in comparison to these. As I looked, and it lasted long, the tower became a fine mouse hue, and everywhere the vast pendant masses of emerald green, ruby reds, and orange began to drip a slow rain of colors.

"After an endless display of less beautiful marvels I saw that which deeply impressed me. An edge of a huge cliff seemed to project over a gulf of unseen depth. My viewless enchanter set on the brink a huge bird claw of stone. Above, from the stem or leg, hung a fragment of the same stuff. This began to unroll and float out to a distance which seemed to me to represent Time as well as immensity of Space. Here were miles of rippled purples, half transparent, and of ineffable beauty.

Now and then soft golden clouds floated from these folds, or a great shimmer went over the whole of the rolling purples, and things like green birds fell from it, fluttering down into the gulf below. Next, I saw clusters of stones hanging in masses from the claw toes, as it seemed to me miles of them, down far below into the underworld of the black gulf. This was the most distinct of my visions. . . ."[7]

Havelock Ellis, reading Mitchell's account, shortly thereafter tried the drug for himself and was most impressed by the imagery, declaring the peyote experience to be "above all, an orgy of vision." He added that the intellect, in the drug-state, remains unimpaired and that for this reason peyote "is of all this class of drugs the most purely intellectual in its appeal. . . . On this ground it is not probable that its use will easily develop into a habit . . ." Of all the "artificial paradises," thought Ellis, this one "though less seductive, is safe and dignified beyond its peers."[8]

Another noted authority inspired by Weir Mitchell's panegyric to try the peyote was the American William James. What direction peyote research might have taken had James had a good experience with the drug, no one will ever know. The great psychologist consumed one button, was "violently sick for twenty-four hours," emerged with an horrendous hangover and advised brother Henry that "I will take the visions on trust."

And so the possibility of serious American study of peyote was all but extinguished, and until recently, anthropologists studying Indians have provided almost all of the data concerning this drug. Since 1954, the writings of Aldous Huxley concerning his mescaline experiences have reawakened interest in the cactus and launched its widespread use among artists and intellectuals. Not, however, among very many scientists, since the more potent LSD was by then available and could be taken without the preliminary physical distress of peyote. Synthetic mescaline has been available since 1920, but this psycho-chemical, suffering from the bad and false impressions about peyote, was not widely used in experimental work in the United States until the advent of LSD, psilocybin, and the other new synthetic psychedelics. Some mescaline research of importance was accomplished in Europe in the first decades of this century; but it is only with historical aspects of peyote that we here have been concerned.

LSD-25, in part a derivative of the fungus ergot (*Claviceps purpurea*), is an immensely powerful psycho-chemical, one ounce of which would provide a psychedelic experience for 300,000 adult persons. A dose so miniscule that it measures no more than 1/700-millionth of the weight of an average male will yield significant mind-altering effects. As Sidney Cohen has noted, enough LSD could be carried in a two-suiter piece of luggage to temporarily incapacitate the entire population of the United States.[9]

As regards usual dosage, this varies widely from one therapist or researcher to the next and depends upon the aim of the session as well as upon decisions made on the basis of individual experience and generally established criteria. For example, psychotherapists frequently have worked with doses as small as 25 micrograms and very often work with doses no larger than 100 micrograms. On the other hand, in treatment of specific types of patients, dosage may be greatly increased. Alcoholics, for instance, have been given LSD in doses of as much as 600 micrograms and even up to 1,500 micrograms—an enormous amount and a dose that should never be administered for other than therapeutic reasons.

In the case of experimental volunteer subjects, some researchers prefer a dose of about 100 micrograms for the subject's initial experience; but others customarily employ doses of 300 or even as high as 600 micrograms (too large a dose in our opinion). Probably most workers in this field take into account the body weight of the subject, giving one to two micrograms for each kilogram (2.2 pounds) of body weight. Experienced subjects who have proved themselves well able to handle the doses already administered then may be given larger amounts of the drug, if this seems desirable, in subsequent sessions. Also, a dose administered at the start of a session is sometimes augmented with a "booster" given when the subject is, say, two or three hours into his session. Along with LSD, such other psychedelics as mescaline, psilocybin, and DMT (dimethyltryptamine) have been given. Tranquilizers, amphetamines, and other drugs also have been used in conjunction with the psychedelics, and for a variety of purposes.[10]

The LSD effects ordinarily begin thirty minutes to an hour or so after the drug has been orally administered and then last for from eight to ten hours, the effects diminishing gradually toward the end of the session. Intramuscular injection of the drug produces a quicker onset of the effects. As distinguished from peyote, unpleasant physical symptoms occurring at the start of a session are mild or absent in most cases when the subject is not unduly anxious. Yet to all of these statements there are fairly frequent exceptions—the drug taking more or less time than that mentioned above to produce its effects; the effects lasting for substantially shorter or longer periods of time than the average just cited; the effects terminating abruptly rather than gradually; and distressing physical symptoms being experienced in varying degrees for varying periods of time in some cases.

LSD first was synthesized at the Sandoz Research Laboratories in Basle, Switzerland, in 1938, by A. Stoll and A. Hofmann. However, it was not until 1943 that Hofmann discovered the hallucinogenic or psychedelic properties of the drug. Having concocted the LSD-25, Hofmann experienced "a very peculiar restlessness which was associated with a slight attack of dizziness." He had to stop working, returned to his home, got into bed, and there experienced "a not unpleasant state of drunkenness which was characterized by an extremely stimulating phantasy." When he closed his eyes, he saw "phantastic images of an extraordinary plasticity. They were associated with an intense kaleidoscopic play of colors." The symptoms went on for about two hours, then disappeared.

Hofmann's curiosity now was aroused. He supposed he must somehow have ingested or absorbed through his skin an unknown amount of LSD. Later, he returned to the laboratory and took what he considered at the time to be a minute amount, about 250 micrograms. However, as he soon was to learn, he had discovered the most potent of all psycho-chemicals known to man, and even 250 micrograms were more than sufficient to produce a full-blown psychedelic experience.

About forty minutes after taking the drug, Hofmann began to experience once more the familiar restlessness and dizziness; but these symptoms were followed this time by more formidable disturbances of vision, inability to concentrate, and then by fits of uncontrollable laughter. It was during World War II, there were no automobiles available, and Hofmann set out on the four-mile bicycle ride to his home, accompanied by an assistant. Along the way, the symptoms intensified, coherent speech became a near-impossibility, the field of vision was increasingly distorted, and he had the impression that his bicycle was not moving, although his assistant assured him that he was traveling at a fast pace. Reaching home, he sent for a physician.

Hofmann now was thoroughly frightened, fearful the drug had precipitated a psychosis, and this anxiety gave a negative direction to his experience. Faces of persons present around him resembled grotesque, brightly colored masks. He reported "strong agitation alternating with paresis; the head, body, and extremities sometimes cold and numb; the tongue metallic-tasting; throat dry and shriveled." There was a feeling of suffocation and intervals of confusion alternated with periods when his thoughts were orderly. He seemed to be standing outside his body, looked back at it as "a neutral observer," and listened to himself as he raved incoherently and sometimes screamed.

The arriving physician found his pulse to be weak but circulation was generally normal. After about six hours, Hofmann found his condition very much improved. He noted that the perceptual distortions remained, with objects seeming to undulate and "their outlines were distorted and resembled the reflections one sees on choppy bodies of water." Colors continued to change in an unpleasant way and with the eyes closed he saw phantastic images undergoing constant changes of form. He noted that sounds were translated into vivid colored images.

Finally, Hofmann fell asleep, and next morning found himself tired, but altogether recovered. The hallucinogenic or psychedelic properties of the drug now were clearly recognized and Hofmann and his colleagues initiated the work that has attracted the attention of much of the world.

Following publication of the first reports on LSD, research began rather slowly and the volume of scientific papers published previous to 1950 was not large. After that, however, this research and the publications it produced soon gathered such momentum that the scientific bibliography alone contained thousands of items by 1965; and medical and other journals then were reported to be stocked with such backlogs of material that several years would be required before even the supply on hand could be published. Accompanying this torrent of scientific publications has been another eruption of printed matter—in books, newspapers, mass-circulation magazines, scholarly and literary quarterlies, etc.—ranging from first-person accounts of psychedelic experiences to sober analyses of the social, political, religious, philosophical, and other implications of the drugs. This latter, more generally accessible literature, has flourished along with and helped to promote an increasingly heated debate concerning claims made for and against the drugs and concerning, too, such questions as who should have access to the psychedelics and for what purposes. Much fuel has been added to the flames of this debate by the emergence of a large-scale psycho-chemical black market and what has come to be known as the Psychedelic Drug Movement—a "movement" in which scholars and thinkers of some eminence find themselves marching more or less in step with such diverse elements as artists, clergymen, beatniks, and a host of youthful adherents whose motives range from a frivolous quest for kicks to a high-minded search for union with deity. Bizarre though it often has been, this debate is of real and major importance and the present volume is, to some extent, an effort to throw light on some of the questions it has raised.

Both scientific disagreement and journalistic error and excess have been instrumental in creating public confusion with regard to the psychedelic drugs. In discussing these drugs with "the man in the street" we have encountered, again and again, the beliefs that "LSD makes you crazy" and, at the opposite extreme, that LSD is a cure-all for mental ills that psychiatrists are keeping off the market lest it put them out of business. While neither of these beliefs is valid, one has no difficulty understanding how it is that such ideas have gained currency. And neither is it difficult to understand how, with such polarities as psychosis and panacea involved, what should have been serious discussion has been very often debased to the level of irrational polemic and assertion of proprietary claims.

The widely held belief that "LSD makes you crazy" is primarily derived from both medical and lay misinterpretation of the psychiatric hypothesis that the "hallucinogenic" drug-state is a psychotic or psychotomimetic one, resembling if not identical with schizophrenia. This hypothesis, since much modified, and by many or most abandoned as erroneous, emerges repeatedly in the press and elsewhere as a flat declaration that the LSD subject becomes temporarily insane. Publications carrying first-person accounts by former LSD subjects who had painful and grotesque experiences then do much to reinforce this belief.[11]

That almost any LSD subject may experience, under certain conditions, a transient psychosis or psychosis-like state, is a fact. However, it is also a fact that a "psychosis" rarely ever will occur in a reasonably healthy subject who has not been led to expect it and who has not been exposed to stresses precipitating the "psychotic" episode. Not LSD, but mishandling of the session, is with few exceptions the key factor when a normal subject experiences an LSD "psychosis" that was not intentionally brought about.[12] As this has come to be generally understood, and as session-guiding techniques have improved, the occurrence of drug-state "psychoses" has diminished accordingly.

While the LSD-state is not, with rare exceptions, a bona fide psychosis, it does include many phenomena which bear a more or less close resemblance to symptoms commonly encountered among psychotics. For example, the drug subject may experience a variety of hallucinations, delusions, abnormal body sensations, ego disturbances (de-personalization, derealization, deanimation), time and space distortions, and other deviations from normal consciousness; and the study of these sheds some valuable light on the experience of psychotics. This, however, has proved treacherous ground where hanging psychiatric labels on superficially similar drug-state phenomena often has been unwarranted and probably harmfully misleading. A key point here would seem to be the great difference between a psychotic's and a "normal" subject's *reactions* to the various "disturbances" of consciousness—the healthy subject often thoroughly enjoying what, in the psychotic, may be productive of torment and panic.

In any case, one must be wary of equating experiences which may have only surface similarity. For example, the subject who has a "mystical experience" may feel, as in traditional mysticism, that his physical body has dissolved; but to call this "somatopsychic depersonalization," and thereby "prove" that a psychosis exists, is to make an equation that much historical evidence suggests is invalid. It is all too easy to observe a few "symptoms" and from these diagnose a "psychosis"—as, for instance, one might regard love as a "psychosis" if considered just on the basis of the "symptoms." Lovers, after all, display not infrequently such "symptomatic behavior" as monomania, *folie à deux*, "paranoidal" suspicion, extreme fluctuations of mood, hypermnesia (as regards the beloved's words), illogicality, delusions, *idée fixe*, ideas of reference, the belief they can read one another's mind, impaired or distorted perception (especially as regards perception of the beloved), physical states ranging from apparent neurasthenic fatigability and lack of zest to apparent hyperhedonia and hyperkinesis, and so on. But if love is a madness, then we all carry within us a powerful desire to be mad—at least once.

As to the question of whether the LSD state is identical with schizophrenia, we have it "from the horse's mouth" that it is not. A group of schizophrenic patients given LSD declared the two states dissimilar.[13] With this verdict, many scientific investigators are in accord, noting important differences between schizophrenic and drug-state "symptoms."[14]

As regards the opposite pole of popular belief concerning the effects of LSD, some startling psychotherapeutic results have been reported in the treatment of particular groups of patients. This has been most notably true of therapy directed at alcoholics who, in some cases, were selected as LSD subjects precisely because they had proved intractable to all previous therapy.

In four Canadian studies, for example, seventy-two per cent of the alcoholics treated either remained abstinent (over fifty per cent of the total number treated) or reduced their alcoholic consumption throughout the post-session assessment period of about one year. Members of control groups (used in two of the studies), treated identically but without psychedelics, showed similar improvement in only twenty-three per cent of the cases. These results were achieved in most instances with a single drug session; and the subjects, as in other, similar studies, frequently attributed their improvement to increased self-awareness, self-acceptance, religious feeling, and reorientation of values. Dosages generally ranged from 200 to 1,500 micrograms of LSD.[15]

Good results have also been achieved, for example, at hospitals in British Columbia and Maryland, where some twenty-five per cent of the alcoholic patients were reported totally abstinent or much improved after LSD therapy. In the case of the former institution, the LSD results were compared with results of other treatments then in use which yielded abstinence in only five to ten per cent of all cases. The abstinence rate claimed by Alcoholics Anonymous is fifteen to twenty per cent.[16]

Some impressive results also have been claimed in the rehabilitation of criminals. For example, Timothy Leary and his associates treated with psilocybin a group of 33 prison volunteers due for parole. Ten months later, only twenty-five per cent of this group had been returned to the prison and then only for technical parole violations. This compared to a usual return rate of fifty to seventy-five per cent after eight months.[17] And at Everdeen, The Netherlands, outstanding results in the LSD treatment of "psychopathic criminals" have been reported by Dr. G.W. Arendsen-Hein. Subjects received 50 to 450 micrograms LSD once a week or every two weeks and treatment continued from ten to twenty weeks.[18] As Arendsen-Hein's work was capsulized in *Lancet*:

"Criminal psychopathy is an . . . obstinate (and dangerous) condition, and the work of (Arendsen-Hein) . . . is of particular importance. A modern therapeutic regimen had helped many of his cases, but systematic LSD treatment had been started for those who, being physically fit, non-psychotic, averagely intelligent, and anxious for recovery, were of longstanding severe psychopathic criminality and quite untouched by ordinary therapeutic contact. Under this (LSD) regimen, abreaction took place, conflicts were revealed, resistance fell, and introspection and insight increased: a new capacity for human relationships was formed. The subjects showed less fear of LSD than of other treatments and cooperated well. Fourteen of 21 cases were clinically improved though a longer follow-up was awaited. Dr. Arendsen-Hein was sure we should re-think our belief in the intractability of psychopaths: this method enables us to penetrate deeply and bring about changes in personality formerly thought impossible."

Among these criminal psychopaths the psychedelic experience frequently was productive of "cosmic-religious experiences," reorientation of values, and consequent feelings of "great enrichment" and increased "self-confidence." These and other therapeutic effects of the drug yielded, in turn, "marked improvement of behavior."

Treatment of sexual disorders—frigidity, impotence, homosexuality and fetishism—and some other neuroses has many times been described as both drastically shortened and made more effective when LSD was used as an adjunct to psychotherapy. For example, a London psychiatrist reported, after twelve years experience with the drug, that the average number of treatment sessions required was only 25, at a cost of about seven hundred and fifty dollars. This compared to psychoanalytic sessions spread over several years at a cost to the patient of thousands of dollars. The unique and valuable tools made available to therapists through the psychedelic drugs will be discussed in some detail throughout this book.

LSD has, additionally, been used to produce marked improvement in mentally retarded and schizophrenic children and also in psychotic adults. Diagnostically, too, the drug is of value since, for example, at the start of a psychosis, what are to become major symptoms may appear in magnified form under the influence of the psychedelics. It is of interest that Czech psychiatrists, when psychotic symptoms (such as suicidal tendencies) appear in the drug-state or afterwards, do not discontinue the psychedelic therapy as do most of their European and American counterparts. On the contrary, a subject who manifests such symptoms is given LSD again two or three days later and "the symptoms clear up."[19] Czech psychotherapists administer LSD to patients once a week for as many as 25 to 35 weeks—much more frequently than is usually done in this country. Subjects in the Iron Curtain countries have mystical, religious, transcendental, and aesthetic experiences, just as do subjects in the West. Such experiences are considered to have a certain transitory therapeutic value—increasing self-esteem and feelings of oneness with other people and with nature; but such transcendental experiences are regarded as having "no real content—the patient. . . [is] completely detached from reality." After the gains from the "tran-

scendental" experience are thought to have been consolidated, the patients are encouraged to become "more interested in what they will do
with their real lives," and become "able to see reality with new eyes."
The Czechs appear to believe that LSD is administered in the United
States primarily for the purpose of inducing mystical experiences.

Returning to LSD work in the United States, in the case of terminal
cancer patients the drug has been found to relieve intolerable pain for
substantially longer periods of time than do such powerful analgesic
drugs as meperidine and dihydromorphinone. Here, LSD's psychological effects appear to contribute in a major way to its analgesic effectiveness, permitting the patient to ignore his illness or to view it with
philosophical detachment—sometimes retaining the improved emotional outlook for as long as two weeks after the analgesic effects have
worn off.[20] It has been suggested that LSD here reduces the ability to
anticipate suffering and death—the anticipation of which itself intensi-
fies pain—but this seems to us doubtful. However, the hypothesis receives some support from the successful use of LSD as a preanesthetic
agent in preoperative situations (100 micrograms LSD administered
two hours before abdominal hysterectomy as the only premedication
except atropine).[21]

While assertions that LSD lacks therapeutic value are now heard
less often than in the past,[22] the drug continues to be described by
some authors as too dangerous to be used in therapy—since it may
produce psychoses, attempted suicides and panic episodes. So it may,
with certain types of patients, but in the vast majority of cases it does
not; in any case, this should not be understood to mean, as it often has
been taken to mean, that the dangers are the same for normal persons
serving as volunteer subjects in various types of potentially important
research programs. Certainly, any view that there are grave risks to
normal persons is not borne out by the experience of most researchers
working with volunteer experimental subjects.[23]

On the basis of a survey of a great mass of literature concerning the
use of psychedelic drugs in psychotherapy, it seems safe to conclude
that for certain kinds of patients, and also for certain kinds of therapists, these drugs have present value and an enormously greater potential value. However, not every therapist is able to use the psychedelics
effectively or even without some danger to himself as well as to his
patients. And while, for example, alcoholics, some sex deviates, and
persons with anxiety problems often have been helped by LSD and
similar drugs, the psychedelics are of little use with highly dependent

individuals, persons of low intelligence, or in the treatment of compulsion neuroses. These drugs are regarded by some therapists as specifically contraindicated in patients with deep depressions, with conversion
or fixed neuroses and, in almost all cases, with psychotics. Thus the
psychedelic drugs are no more a panacea for all mental ills than an
agent that "makes people crazy."

The foregoing by no means exhausts the range of psychedelic drug
research. An immense amount of work has been done with a great
variety of animal organisms other than man. A large number of neuro-
pharmacological studies have led, for example, to fresh hypotheses concerning the pathogenesis of schizophrenia. Physiological changes produced in man by LSD and other psychedelic drugs have been enumerated in considerable detail. Among the results of these neuropharma-
cological studies, we have learned at least something about how LSD
works to produce its characteristically psychedelic effects. Concerning
this, Sidney Cohen remarks:

"After an average dose has been swallowed, about two-hundredths
of a microgram (0.00000002 gram) passes through the blood-brain
barrier. This would mean that only 3,700,000 molecules of LSD are
available for contact with the twelve billion brain cells, and then for
only a very few minutes. Such infinite sensitivity of the nerve cells to a
transient exposure to LSD can only mean that the drug acts to trigger a
chain of metabolic processes which then proceed to exert an effect for
many hours afterward.

"From the existing evidence it appears that the entire brain is not
involved. It is in the diencephalon, or midbrain, that the extraordinary
events occur. This region contains the limbic system, which modulates
emotional responsivity; the reticular formation, which regulates awareness; and the sympathetic and parasympathetic centers, which control
dozens of physiologic functions, from pupil size to body temperature."[24]

That LSD affects the responsiveness of the reticular area to sensory
stimuli (so enhancing the importance of environmental factors) has
been shown by electrophysiologic experiments. LSD action also has
been closely linked to central nervous system mechanisms regulating the
way the brain filters and integrates sensory information. About these
mechanisms, only very little is known.[25]

Apart from this strictly scientific work,[26] to which should be added
programs in psycho-chemical weapons research and development, much
additional work of importance has been carried out in a great many

areas. For example, still other psychedelic drug work has involved suggestive, if not very conclusive, investigation of effects upon creative (mostly artistic and technological) process and upon problem-solving and learning. Studies in the mythopoeic process and in the origins of religious ideas, investigations into the broad philosophic areas of epistemology, ethics, aesthetics and axiology, and even parapsychological experimentation all have been conducted during recent years. Some of the most controversial work has involved the attempted artificial (chemical) induction of mystical and religious experiences; and to this we have given a lengthy chapter, describing and evaluating our own work and also that of others.

Having supplied this background information concerning some of the psychedelic drug work to date, we will turn our attention to some of the other factors involved in the controversy and confusion that unfortunately permeate this field.

Notes from the Psychedelic Underground. A substantial contributor to the aforementioned controversy and confusion is the so-called Psychedelic Drug Movement which, in a general way, might be defined as consisting of the uncounted thousands of persons who make occasional use of psychedelic drugs "illicitly" and who insist upon the rectitude and value of what they are doing.

This movement and its members are far removed in almost everyway from the ranks of the socially outcast narcotics addicts with whom they sometimes are confused. Participants are mostly students, artists, intellectuals, clergymen, scientists and, in general, representatives of the more intelligent and better educated segments of the population. Drugs are obtained from friends or are purchased on the black market. The psychedelic experiences are had without medical or other professional supervision and for reasons having nothing to do with therapist-patient relationships or official research programs. The persons involved tend to feel very strongly that their motivation is healthy and ethical. The society, in their view, errs in not making the psychedelic substances more easily obtainable—so, one is justified in obtaining the drugs from black market sources. As regards Drug Movement motivation, Dr. Richard Blum, who has made extensive studies in this area, comments:

"The movement is composed of people who have taken LSD and/or other hallucinogens and see in these drugs a tool for bringing about changes which they deem desirable. The emphasis is on the enhancement of inner experience and on the development of hidden personal resources. It is an optimistic doctrine, for it holds that there are power and greatness concealed within everyone. It is an intellectual doctrine, for it values experience and understanding more than action and visible change. It concerns itself with areas dear to the thinker: art, philosophy, religion, and the nature and potentials of man. It is a mystical doctrine, for it prizes illumination and a unified world view with meaning beyond that drawn from empirical reality. It is a realistic doctrine as well, for it counsels compromise and accomodation between the inner and outer worlds. 'Play the game,' it advises, 'don't let the Pied Piper lead you out of town.' And it is, explicitly, a revolutionary doctrine, although the revolution it proposes is internal, psychological, and by no means novel. It calls for freedom from internal constraints, freedom to explore oneself and the cosmos, and freedom to use LSD and other drugs as the means thereto."[27]

Most of the people making up this movement have never been seen as presenting a "social problem" for the reason that the society generally has no knowledge of their activities. The main exceptions to this are the less discreet students and a "bohemian" or pseudo-beatnik fringe, which also includes some student representatives. It is in this latter group that most of the psychical casualties and the more spectacular incidents occur. They, and a few well-known individuals who have made the expansion of consciousness their cause, account for most of the extraordinary amount of publicity and other attention "extracurricular" use of the psychedelics has received.

Even on the pseudo- or, if you will, meta-beatnik fringes of the Drug Movement intentions are usually thought of as being serious and constructive—self-understanding, religious enlightenment, mystical experience, harmony with the universe and with other persons: these are the stated goals of the drug-takers and there is rarely much reason to doubt their sincerity. If primarily hedonic use of drugs is reprehensible, the fact has little to do with this group. What we do find, however, is a lack of respect for the potency of the drugs and a consequent carelessness about who takes them and under what conditions. Thus, since proselytizing is rather common, psychedelics are sometimes passed along to badly disturbed individuals who certainly would have been rejected as experimental subjects by any responsible researcher. Also, failure to provide for a proper setting sometimes results in very bad drug experiences even for those who are not seriously disturbed. Yet, and totally committed as we are to the position that sessions must be adequately guided, we find it impossible to say on the basis of our many interviews and other studies of the Drug Movement that casualties have occurred among its members with a frequency as great as that among participants in many programs directed by medical and other scientific personnel. What this means is only that in the case of the latter nonsupportive (including inquisitorial) experimenter attitudes wedded to a psychotomimetic expectancy have proved to be even more damaging than the most haphazard drug use occurring in a basically friendly and supportive setting.

On the other hand, the meta-beatnik fringe does display one type of behavior not found among subjects whose drug use has been limited to controlled situations—a type of behavior which, for this group, probably constitutes the best single argument against their free access to psychedelic drugs. This is the tendency to become increasingly involved, as do many Eastern occultists and "holy men," in introspective "spiritual" pursuits to the neglect of the external requirements of daily life. The Pied Piper does lead many such persons out of town; and he leads them into small cultish units of fellow true-believers where the interior pursuits are followed to the exclusion of almost everything else. Here, there might seem to be a kind of addiction; but, if so, it is not an addiction to drugs—rather, to cultist activities which, in this case, happen to include the use of psycho-chemical substances. Certain food fadists and adherents to mental healing and spiritualist groups, for example, display the same sort of exclusive absorption with consequent withdrawal from larger social involvement.

The following case of a twenty-three-year-old male university student (S-1) is representative of attitudes and behavior to be found on this meta-beatnik Drug Movement fringe—except that in this case there does seem to be the fact or potential of psychological habituation to drug use (the only such case of possible "addiction" we have found).

When first interviewed S was a member of an Eastern (Zen, Yoga, Subud, etc.) -oriented group also making free use of psychedelics. These were purchased on the Greenwich Village black market at a price from five to ten dollars for an LSD dose that might range from 100 to 250 micrograms (according to the word of the seller and also to estimates based on the drug effects). Similar prices were being paid for mescaline, psilocybin, and other psychedelic drugs. S, by "rough estimates," had taken during a period of about one year: LSD, 6 times; mescaline, 5 times; DMT, 15 times; peyote, morning-glory seeds, and marijuana, "many times." He had discovered that the drug-state enabled him to "feel unusually secure" and to overcome marked anxiety and inferiority feelings. Thus, he found himself "wanting to stay there" and described himself as being in danger of becoming "psychologically addicted" to the drugs. This is exceedingly rare, and his account of his emotional response much more closely resembles those described by heroin-users than those taking psychedelics.

S felt that, outside the drug-state, he had become "less responsible" than he had been previous to his psychedelic experiences. He had become more "carefree" and "happy-go-lucky" than he had been before. But this "carefree" state had not really made him happier and he certainly was not better adjusted. It was reflected mainly in his feeling free to cut classes and in a lack of concern about the grades he was making, and his schoolwork had suffered accordingly. He had achieved states of "mystical consciousness" and religious "illumination" (with mescaline, but not with the other drugs)—something he had failed to do in the past despite much strenuous work with various Eastern disciplines. But these had not produced the beneficial self-transformative effects he had hoped for and confidently expected.

Against this background we reproduce his own statement, written some six months after the first interview. It is one that might just as well have been written by any of a score of other, similar young people we have interviewed. S writes:

"LSD and other psychedelics emerged into my surroundings about the same time as Yoga and other Eastern teachings. Shortly thereafter followed my first inklings of the vital importance of modern science. . . . I have had the drugs many times. As they become more and more available to me, I avail myself of them more and more. The high is not in the drug, but in me. Each trip I take takes me to a new place; I never return the same. Pieces of music with which I thought I was thoroughly familiar, having heard them hundreds of times before, I hear as if for the first time during an LSD trip.

"Before taking the drug I feel apprehensive about the possibility of 'flipping out,' but during the high I am afraid I won't flip out enough. Like an organic computer I program my brain with Vedanta, *I Ching*, ragas, Bach, Tibetan scriptures, all kinds of 'Art,' and then turn on the metabolic switch. Presto, the ego wastes away for an endless spell, and an identity-less 'I' lets go in order to hold on to 'the clear light of reality.' Usual dose 250 to 300 micrograms. Almost always take it with another person or group of persons. The one time by myself on LSD was very negative, communication impossible, sidewalks of New

York very poor set and setting, all around frightening trip and waste of me and LSD both.

"With all psychedelics, but especially the combination of LSD and DMT, I enjoy the vision of beautiful patterns in motion everywhere: on plain cloth, on walls, in clouds and dirt yards. I seem to be able to project the pattern of my own pulsing eyes on any field. I don't feel as if this is pure hallucination since what I see is really there when I see it, and remains there, even if I leave and return later to look again. But when the LSD wears off the pattern fades back into plain field.

"During the high, there is nothing that is not symbolic, considerable, miraculous, accept-worthy (except occasionally my selfish self). All senses are heightened; touch becomes really pleasant and comforting; sexual inhibitions seem nonexistent, or rather unnecessary in the first place. A feeling of complete communication on all levels, such as eye gestures, mouth gestures, hand gestures, verbal and tonal messages.

"The basic problem LSD makes me confront: How to be high like that all the time without drugs? How does one leap from externally induced temporary ecstatic union (or self-acceptance) into the permanent mystical being-at-one with the whole working works? It seems like an idiotic misprocedure to sustain almost-heights of ecstacy from dose to dose, yet there has been nothing like it without these doses. The ecstacy came as a byproduct of not having to worry about my self, of selflessly serving others instead of trying to rule or dominate."

S was seen again briefly about one year after the initial interview and continued to be very much involved in the Drug Movement. He now was enthusiastically participating in a number of projects—making an avant-garde film, working as a musician from time to time, continuing his Eastern studies and such practices as hatha yoga exercises and meditation, traveling to visit others with similar interests, and he was planning to return to school in the fall. Psychedelic drug use was regular and he reported having taken, while alone in a forest, a 1,250 (!) microgram dose of LSD. This had produced, as one might expect, some very bad moments for S. For a time, he panicked and lay under a tree screaming. Afterwards, however, he regained control and when the experience was ended felt that some of his conflicts had been resolved.

What the overall effects have been in this case is something we are not in a position to evaluate. It is, indeed, difficult to evaluate the impact of regular psychedelic drug-taking on many of the Drug Movement people we have interviewed. Whether they have, as so many claim, become more creative and have improved their relationships with others often is dependent upon a rather arbitrary view of what constitutes increased creativity and improved relationships. Especially among the bohemian fringe group the tendency is generally toward more artistic and spiritual interests and away from the more practical concerns our society traditionally has sanctioned. But is this disengagement from "the rat race" and the "social games" and concomitant engagement in less orthodox pursuits, to be considered a good or an evil; a healthy advance or a sick retrogression; a finding of one's proper goals or a losing sight of them?

The same questions arise when one attempts to evaluate the rather similar aftermaths of psychedelic experience we have found among a number of other Drug Movement people who are far removed, at least on the surface, from the bohemian fringe groups. A prominent professor of theology told us that, since taking LSD on several occasions, he has come to seriously question whether he would not do better to abandon the teaching of theology, in which he has long since lost most of his interest, and devote himself exclusively to painting, which he much prefers and for which he has demonstrated real talent? His lectures now seem to him to be of questionable value and preparing them has become a tedious task that he undertakes with increasing reluctance. The economic rewards of academic life are, in this case, considerable: "But what does it profit a man if he gains the whole world and loses his soul?"

Do the psychedelic drugs in fact pose a threat that a significant number of presently productive individuals will, if exposed, abandon their posts as bank presidents, manufacturers, clergymen, engineers, physicists, educators, in favor of writing blank verse or pondering the riddle of the cosmos? And, if so, do the presumed interests of state and society transcend and override the rights of individuals to dedicate themselves to esthetic or spiritual endeavors? What is really best for the person himself? And is he discovering where his true genius lies or is he succumbing to suggestions owing their exceptional potency to chemical effects and yielding subsequent self-delusion? We will not attempt to answer these latter questions, but think it extremely improbable that the psychedelic drug experience could ever make another India of a country whose citizens are so overwhelmingly rooted in Western traditions.

While the incidence of psychotic episodes and lesser but still serious mishaps is not nearly so great as some of the alarmists would have us believe, these do occur often enough among the Drug Movement people to make it quite clear that access to the drugs must be controlled and that psychedelic experiences need to be guided by persons who have been trained for that purpose.

A dramatic illustration of this occurred in one case that could have ended in a suicide. S-2, another representative of the movement's meta-beatnik fringe, is a writer and painter in his mid-thirties. A university graduate, he traveled extensively in the Near East where he studied mysticism and experimented with hashish. Returning to this country, he associated with a group of students and ex-students seriously interested in and using psychedelic drugs. S had several LSD and mescaline experiences with members of this group and then decided to have some LSD while alone in his apartment. He took 150 micrograms and then, about an hour later, another 100. The drug effects seemed easily manageable and he decided to go out for a walk.

About a mile from home S began to experience severe anxiety accompanied by frightening hallucinations. He thought that taxi-cab drivers resembling grotesque charioteers were trying to run him down. Glass buildings exploded before his eyes and the air around him became filled with countless fragments like flying crystalline needles and knife blades that he feared would slash him to ribbons. The hallucinations ended, but the people around him seemed to become increasingly menacing and, recognizing his paranoid ideation, he hurried towards home and managed to get there without incident. He locked himself in his room and lay down on the bed where at once he was assailed by a torrent of chaotic and terrifying ideas and images. These, just after the drug effects had worn off, he reconstructed (in part) as follows:

"Floor a tempest. Sanitorium. No keys, no doors, walls or locks. Who are you? Roshomon swirling on sheets of torture beach. OK, begin. Trilogy of life faces sea of death. Battalions begin their march down the brain stem. Spears of red sashes helmetted in Tibetan black. They bend the kundalini sacrum. Ant out of my behind and climb back in. Demons. Demons, a million of them. I start to sing: 'My Mother is God, My Father is God, My Brothers My Sisters all are God. God to the Right, God to the Left, God overhead and ahhhhhhhh,' now the battle begins. Black archer stretches my flesh and snaps lining of my stomach. I fire back but can't touch him. Six thousand streets pour with phlegm, each helmet holds a face, each spear holds a tear. Is this masochism? Where else can I go, can you go? I rip off my shirt and start to sweat. All those karmas. Death house walls me in. Battling eunuchs cut off their legs and roll up their pants, impale catastrophes.

Let's have it. Smell like cheese in a gym, women hiding stained socks. No love. No love. Not anywhere. Three kabuki non-actors take karate stance, grimace, prepare fingers for attack. Slot machines and bubble gum. Can't do the concentration camps in this incarnation. Need whole session, and besides I did them. AIEEEEEE! I'll never look away again. He plunged his fingers into my liver, splattered grin with blood. Knife scars Beirut face, coagulates black sand. Child beats my insides with a whip, then hangs by his hair. Feel him squeezing my blood. Start my chants, 'OM NE MASHA VAYA' but can't find a battling mantra. Find one quick, hold on. AIEEEEEE . . . EEEEE . . . E . . . E . . . E! Cosmic opera not sung. He is looking at you. He is rolling up his sleeve. He is hideous formed and fast. He is hissing at you. Watch the ant army, phalanxed thoughts and his circling steps. My teeth are bleeding to death. Go mad is better thought. Go mad, cop out on consciousness. Ain't no proof it even exists. AEEIIIII . . . III! He leaps on my lungs. I don't even want to redemption this self. Am I that crumby little nigger street, sick with ape laughter, cockeyed and thin? You bet you are, baby, and more of that to come. Stop playing kid. Third one leaps onto my head throwing out all the books I had read. You're no enemy, friend. Then he dumps everything I've written, every word I know, down my throat. Vegetable soup. Army cheers as its being fed. They pierce pages with their spears, then start victory dance. Old faggot being beaten to death by King of Mohawks. Forty-second Street being beaten to death by naked girls. Girls, Girly Shows, I hate all this crap, B-29, Cowboys and Indians, Alabama, high school dreams and block sweaters, reductio ad absurdum . . . Football. Laughter-pain and Laughter. I'm copping out of this come down culture. It's back to hustling and selling hash. Greece baby, I hear you call. I want to die there on the bed of your womb. Sea ash, sea ash and AAAIIEEEEEEE! Black archers stretching my flesh, tear open my wounds. It's a belly bacchanal. My head hanging with blood, pain, remorse. All the evils. I try to cut loose but I'm too tired now. My hands clutch my skin. I kiss myself all over. I catlick. I want out of the time knot. I plead for help but there's only one sound and I can only dump that out the window. But it's not even high enough. Shiver. Groan. Try not to scream too loud or you'll get yourself busted. Oh, what a flesh saving phony. The phone."

What S has tried to recapture with the above is a series of images and ideas that became progressively more unendurable until he felt that he had to "get out of the time knot"—i.e., die. He considered jumping out of the window but was uncertain whether it was high enough. He says that he was caught up in powerful suicidal impulses on which he might well have acted had the phone not rung at the time that it did. This phone call, from a friend, resulted in an abrupt change of mood and ideation. He went over to the friend's house, which was nearby, and describes the remainder of his "session" as pleasant. But he feels the psychosis, as he himself regards it, would have continued throughout the session and probably worsened had it not been for the call. S doubts that he could have "hung on." Yet, looking back on this experience, he describes it as "very worthwhile" on two counts: It was a "catharsis," and afterwards he had "a sense of pride at having survived the psychosis."[28] He has since had several other drug experiences without any recurrence of the suicidal impulse or of the other painful phenomena— no guarantee, of course, that these will not recur in the course of some future drug experience.

Since a Drug Movement census is scarcely feasible, no accurate estimation of the number of persons involved can be made. However, it seems evident that a substantial majority are under the age of thirty and that probably at least ninety per cent are clustered on the East and West Coasts. Psychedelics have been rather easily obtainable in New York City for six or seven years and Los Angeles and Boston have had their black markets at least since 1962. The Drug Movement appears to have its heaviest student representation at Harvard and Columbia Universities. However, at some other colleges and universities as well the use of psychedelics has become a "status symbol" and is fairly widespread. Because of this factor, it is likely that many persons claim to have tried the drugs who in fact have not done so. According to one recent report, many people in New York City were purchasing and placing on their shelves a rather "Far Out" book about the drugs—their aim being to convince their friends that they, too, had "made the psychedelic trip."

Since LSD and some other synthetic compounds can be rather easily produced without expensive laboratory facilities, it is possible that the black market supplies may be coming from a number of small local producers. However, at least some of the drugs are probably being imported from other countries. When black market psychedelics first began to be sold, an LSD-soaked sugar cube could be had for one dollar and profit may not have been the main motive behind manufacture and distribution. Over the last year, however, prices in the New York City area have fluctuated between four and twelve dollars for a capsule claimed to contain about 200 micrograms. Most buyers probably paid eight to ten dollars. Since LSD, if it were legally obtainable, would retail for something like two cents a dose, it is evident that very large profits now can be made.

Some expressions of concern that buyers might be poisoned as a result of taking the black-market chemicals seem unwarranted. A clergyman has told us that an "LSD" capsule he obtained from a black-market source was taken to a chemist for analysis and was found to contain "mescaline and a little bit of heroin." However, if the capsule actually contained heroin, the most plausible explanation is that it got there by accident. This might indicate, then, that criminal narcotics interests have moved in on the psychedelic market—presenting some new and obvious dangers. Some purchasers have found that their capsules of "LSD," "mescaline," "psilocybin," or whatever, contained only sugar or talcum powder, a much more likely ingredient than heroin. In a few cases we have heard of, the dosage appears to have been considerably lighter than that bargained for. Inept or careless measuring might explain this and would also raise the possibility of exposure to dangerously high dosages should the error lie in the opposite direction; but we have yet to hear of this occurring.

One result of the drug black market and also, it seems clear, of poor medical and political judgment, has been stringent Federal Food and Drug Administration action that has drastically curtailed psychedelic research in this country. So stringent have these regulations been that since October, 1962, the drugs have been available only to those few individuals or groups of researchers working under federal (only 13 in 1965) and certain state grants. Some persons already possessing a supply of the drugs continued their work—but in what has been described as a "legal limbo" with the possibility of prosecution always present. And, in mid-1965, that work, too, was made clearly unlawful. Thus, we have the ironic situation that while almost all therapeutic and experimental work has been made impossible, there is a growing Drug Movement and a flourishing psychedelic black market supplying just those persons who use the drugs under conditions least likely to prove of real benefit to anyone.

Three:
Experiencing the Body
and Body Image

Throughout the psychedelic experience the subject from time to time is concerned in a remarkable variety of ways with his body. In the earliest stages of the session the awareness of the body can involve mainly the presence of disagreeable and sometimes alarming physical symptoms. This is particularly the case when the substance ingested is peyote and some of the physical symptoms are direct reactions to the toxicity of the alkaloids. In the case of LSD-25, where the symptoms are psychogenic or emotionally based, the discomfort is usually comparatively mild and may go almost unnoticed.

With peyote any of a cluster of distressing symptoms appear as the drug takes effect. These may persist from around thirty minutes to one or two hours or even longer. The best known and most troublesome of the peyote symptoms is nausea, often with vomiting. However, the nausea may be reduced and vomiting avoided in many cases with the aid of such a drug as Dramamine.

Other frequently encountered symptoms are feelings of being too hot or too cold, excessive salivation or dryness of the mouth, and dizziness—all possibly attributable to disturbances of autonomic functioning.

Subjects complain, too, in some cases, about difficulty breathing, stiff neck, tremor, headache, pressure around the head, or pains in the vicinity of the heart with consequent fears of heart attack, say, or suffocation. There is very often a feeling that the body's surface has been mildly anesthetized, with the flesh becoming "rubbery," as it is frequently described.

Many researchers agree that most of the unpleasant physical symptoms occur more often and are felt more keenly in a medical setting and with those subjects who are anxious or expect that symptoms will appear. That the LSD and some of the peyote symptoms are nonexistent or much less severe in the case of experienced subjects reinforces the belief that the symptoms are very largely psychogenic.

Disturbing physical symptoms tend to disappear or be readily manageable after the first hour or two of the session, when the subject has had time to gain confidence in his ability to handle the novel situation. These distressing symptoms at the outset have led to the oft-repeated observation that with these substances, and unlike alcohol, the "hangover" comes at the beginning instead of after the intoxication.

It is usually only after the passing of the more unpleasant physical symptoms that the subject experiences those drug-state awarenesses of the body and body image which are the main concern of this chapter. These altered awarenesses are extremely diverse and may be entertaining, instructive, frightening, and even therapeutic. They may occur sporadically or more or less continuously throughout the remainder of the session.

The subject may, for example, experience slight or drastic changes in the size, configuration, substance, weight and other attributes contributing to definition of the body. He may seem to himself to assume the form of some animal or even some inanimate object; and he may be reduced to a sub-atomic particle or expanded to the proportions of a galaxy. He may experience his body's dissolution and the sense of having no body at all—the so-called somatopsychic depersonalization.

Some of the changes in body awareness resemble similar experiences reported by psychotic individuals. However, considerably different are the *responses* made to the changes by psychedelic subjects on the one hand and psychotics on the other. It might be added that the drug-induced changes also resemble those experienced by hypnotic subjects, practitioners of yoga and spiritual disciplines, mystics, ascetics, occultists, spiritualists, and a whole host of other persons who cannot be reasonably branded as in every case insane.

The altered awarenesses induced by the drugs may involve the whole body or a part or parts of the body. Of considerable therapeutic import, not only may a normal body image be distorted, but a previously (pre-drug) distorted body image may become normalized.

Recognition of the altered state of the body or body image comes to the subject in various ways. He observes the altered image in a mirror; he has an altered "feeling" of his body's contours; he looks at some part of his body—say, a hand—and observes an apparent transformation; he "feels" that his body is heavier or lighter, has greater or lesser density, and so on. There is also an "internal awareness" of the bodily functions, particularly of the flow of blood through the veins, the receiving and transmitting operations of the nervous system, and of the activities of the brain.

In addition to changes in the awareness of the body as a physical entity with a certain size, shape, color, organs and other components and attributes, there may be altered attitudes towards the body or emergence into consciousness of attitudes presumably not new but previously not conscious. These attitudes may be directed toward either the normal or the altered body or body image.

Attitudes toward the own body commonly verbalized by subjects are numerous. Among the more typical are the following, one or several of which may be expressed from time to time by a subject during the course of one session:

The body is variously regarded by the subject as an instrument or tool, an operated vehicle, a plaything, an encumbrance, a source of pain and pleasure, a regrettable necessity, a source of wonder, a source of contempt, as the "temple of the spirit" on the one hand, or as a "mere machine" on the other. The body may be thought of as a prison or a trap; as a traitorous agglomeration of imperfectly operating parts (not uncommon when there is chronic illness or sexual malfunctioning); as interactive and co-operative with, or as dominating or dominated by the mind. Keen awareness followed by articulation and analysis of these attitudes can lead to a coming to terms with the body and a strengthening new feeling of at-homeness in the body.

The altered body awarenesses result from a variety of triggering factors: mood, ideation, perception of various external stimuli, along with inferred unconscious factors. For example, a subject may experience his body as abnormally heavy because he is depressed, because he has begun to think of himself as being too fat, or because he is "thinking weighty thoughts"—in this last case, the verbalization "weighty" being applied first to the thoughts and then to the body; or, as sometimes happens, only to the head which "contains" the "weighty thoughts." The heaviness associated with depression is also sometimes the product of a verbalization, as when the subject thinks of himself as "burdened with grief" or "weighted down by sorrows."

Should a subject believe that his substance has been altered so that, for instance, he seems made of glass, the guide's probing may uncover the cause of this transmutation in the subject's feeling that his thoughts are transparent to the guide. Or it might derive from the subject's feeling of fragility; from his having "become" some nearby glass object; or from, as one subject put it, his sudden recognition of himself as being "a pretty cold and slippery sort of fellow."

A subject may experience herself as beautiful or ugly in terms of what she conceives to be the impression she has made upon the guide; as a consequence of anxiety or euphoria; or as a response to a recollected estimation of her appearance made by some other person at some time in the near or even the very distant past.

The triggers producing the altered body awarenesses—some of them traceable, some of them not—along with the subject's responses to the changes, will be considered in greater detail in the following survey of some of the more typical varieties of experience of the body and body image within the context of the psychedelic state.

A *Taste of Wonderland.* Having fallen into one of literature's more celebrated holes, the young Alice tipples from a bottle labeled DRINK ME and soon finds that she has dwindled to a height of ten inches. A little later, she eats some cake and grows to a height of more than nine feet. These effects, while they seem awfully curious to Alice, appear modest enough when compared to the contractions and expansions reported by some psychedelic voyagers from the depths of their chemically-induced Wonderlands. Time and again these subjects remark of their alternating growths and shrinkages that they feel "just like Alice in Wonderland."

S-1, a twenty-six-year-old male then working as a clerk in a book store, ingested about 80 micrograms of LSD. He experienced only shrinkage, no growth, and reported that he felt himself to be six inches in height. Curiously, the objects in the room underwent a similar and proportionate transformation, while the guide and another observer retained their normal dimensions, appearing to him to be giants.

Although an inch taller than the guide, S tilted his head back to look up at her, stating that he felt as David must have felt looking up at

Goliath. He also compared himself to Alice after she had taken a drink from the bottle.

At one point S was given a box filled with many miniature Japanese figures. He greeted these with expressions of delight announcing that they were more his own size. Then he clutched the figures to him as if they might help to protect him from the onslaughts of the giants. When the guide approached him he seemed to shrivel and attempted to hide behind one of the figures, which was little more than one inch high. Later, he sat "hand in hand" with one of them, the doll's hand being perhaps an eighth of an inch in length. He claimed that he felt the doll's hand as completely filling his own.

Taken outside, S expressed the fear that someone might step on him and crush him. He seemed to take comfort in comparing himself to Stuart Little, the six-inch-high mouse of E.B. White's story, who lived the life of a little human being. If Stuart Little could live a fairly normal life and avoid being stepped on, then so, he thought, might he. But the prospect of crossing the street caused him much anxiety and he requested the guide to pick him up and put him into her pocket.

The unusual extended shrinkage experienced by this subject seemed to be a clear reflection of the condition of his ego and his overall life situation: Although gifted and possibly quite brilliant, S had never been able to fulfill his potentials. At the time he was working at a job he considered to be dull and far below his capacities. He felt that his employer and others "looked down on" him; and he was married to an enormously egotistic and narcissistic woman whose behavior intensified his feelings of comparative inadequacy.

While, as noted, in this case the subject's shrinkage seemed a clear reflection of the state of his ego, in most cases the phenomenon either remains inexplicable or seems to have little relevance to individual problems or psychopathology. Quite a few subjects expect to have this particular experience—because they have heard that it occurs so commonly in psychedelic sessions. Others compare the "drug world" with Alice's Wonderland and proceed to have their ups and downs on the basis of that analogy. It has not been our observation that, generally speaking, experiences of growth and shrinkage result from either transient or basic feelings of inferiority or superiority on the part of the subject.

In the case of S-2, a forty-one-year-old male, a drastic reduction of body size was accompanied by an equally remarkable inflation of his already considerable ego. Dwindling to "micro-nuclear" proportions, he first reported his "atomized" state, then grandly announced: "I am the nuclear image of eternity. . . . I am the original stuff. All universes find their pattern in my being for I am the cosmic infinitesimal." Looking at the guide in a patronizing way, he said, "You are merely an aggregate of me. I am the source, the fountain, the stuff before stuff. Ahhhh it is glorious . . . glorious to be alive *here* . . . here with Me in Micro-infinity." At that moment the sun came through the window, casting its rays on S, who stretched luxuriously and declaimed, "Ahhhh, you see. A wave-length shower!"

An hour or so later this same subject, body size now normalized, seemed to regard himself as the Godhead or source of creation. The guide noticed him grandly flinging out his arms and inquired what he was doing, to which S replied: "Creating universes . . . making suns . . . Can't you see? With a flick of my wrist a new cosmos begins. Not that I have to [make an effort]. As anyone can see new worlds are bursting from me all the time." He pointed to the "whirling radiance" which, he said, he could see enamating from all over his body. "A while back I was just the essence of everything. Now I am also the existence." And he returned to flinging out stars and planets.

Similar typical "macrocosmic" statements from subjects take the form of "I am Everything . . . It is Me . . . I am It . . . I Am the Universe . . . The Universe and I are One . . . We are the same . . . It is One . . . One is All . . . I am the It, the One, the All." And so on.

One theory has it that the psychedelic drugs tend to caricature the personality traits of the subjects. In the case of S-2, then, it might be supposed that his feelings of grandiosity were simply an exaggeration of his normal egotism. But why the simultaneous shrinkage of his body in the initial instance (when a great many other subjects, claiming similar omnipotence, assume the proportions of universes, galaxies, etc.)? We could arrive at no satisfactory explanation for this apparent contradiction.

With regard to this, we might add that we have met with numerous instances of persons becoming galaxies, sometimes at the suggestion of the guide. Being a galaxy is invariably described as "very hard work." In two of these cases the subjects described themselves as creating new matter and new suns from the "galactic center" and the "galactic nucleus." This hypothesis for the creation of matter and of suns has been recently advanced by leading astrophysicists.

S-3, a twenty-nine-year-old housewife, dwindled to molecular proportions and said she was afraid of falling through the "vast spaces between the atoms. You know what it all is out there? It's mostly space!" When she walked across the floor she insisted on clinging to the arm of the guide, lest she fall through these spaces. When the guide suggested that the arm she was clutching was also composed of atoms whirling about in a vast emptiness, the subject simply ignored the paradox.

Occasionally, body shrinkage is encountered as an aspect of regression to an infantile or even fetal state. With fetalization, there then may occur an experience of rebirth. In a few cases, rebirth is followed by a condensed revivification of the subject's life, the body being experienced as passing through the various stages of growth and development until the subject regains his normal body image at the present point in time. We are familiar with one such case, not our own, where an economist in his mid-thirties regressed to an infantile state. He tore off his clothing and defecated. Then he tried to "get into the womb" of his girl friend, who was an observer at the session. He became rather violent in this endeavor and had to be forcibly restrained. He then began to sob, voided some more feces, and seemed to be unable to comprehend the language of either his girl friend or the physician-guide. Finally, an antidote—in this case Thorazine—had to be administered. In the great majority of cases, however, the experience of rebirth leaves the subject relaxed, tranquil, and happy, and may be a means by which the "reborn" subject "leaves behind" him various of his problems.

S-4, a thirty-five-year-old male, utilized a part of his session to hold a "conversation with God." During this conversation, he experienced "an intense awareness of God's presence." At the same time, he felt his body becoming elongated and angular, an El Greco-like figure with features ascetic and priestly. He estimated the increase in his height as from five to seven inches and reported, as many other subjects have done, that his perception of the room was that normal for a person of the height he seemed to be. In these cases, when the effects of the drug have worn off, the subject may be asked to ascend a ladder and stand on the rung that would enable him to look down from about the same height as he had seemed to look down from when his stature was increased. These subjects insist that they then perceive the room as it was perceived in the body distortion situation.

S-5, another male in his mid-thirties, became a giant and, like Alice, was afraid that the room would be unable to contain him. S feared that his expanding body might crush the guide's body, and solicitously urged that the guide leave the room. Then, however, S chuckled and remarked that "Of course, I'm not really all that big, I just seem to be growing, and I know that it's the drug affecting my mind in some way."

This experience lasted only a few minutes, but during it S described imaging himself as engaged in an awesome gigantomachia with other beings of his own size. In this war of giants, he was "very ancient" and belonged to "a breed of giants that walked the earth long ago." While experiencing his vision he stood with eyes closed and arms folded, face serene, and voice calm. The giants, he said, wore caveman-like garments fashioned from the skins of animals, possibly mastodons; and they fought with huge gnarled clubs and with their hands in a strange style of wrestling. Once S picked up another giant and hurled him over the edge of a precipice. S expressed uncertainty as to "whether my people are fighting among themselves, or we have been attacked by a hostile clan." He thought the scene of the conflict was probably Ireland or Scotland, though it might have been to the south in the British Isles, or possibly someplace in Europe. He could not fix the incident in time, explaining "We had no calendar and thought only in terms of night and day, the waxing and waning of the moon, the changes in vegetation, and the seasons." The gigantomachia was rather quickly followed by a vision of "exquisitely sculpted swans, made of something like ivory and mechanically propelled across a deep blue lagoon that is flecked with gold by the sunlight." Then S found himself restored to normal size.

The experiences of growth, while they sometimes give a feeling of physical strength and self-confidence, are never as dramatic as the shrinkage and seem to be of comparatively slight psychological interest and importance. Subjects find them entertaining, but rarely in any way significant or productive of anxiety or other strong emotional responses. We are speaking here of experiences of bodily expansion, not of the macrocosmic experience of being a universe, which may yield an intense euphoria or transient feelings of omnipotence. Again, a familiarity with *Alice in Wonderland* along with expectancies based on knowledge of the previous experiences of others often provide a sufficient explanation for what occurs.

Interestingly, the body does not gradually grow or expand into the macrocosmic state; neither does it dwindle away to nothing to permit the having-no-body experience. These conditions of non (physical)-being and ultimate, total, or plenary being, are preceded by the dissolution of the human body or, in the latter instance, sometimes by a kind of explosion into the macrocosmic state. Alice's fear that she might go out altogether, "like a candle," has never been fulfilled in the experience of our subjects—perhaps because it didn't happen to Alice?

In the case of growth and shrinkage, as with a good many other experiences reported by the psychedelic subjects, it is always difficult or impossible to separate the consciously fabricated events from those occurring on some other level. A subject may, for just a few moments, seem to himself to have dwindled to miniscule stature and then go on for quite a while afterwards having fun inventing adventures for this miniscule body although he has long since ceased to experience his body as actually being the size described. This temptation to "make a good story" seems one to which a great many persons fall prey, despite their wish to make an honest contribution to the guide's research. True, even such persistent fantasies may prove instructive in some sense; but they are less instructive than are the authentic body image distortions.

Being Non-Human. Transformations into animal forms, becoming inanimate objects or "pure energy," and dissolution into the no-body state are experiences subjects find entertaining, but which they also believe provide them with helpful insights and contribute to their self-understanding and education generally. In the case of the psychotherapist these experiences, which often may be induced by suggestion, are of great potential value. The experiences also may be instructive to such persons as anthropologists studying the animal metamorphosis rites of preliterate peoples; and, indeed, to almost anyone concerned with the study of human behavior, culture and customs. In this chapter we can do little more than hint at the barely tapped wealth of possibilities afforded in this area by the psychedelic drugs.

Of the metamorphoses into animal forms, one of the most common is the chicken-in-the-egg transformation encountered as one variety of the experience of rebirth. Here the subject becomes a baby chick, breaks out of the egg, and typically beholds a fresh "new world" all around him. He then rather quickly resumes his human form, and will often report that he is seeing this world "with the eyes of a child." Everything looks new and fresh and objects and persons are perceived, in one subject's words, "as a child must perceive them, unblinkered by convention, his vision not yet limited and distorted by conditioning."

S-6, a thirty-seven-year-old anthropologist and author, had a long-standing interest in animal metamorphosis rites as practiced in various parts of Africa and the Caribbean. After several LSD sessions with various guides, he managed to obtain about 500 micrograms and took the LSD in the privacy of his apartment with no one else present. He experienced transformations into goat and lion forms, but the most impressive of his changes involved becoming a tiger:

"I had obtained some appropriate ritual music and lay down and soon became totally absorbed in the recording. I expected (or hoped) that the metamorphosis would take place, but my expectancy was surely no greater than that of those who participate in these rites.

"The first phase of my experience was on the human level. As I managed to scribble, before again abandoning myself (appropriate term!) to the recording, this was my first authentic experience of the orgiastic. I was totally *there*, totally a participant, and what I participated in was a frenzied dionysiac union with a multiplicity of others: the forging of a single will or emotional state, I cannot say which, but perhaps a will to yield utterly to a wild, animalistic sensuality and emotional outpouring—an ecstacy in which particular bodies were abandoned for a single body constituted of us all, a body writhing as if in the throes of an almost unbearable onslaught of sensuality.

"I have no idea how much time elapsed—surely not more than ten or twenty minutes as the clock would measure it—before I became conscious of myself moving across the floor of the apartment, moving as best I can recall by propelling myself along on my knees with my flattened palms also pressed against the floor. At about this same instant I found myself before a full-length mirror and, looking into it, was confronted by a huge, magnificent specimen of a tiger! Simultaneous, I think, with my perception of this image I became aware of my tiger's body, of emotions that seemed to saturate my being, and of a narrow or compressed kind of consciousness that focused only upon what was being perceived and upon the emotional state on the one hand and basic physical sensations on the other. I was *in* this body, and *felt* this body, as I never have been in or felt my own.

"Yet even with what seemed my complete immersion in my tigerness, I did retain some infinitesimal human awareness—as if some minute segment of myself continued to stand guard over this strange event and would not permit me to escape entirely from my human self. I seem to recall a kind of pull back toward the human condition exerted by this fragment and that I resisted the pull with all the force at my command.

"Confronting the image in the mirror, I knew and yet did not know that this image was my own (although, oddly, it seemed to me later that there was, in the face of this tiger, something of my face). I reacted to the image, partly anyhow, as if it might be another tiger with whom I had come unexpectedly face to face. Yet something in me questioned the reality of the image, and I recall my bafflement when I ran my claws across the glass and touched the hard, flat surface. All the while I was making spitting and snarling noises and my muscles were tensed in readiness for combat. Finally, I turned away from the mirror and padded restlessly around the apartment, still making those sounds that somehow indicated to me bafflement and rage.

"God knows how much anthropomorphizing I was doing at the time, or how much the experience has been distorted in the attempt to recollect it. But it seems to me I looked at the room with incomprehension and a sense that this environment was alien and not at all where I belonged.

"Still later, how I got there I haven't the slightest notion, I was locked up in a cage in some zoo. It seems that I paced interminably up and down within the barred enclosure, looking out with a kind of flattened vision at people like paper cutouts who stood peering into my cage.

"The return to a human consciousness was by gradations, but fairly rapid, bringing with it a kind of regret. I hadn't been, if one may put it that way, very happy as a tiger; and yet, in some way I won't try to define, I felt that the tiger represented some valid and essential aspect of what or who I am.

"My return to being a person seems to have occurred while I slowly got up off all fours and very slowly straightened my body until I was standing erect. Then I went over to my desk and wrote down a paragraph that, however bizarre sounding, does have, I believe, its grain of validity and meaningfulness for me:

" 'I am a tiger who has learned to turn himself into a man; but the tiger still spends more time as a tiger, emotionally at any rate, than as a man. The tiger will have to become more of a man and less of a tiger if he wants to fulfill his human destiny and realize happiness.'

"Reflecting upon my experiences in the zoo, I jotted down a few other memories and words of wisdom for posterity:

" 'The lion is as strong as the tiger and is less the victim of rage and fear. Therefore he, not the tiger, is the King of the Beasts despite his lesser physical beauty. It is his lack of anxiety or lesser anxiety that makes him regal and the proper claimant to his title.

" 'The tiger, in the cage, gives always the sense of being imprisoned.

He never ceases to rage against his imprisonment and this passion for freedom invests him with, or contributes to, his dignity. But the lion, somehow, seems much less a prisoner. It is not that he has, like certain other creatures, placidly accepted being caged. Instead, he has managed somehow to transcend the fact of his captivity, and this the (more feline) tiger can never do.'

"Those who have witnessed the transformation rites in such places as Haiti and Rhodesia say that the person who believes himself transformed into a certain animal takes on the aspect of that animal. For various seemingly sound reasons this perception by the spectator does not seem to be exclusively the end-product of suggestion and whatever responses are induced by the ritual. Would I have appeared to an observer to resemble in any way a tiger? Somehow I think the answer to that is 'Yes.' But probably, I now feel obliged to add, I would only have looked like a silly anthropologist, 'out of his skull' on hallucinogens, foolishly crawling around on the floor and making idiotic noises.

"Looking back from the perspective of several days, I have a few additional words to say. I now seem to have a recollection of a dance in which I participated dressed, like the others, in a tiger skin. Whether this is an afterthought, I can't say with any certainty. The final (for now) term I would apply to the experience is *enriching*. I am too confirmed a skeptic to let myself go beyond that. But I think I *will* suspend my judgment about what occurs at these transformation rites until such time as I have witnessed some of them at first hand and, I hope, have participated actively in them as well as observing."

This experience is much more vivid than any of its kind occurring in our guided sessions. This fact might be attributed to a variety of factors: the subject's knowledge of and interest in transformation rites, as well as his strong wish for the experience and the recording he had available to induce it. In much more typical metamorphoses, at the guide's suggestion subjects have often become bulls in the ring at Knossos or Madrid. They have vigorously pawed the earth, snorted, and one seemed about to charge, but he promptly and amiably responded to the guide's command that he resume his human form.

Other subjects, receiving similar suggestions, do not participate actively with their bodies but recline or sit and experience the transformation and subsequent events only cerebrally. A few of the LSD subjects, spontaneously or in response to suggestions, have undergone a kind of series of evolutionary metamorphoses carrying them from protoplasm up to man—then claiming to have experienced all the stages on life's way. Animal transformations are usually regarded by the subjects as a kind of mental game-playing and minimal significance is attached to them. In fact, this kind of shallow or playful reaction, and similar reactions to certain other phenomena, provide a useful tool for the guide who may employ them to divert the subject or lighten his mood.

The experience of having-no-body is one that psychedelic subjects tend to place in the category of the ineffable. And how much may be said, after all, about a body one doesn't have? Having-no-body may occur within the context of a "mystical experience." As a physical state (or non-state) it represents, as noted, the end-stage of a process of dissolution, the body breaking down into minute particles which dissipate or dissolve. The experience tends to be pleasurable, when not mystically rapturous.

"Thingification" or becoming an inanimate object takes various forms and the subject reaches his condition of thingness or object-being by traversing one of a variety of possible psychical routes. In the most common forms of this experience the subject either identifies with and "becomes" some actual object present in the room, or he finds himself transmuted into some imaginary object. When he effects union and oneness with an actual object, he usually does so by fixing (usually spontaneously, sometimes intentionally) on the object and emphatically merging with it. As object, he retains consciousness but is rarely aware of any incongruity in that fact. It appears to be an *as if* sort of consciousness—the subject unreflectively thinking and feeling as he supposes the particular object would think and feel: he anthropomorphizes the "consciousness" of the object. When the object he "becomes" is an imaginary one, he behaves in an approximately similar way, although in this case he may place himself as object in the actual environment around him or fabricate another environment to contain the imagined object that he has become. In general, but allowing for numerous exceptions, the imaginary object-self is more revealing of the deeper strata of mind; when an actual present object is chosen, it tends to be more revealing of what is in or near the surface of consciousness.

Relatedly, the subject may become an animate but presumably non-conscious object, such as a plant; he may become earth, fire, water, or air; he may become a humanoid object such as a robot or mechanical man;[1] and so on.

Since robotization is a fairly well known phenomenon occurring in schizophrenia, it may be well to point out the differences in schizo-phrenic and psychedelic subject response to the experience. With the schizophrenic, robotization is experienced as a painful deprivation of autonomy and terrifying dehumanization. Of six robotized psychedelic (peyote) subjects observed, four found the identification amusing and entertained themselves for a little while by walking and gesturing stiffly, inquiring as to whether they "clanked," their motors sounded all right, or they needed refueling or winding.

One subject said "I don't want to be a robot"—and at once stopped being one. Only in a single case was there any strong negative reaction.

S-7, in her late twenties, the wife of a Navy lieutenant, became a mechanical woman—a "metallic automaton." She is a small, attractive woman with an appealingly elfin and otherworldly quality about her. She is "very religious" and takes an avid interest in such things as visitors from outer space and the lighter side of the occult. S reads a great deal, mostly fantasy, fairy tales, science fiction and nonfiction related to her interests. She is a warm, happy person who has excellent relationships with her husband, two small children and friends. She is active in her city's cultural affairs, especially the theater. Any criticism of her by friends is confined to the affectionate observation that she is "a bit of an oddball."

Becoming a mechanical woman, S described herself as reacting with instantaneous and profound aversion "to this thing I have become." She explained that her "only neurosis," with her for as long as she could remember, consisted of a very deep-rooted and almost phobic dislike of machines. She wondered why, since this was so, she should now have become one; and went on to express her strong opposition to such ideas as "a mechanical universe" and "man is nothing but a machine." She was particularly distressed at the thought that "this mechanizing of myself may mean I don't believe what I've always thought I believed. Maybe this is the way my unconscious has of telling me that I *am* a machine, or that deep down I think I'm one." Further speculations along these lines increased her distress and she resisted the guide's efforts to divert her, insisting, "No, I have to find out what this means." She sat stiffly in her chair and spoke in a monotone quite different from her ordinary way of speaking.

The guide was able to terminate this experience, which lasted ten to fifteen minutes, by smiling and merrily telling the subject, "I know who you are. Why, you're the Tin Woodman of OZ." He then went on to describe the Tin Woodman, Dorothy, and the Scarecrow as they skipped down the famous yellow brick road. As this narration—an appeal to the subject's affinity for fantasy—proceeded, S was caught up in the story and identified with the Tin Woodman. Soon, she was happily looking at some flowers in a vase and seemed to have forgotten the experience that distressed her. She enjoyed the remainder of her session but did not have the mystical experience she had hoped for.

Contact with S was maintained for more than one year subsequent to this session. She herself eventually initiated a discussion of what had occurred and remarked that "It was pretty stupid of me, getting so upset. I guess these drugs can turn you into just about anything." There was never any indication of adverse aftereffects of her session.

Such identifications as with earth, fire, or water are explained by some subjects as deriving from mythic and theological sources—the burning bush, pillars of flame, the creation of man from earth or clay, the notion of elemental spirits, to name but a few. But we have also traced the impetus for "being an ocean" to the subliminal perception of a dripping faucet; and "being a holocaust" to the subject's peripheral perception of a candle flickering in a corner of the room.

The subject, as fire, may be concerned with the fire's warmth—or with its capacity to consume. As water, he may think in terms of a primordial life source—or of floods. One subject said: "I am the oceans. I will inundate all. I will obliterate man and all his works. These do not deserve to survive." But then he smiled and jokingly complained about "constantly being tickled by fishes."

Subjects who become inanimate objects claim to have gained insights of various sorts into the nature of the object. They may say that they know how the object "feels"—and if told that an object doesn't feel at all, will dispute this or say that they know how the object would feel if it could. Subjects appear to enjoy these dialogues; the guide very quickly finds them boring. What may be of importance is *why* the subject has chosen to identify with this particular substance or form or combination of the two. Psychedelic subjects, when willing to co-operate, provide insights concerning human-object relationships that will be of considerable value in the development of a "psychoanalysis of things."

The Reflected Image. Psychedelic subjects, looking into mirrors, have many interesting and sometimes enlightening experiences. The image reflected in the mirror may be determined by the subject's physical or emotional state or by what he is thinking. The mirror image is susceptible to some manipulation by either the subject or the guide and the mirror thus becomes in this context a possible therapeutic instrument.

A subject looking into a mirror may "think" serenity, anguish, rage, joy, sadness, or whatever; and, although his face remains expressionless, the mirror will seem to him to reflect what he is thinking.

The mirror may, without any effort on the part of the subject, seem to him to reflect his anxieties, wishes, or beliefs about himself. Some religiously guilt-ridden subjects and those who think of themselves as daemonic may find a devil or demon peering back at them from the mirror. Subjects with slightly porcine or equine physiognomies have found staring back at them the faces of swine and horses—peyote or LSD + mind maliciously completing the development of what a more charitable nature only hinted at.

S-8, a twenty-three-year-old university instructor, ingested 100 micrograms of LSD and, looking into a mirror, "aged 2,000 years." It was, she said, "a steady progression of aging. I quickly aged through decades until I was a haggard and white-haired seventy, and then the deterioration really set in. Hundreds of years of ruinous decline made their horrid inroads on my face and figure until at the age of 2,000 I was reduced to a wizened, waxened mummy, eyeless, toothless, and brainless."

S says that she has a morbid fear of aging, feeling that "aging is about the worst thing that could happen to one." Further probing of possible causes of this subject's experience elicited the facts that she had read and seen as a child a film version of Rider Haggard's She, and that these had made a powerful impression upon her. Her mirror image experience, she thought, may have been a visualized recall of the similar scene in the novel and film. A few other instances have been observed where a subject visualizes memory material but cannot recognize it as familiar until the material has been dealt with on a verbal level.

Among the drug-induced changes in physiological functioning are changes affecting visual perception, among these dilation of the pupil of the eye. These changes alone produce some mirror image distortions. For example, the face is likely to be seen as blotchy and with the pores seemingly much larger than usual. It is somewhat as if the subject were looking into a magnifying mirror—where few faces ever appear to good advantage. Difficulties in maintaining focus may be experienced, giving the image an unpleasant fluidity. But the psychogenic mirror image distortions are, of course, the more extreme ones.

In our experience every subject who looks into a mirror experiences a certain amount of distortion; and it would be a conservative estimate to say that ninety percent of the subjects experience at least some of the distortions as unpleasant. Such reactions range all the way from a mild displeasure or distaste to strong feelings of fear and revulsion.

Caricaturing oneself and others, face or whole body, is a commonplace. This exaggerated emphasis on selected physical characteristics may make a plump man appear to be grotesquely obese, transform a face with semitic features into a Julius Streicher cartoon, and so on. The suggestion in a face of slyness, sensuality, or cruelty may be magnified to rival the creations of a Hieronymus Bosch. The subject is frequently amused by his caricatured perception of someone else; he is rarely similarly amused when the ugly, vicious, or ludicrous countenance reflected by the mirror is his own.

Perceiving such a travestied version of someone else, the subject will usually say to himself, "This is just the effect of the drug. He doesn't really look anything like that." But, seeing his own distorted image, he wonders, "Am I now seeing myself as I really am? Is my actual character, if not my actual face, being seen?" And: "Are others able to see in me all the time what I now, the veil ripped away, am able to see in myself?"

The guide reassures the subject, who might otherwise go on to develop further paranoidal ideation, by telling him that this is a very common or universal occurrence among psychedelic subjects. Or the subject may be told that every kind of tendency is latent in all human beings and visualizing a latent tendency under the present conditions in no way implies that it will become overt. Or the guide may remark that a great deal of experience has shown that these distressing images reveal nothing about the person's character but are only symptomatic of a natural mild anxiety he feels in a psychical environment so different from the one that he is used to. Without such help from the guide the subject will in any case soon go on to something else.

Unpleasant mirror image experiences are almost as various as they are frequent, and one wonders why the distortion of the image is so often in the direction of ugliness and emphasis on character deficiencies rather than fulfilling the wishes of most subjects to be beautiful and healthy and virtuous. Certainly there is no overall tendency on the part of the subjects to produce mainly painful phenomena or to engage in self-derogation. Nor, with rare exceptions, do the mirror images seem to be very closely related to the "unconscious body image" as it is hallucinated by disturbed hypnotic subjects in psychotherapy.

One hypothesis might be that the visual perception of any kind of distorted self-image creates doubts in the subject concerning his identity; or magnifies doubts already created by some of the other drug effects. These magnified doubts, generating additional subject anxiety, might then cause the reflected image to be distorted in the direction of the ugly image or the image that threatens by suggesting revelation of character faults or repressed perverted or criminal tendencies. But that is only an hypothesis and further investigation is required.

There are also some pleasant experiences to be had with the mirror image. Some subjects report perceiving a succession of comical distortions similar to those produced by the image distorting mirrors so popular at amusement parks. Other subjects are able to see themselves, with the aid of a little autosuggestion, as historical personages, film stars, and other public figures. The ability to "think an emotion" and see it reflected in the mirror is a source of entertainment. In a few cases, with and without the assistance of the guide, the mirror image has been useful in contributing to self-knowledge and has even provided insights resulting in amelioration or resolution of long-standing problems. To give but a single example:

S-9. Female in her mid-thirties. 175 micrograms LSD. Several hours into her session, S looked into a mirror and saw a distressing caricature of her face.

In fact, this very intelligent and high-strung woman's face normally appeared to be a kind of caricature. The cheeks seemed drawn and held in by a continuous muscular effort, and pursed lips contributed to the general impression of a rigid, puritanical personality.

After discussing her appearance and accurately appraising the impression she made on others, S indicated a wish that something could be "done about" the face to make it more attractive. She also felt that the face did not accurately express her personality.

The guide suggested to S that she try to work with the mirror image. She should try to fill out the image, not only of the face but of the whole body, which was thin and shapeless. Following the suggestions, S worked successively with various features of the face and then the rest of her body, managing to change the mirror image into something much more to her liking.

The guide then suggested to S that she take this new mirror image for her own image. She agreed and at once her lips relaxed, giving her a softer and more attractive appearance. She then lay down on a sofa and practiced relaxing her musculature and experiencing her body in terms of the mirror image she had created. S was repeatedly exhorted to continue after the session to practice envisioning the new image and identifying with it, and also to practice the techniques of fractional relaxation taught her by the guide.

S adhered to this regimen and several months later presented a much improved appearance. Her cheeks seemed filled out, her mouth and general expression were relaxed, and even her body appeared to have become somewhat more rounded and less angular.

S always had been a fairly heavy eater, but never had been able to gain weight. Now she did begin, gradually, to gain weight without increasing her food intake. She became less high-strung and it seemed as if the muscular relaxation was accompanied by a kind of "metabolic relaxation." Without reducing her overt physical activity, she seemed to be able to "keep" more of her calories and thus to fill out.

When transformations of this kind occur, they seem to have been too easily achieved. But the psychedelic experience provides one context—and there are a variety of others—in which such abrupt and dramatic changes in a person's life do sometimes take place or receive their first decisive impetus.

The ordinary ways of looking at one's body are to look at it directly, seeing those parts accessible to inspection, or to look into a mirror or mirrors where larger body areas may be seen at a glance and where some parts of the body may be seen that are not accessible to direct observation.

Direct observation of the body, which cannot of course include observation of one's own face, is rarely if ever as disturbing or as interesting as the mirror image may be.

With direct observation one's own body is seldom rendered more aesthetically delightful by the drug-induced distortions. A subject may perceive the hand or some other part of the body of a loved one or a friend as exquisitely sculpted from ivory or alabaster; but the subject's own hand is much more likely to appear coarse-textured, fattened or shriveled, and crudely made. One wonders if the unpleasant sensations experienced early in the drug session might not partly account for all this implied hostility to the own body and the perceptual revenge wreaked upon it?

Distortions of spatial perception when applied to the body sometimes are amusing. A subject may lie on his back and look at his feet—which may seem to be five yards away or just under his chin. Such a distortion may or may not be accompanied by a sense of the body's elongation or foreshortening. An arm may also be perceived as absurdly long or short—so that if the subject relied on the visual evidence alone, he would think himself capable of reaching the whole length of the room to pick up some object 20 feet away. But this sort of distortion is almost always accompanied by an intellectual recognition that the perception *is* a distortion and such a feat therefore impossible.

Some psychedelic subjects "see" their own body by spontaneously or intentionally employing means other than direct observation and looking into reflecting surfaces. Some are able to project an image of their own body on a wall or into a crystal; or they may close their eyes and envision their own body image. The image projected on a wall is usually perceived as "flat," as in a painting; the image in the crystal is seen as dimensional, having depth; the image seen with the eyes closed may be perceived as either flat or dimensional, the subject often expressing uncertainty as to which. A few subjects spontaneously see, or claim to be able to project, an image in space—for example, an image that stands next to them or confronts them and may or may not possess some degree of solidity. One subject claimed to be able to "multiply" himself several times, simultaneously perceiving several images, replicas or doubles of himself that could occupy any position within his field of vision.

There is also a fairly common experience where the subject seems to himself to project his consciousness away from his body and then is able to see his body as if he were standing off to one side of it or looking down on it from above. A few subjects feel that they are able to leave the "material body" and move about in something like the "astral body" familiar to occultists. This astral body is described as being diaphanous and almost, but not quite, immaterial. It may be composed of "energy," "electrical impulses," and so on. Some identify this astral body with an "aura" they earlier had perceived as radiating from them, an "energy force field" surrounding the body. The perception of the aura by psychedelic subjects is very common.

One subject, having silently reclined with eyes closed on a couch for several minutes, sat up and reported himself able to travel in his astral body and to pass through walls and other solid obstacles. He had just been down on the street, he said, and described very vividly what he had seen there. But asked to pass through the wall into the neighboring apartment, with which he was not familiar, and to describe its furnishings, he declined. He found the request insulting and said that it impugned his integrity.

The experience of observing the body as if from a distance is, however, real enough and is common in the drug-state. It occurs in non-drug situations too—with both psychotic and non-psychotic persons—but with the drug subject it ordinarily generates none of the anxiety felt in certain other contexts. The experience may involve a whole series of self-images, the subject looking at his body looking at his body looking at his body, and so on. It is the familiar picture within a picture within a picture effect, sometimes achieved by employing a series of mirrors.

Body Alchemy and Other Wonders. The psychedelic subject may "feel" that his body has been altered in a variety of ways. He may feel, for instance, his normally flesh-and-bone body transmuted into some other substance, as if by a psychedelic alchemy. Then he will experience himself as made of wood, of metal, of glass, or whatever.

Experiencing such a transmutation of substance, the subject will, however, continue to regard this body he occupies as his own. To experience one's body as metallic in substance may thus be a thoroughly different experience from that of robotization previously discussed. That is, the robotized man may become something other than himself: he may be a thing. He has lost his autonomy and must exist in accordance with whatever restrictions govern the existence of what he has become. The "metallized" man, on the other hand, continues to function largely as before. Rarely does being metal (or whatever) interfere even with the flexibility of his body. It is simply a feeling as to one's substance—probably impossible to convey to one who has not experienced it or at least observed a subject experiencing it.

Any perceptual distortions will be tactile. Picking up an object, the subject may feel as if the contact were that of two hard objects touching. The subject may, if metallized, feel that the surface of the body is colder and slicker, as well as harder than before.

The symbolism of these particular transformations is usually readily accessible. Subject and guide discuss and analyze the significance of the substance and why it was selected by the subject. The transmutation is rarely experienced as unpleasant, but the subsequent analysis proves disturbing in some cases. Substance transmutations not suggested by the guide have occurred in less than five percent of the subjects.

Subjects very frequently experience the body as slightly heavier than usual. This feeling of heaviness may persist through most or all of a session, may be intermittent, or may appear only at the beginning in combination with the other physical symptoms common at that time. Experiencing the body as excessively heavy is infrequent. One subject reported himself unable to get out of his chair, so heavy was his body. He "weighed a ton" and felt as if he were "made of lead"—referring to his weight, not to any change in substance.

Feelings of lightness are often reported. The most extreme version of this experience is "weightlessness," which may be accompanied by a feeling that the body has levitated. Weightlessness sometimes precedes or accompanies ego and/or body dissolution and the religious and mystical experiences.

S-10, in her fifties, with mystical tendencies, reported her progress toward the weightless condition in the following euphoric terms: "——[subject's name] is no more. The small self has departed. Ohhhhhhh . . . my body is lightening. (Much laughter.) Her body is lightening. Now she is egoless. Now she is weightless. Ohhhhhhhh . . . I have finally . . . finally come to MYSELF. And I have another body. It is a body of bliss. A pure body of light and eternity. Ohhhhhhh . . ." and so on.

The experience of a "consciousness" localized in some part of the body—say, in a fingertip—is not uncommon. This localized consciousness may coexist with the subject's usual consciousness or the usual consciousness may have "shifted its place of residence" to the fingertip. When consciousness is localized in some body part, an unusual increase in that part's sensitivity or responsiveness to stimuli is claimed by the subject.

A subject may "feel" the interior of his body, either experiencing his internal structure and processes as he understands them, or experiencing them as altered in some way. "Feeling" the "interior landscape" is one variety of the latter. For example, several subjects have felt the inner body as consisting of trees and vines, streams and waterfalls, hills and valleys. One subject could "feel" his "parental heritage," the respective maternal and paternal contributions to his "cellular structure." This was a "revolting and grisly" experience. He said that "I knew just what in my body came from my mother and what from my father. I could feel my mother and father in my body and I felt that I knew what my mother's body feels like to my mother and what my father's body feels like to my father. I lost for a little while most of my sense of my body as my own. Experiencing so much woman in my body was especially awful."

Occasionally a previously held abnormal "feeling" about the body, as well as an abnormal image of the body, may spontaneously be normalized in the course of a psychedelic session.

S-11, a businesswoman in her forties, had for many years experienced her body and her "mind and brain" as being literally "tied up in knots." She could "plainly feel" this knotting, which she felt to be related to her "tenseness." For more than five years she had been familiarizing herself with literature concerning psychedelic drugs and believed that a psychedelic session was "the only means" by which she could free herself from her tensions and the feeling of knottedness. Hers was an extremely unusual experience.

About one hour into her session, when ordinarily the various distressing physical symptoms would be experienced, S began speaking of a "great but wonderful pain . . . my body is becoming unknotted." One by one, as she described it, the knots in her body "untangled." Later, in a second (LSD) session, the knots in her "mind and brain" also became "untangled." This second "unknotting," like the first, was experienced as "excruciatingly painful . . . also quite glorious." This relief appears to be permanent. Six months later, S had developed no new knots.

In a written report on her experiences, S describes them in a not-too-detailed but interesting way:

". . . they [the LSD sessions] were essentially instinct and emotional level. Also each day since brings something new. In the first experience, the incredible unknotting of my whole body was the outstanding thing. All the fusion of the senses happened too, and I felt whole and full of wonder in nature as I remember feeling as a child. My muscles, nerves, and bones seemed to relax—almost relent—in a way that was infinitely right and to be desired. As you know, there were floods of tears, also right and a 'giving way,' which had to do with grief yet were an impersonal thing as well. The removal of the 'personal' actually made all this physical release possible, I feel. I had no desire—in fact, had a definite antipathy—to disciplined thought of any kind. I simply wanted to be, and flow with the tide. Afterward, my whole body was sore in a delicious way for several days, and I slept as I have not slept since childhood.

"The second [session] was strangely like the first in that it again involved release and relenting, but this time in my head. There was great pain, as though adhesions were being pulled loose, and the pain continued for about twelve hours afterward. I felt no desire to 'cope with' this pain, although, as the LSD wore off, in the late afternoon, it made me almost nauseated. Yet it was good, I knew, and to be welcomed rather than resisted . . . Thinking was not ruled out this second time. WHAT was thought I cannot say. It was more a matter of letting thoughts come and go where they would. It was at times a conversation, but inner, and not needing to be said. I found it a great comfort to be in the room with my husband, although practically nothing was said. I felt a smoothing of both of us, as though we were flowing side by side in a river . . ."

A striking example of normalization of a distorted body image will be given in a subsequent chapter.

Concluding Remarks. The body and body image experiences dealt with in this chapter represent only a small segment of the body phenomena encountered in psychedelic sessions. For the most part the materials just considered might be termed the oddities, the *exotica*, of psychedelic experiencing of the body.

We have been largely concerned, for example, with the body only as it exists for the person himself and outside of other contexts than that of the psychedelic session. Drug effects upon ordinary sense perceptions have been virtually ignored and will be discussed in a future chapter. The body as experienced in a variety of relationships with others and to the world generally will also be discussed in much greater detail in the chapters to come.

In terms of any measure of aesthetic, intellectual and spiritual depth or quality, such experiences as Alice-in-Wonderland distortions of size, metamorphoses into animal forms, and observing image distortions in mirrors, would probably not rank very high. This is not to say that such experiences lack value for the subject or fail to provide important data useful not only to the psychotherapist, but also to workers in many other fields and to mankind generally. But there are, as we will see, available to the subject a great range of other experiences—broader, deeper, and qualitatively of a higher order than those presented here.

Four:
Experiencing
Other Persons

The psychedelic drug subject's experiencing of other persons differs from his normal experiencing of others in a remarkable variety of ways. There are radical alterations of visual perception—of the way the other person is seen—and these are sometimes directly attributable to the subject's emotional state and/or ideation. The subject may find in his awareness of his own psychical complexity a new appreciation and sometimes understanding of the complexity of another or others. The inadequacies of clichés and labels employed to simplify relationships often become apparent. Capacity for empathy seems greatly heightened in many cases. Customary methods of communication may be supplanted by novel, characteristically "psychedelic" methods, including the telepathic if a great many subjects and observers may be trusted on this point. Out of these varied experiences may come significant reorientations in the area of interpersonal relationships.

Visual Perception of Other Persons.   The visual experiencing of other persons is for a majority of psychedelic subjects one of the most dramatic and memorable aspects of the session. How the subject sees another person depends mainly upon: 1)his sensory response to the person; 2)his emotional response to the person; 3)what he is thinking about the person; and 4)inferred unconscious determinants. Sensory and emotional response and ideation, along with unconscious materials, are interactive and apparently any one of the four may hold a temporary ascendancy and determine to some extent the content of the first three. Doubtless this is also true outside the psychedelic drug context, but normally the interaction is not so clear to the person and the effects upon visual perception are much less striking.

Whether the subject sees another person in a positive or a negative way depends upon a great many factors. In general, if the subject is anxious or hostile with regard to another person or persons, he or they will be seen, if visual distortion occurs at all, in some negative way. If another person is liked or regarded as supportive by the subject, then he will be seen, should distortion occur, in a positive way. However, there are always exceptions; the same person may be viewed in a positive way at one time and in a negative way at another; and neither subject nor guide should respond automatically to visual distortions with any *in vino veritas* sort of interpretation.

The guide, when his performance is satisfactory, will only rarely be seen by a subject in a drastically distorted way. Especially, with the same qualification, the guide rarely will be seen distorted in a drastically negative way. The reason for this would seem to be that the guide is required as a kind of "home base," at once constant and yet able to accompany the subject on his psychedelic journey. Additionally, the subject presumably already has come to accept the guide as a trustworthy, authoritative figure upon whose advice and good will he can rely; and the guide, by means of his in-session behavior, continues to recreate and reinforce this role.

Such distortions of the guide as occur thus will be mostly "in favor" of the guide. However, it is always possible that a subject, if sufficiently anxious, will distort the guide in some negative way—a phenomenon the guide may find useful in assessing his own performance and the state of the subject, but should not rely upon exclusively.

In a fairly common distortion the guide may be perceived by the subject as one or more of a variety of archetypal figures. For example, a female guide may be seen as a goddess, as a priestess, or as the personification of wisdom or truth or beauty. Descriptions of some of these "archetypal" perceptions have included seeing the guide's features as "glowing with a luminous pallor" and her gestures as being "cosmic, yet classical." The clothing has been seen by subjects to change and "flow," from the vestments of an Egyptian Isis figure to the robes of an Athena. As a final metamorphosis she has sometimes become some variation of a sort of future space deity, hovering between stars and clad in garments of star dust, glacial ice, and so on. All of these were positive perceptions for the subjects, who possibly enhanced their own sense of security by attributing godly or godlike status and powers to the guide.

However, in a negative variation of this type of distortion the guide was perceived as an Egyptian *bas relief*, a painting of Isis carved on some tomb wall. Perceptually depriving the guide of life, tridimensionality, or freedom of movement, may be a weapon the subject unconsciously wields against the guide to "punish" her, make her less threatening, purchase self-aggrandizement at the guide's expense or otherwise assert a magical supremacy over her. In this case the subject, momentarily irritated, reduced the guide to *bas relief* status and then wrote: "So you are just an Egyptian tomb painting. What a waste!"

Such perceptions as this one, along with similar reductions in which persons are seen as things or even may be denied form and substance, are usually products of anxiety or hostility but also may be rooted in egoism. In this latter case the subject may look out upon a world in which others exist not with-himself, but for-himself. Since this for-himself world is essentially a world of the other-as-object, the perceptual "thingification" of the other is not too surprising. The flattening out of the other—the perception of him as unilinear or as a painting—is often only the first step in an inanimatizing process that culminates in the subject's perception of the other as a thing deprived of all traces of the former identity and humanness.

To examine some more of these distortions the male guide may be seen as a Buddha or Buddha-like figure (positive distortion). The guide was so seen throughout most of a peyote session by a subject who at no time visualized him in a negative way. However, in a subsequent LSD session, this subject was more anxious and produced both negative and positive perceptions of the guide.

S-1, the subject just referred to, participated first in a peyote session that included two other subjects. These other subjects, both good friends of S, were nonetheless negatively distorted by him by means of the caricaturing process previously described. S writes that "Early in my session I noticed a tendency on my part to see people as caricatures of themselves. A minor physical peculiarity would transform itself into a major personality trait. The twitch of a facial muscle became the sinister leer of an evil mind. As the evening wore on this delusion became more pronounced and for a time it was unsettling to realize that I was seeing things as I did, not because that was how they were, but because my mind was shaping them in a peculiar manner—an observation that I think would also find application in my day to day life."

This subject, a businessman in his late twenties, insisted at one point in the session on going out for a walk. Since the dose had been light and the subject was well in control of himself, this was agreed to. Persons in the street then were also negatively distorted:

"Out on the street the cool evening air was chilly but exhilarating. The city, which had seemed from the window cold, grimy and slightly sinister, now was transformed into the wonderland I had envisioned when hearing fables as a child. The rich colors and textures of fantasy, more real than real, were pure enchantment. Walls of buildings had an added dimension to their surfaces. I felt I was walking in a waking dream. It was an all-consuming pleasure, just to see, touch, feel and smell. I had the urge to run and, giving way to the impulse, felt myself propelled along at triple speed, as in an old speeded-up movie.

"The occasional passer-by was also greatly altered in appearance and I saw him as a grotesque distortion of himself. The personality and intentions seemed to be boldly written on his features and reflected in his mannerisms. I found myself laughing openly at these people, a laughter that seemed to be three-quarters sarcasm and one-quarter delight. I believe now that this was a magnification of a trait I ordinarily keep hidden, below the surface, even from myself. It was eerie, how I seemed to be able to divine the intentions of these strangers. I recall also seeing a car, built during the era when much chrome trim was in style. In the bright moonlight it became a blinding mass of glinting silver, overwhelming in its impact. I staggered back and looked with relief on the subtler tones of the city skyline.

"My friend——'s illusions took on a more frightening form. I can still see his expression as he looked down at a caterpillar on the ground and saw it seemingly grow in size to gigantic proportions and start to pursue him. He quickly looked away and never looked back on the creature again.

"Returning to the apartment I saw once more how the others were distorted, as if I were focusing on the dominant quality of each. . . . The guide seemed more and more, as the evening wore on, a kind of benign Buddha, making his own inner judgments of the people present."

Despite the negative visual distortions (generally of persons, but not of objects), S regarded his peyote experience as being overall an extremely positive one. He limited himself mainly to sensory experiencing and found his awareness of color the most memorable aspect of the session. On his way home, "The city was bathed in the first pink rays of the morning sun and was truly breath-taking to behold. The soft greens of the trees and grass of Central Park were beyond belief. The buildings and streets had a warmth and charm hitherto reserved for memories of bygone days . . . That evening I was back in my old familiar world, but with an awareness of and appreciation for colors, hues and textures that I had never had before. This effect remains with me still (some four months later), but to a lessened degree. The scarcely remembered nausea was indeed a small price to pay for the remarkable night and the heightened awareness of the world around me that I still retain."

In his subsequent (LSD) session, S was determined to come to grips with some personal problems and to try to revise his thinking about various key persons in his life. The emotion generated by this effort, along with several unfortunate but unavoidable aspects of the setting, resulted in the subject's being more anxious than during his former session and also resulted in transient feelings of hostility toward the guide. Both the anxiety and hostility were at their strongest early in the session and yielded negative distortions of the guide who appeared to be "younger and more soft and plump . . . (The guide's) hair was hanging down in an unattractive way . . . (and the guide resembled) Little Boy Blue in the Gainsborough painting"—a decidedly negative perception for this subject. Later, S feeling less anxious and no longer hostile, the guide was seen by him as "very firm and massive, mature and authoritative looking"—a strongly positive perception.

This subject's negative visual perceiving and "caricaturing" of strangers encountered on the street is typical. When strangers are seen and visually distorted by a subject, the distortion is almost always negative in one way or another. These distortions, as with the distortions of the guide, are usually products of anxiety and hostility. These last derive, in turn, from a variety of ideas and feelings that frequently have included the following:

Subjects almost always tend to feel ill at ease with persons who are not also taking the drug or who have not had some previous experience of it and so that they might "understand." The subject is uncertain of the extent to which he is able to function normally if need be and so sees those who have no interest in protecting his well-being as threats to him. As with primitive man, there is the sense that "the stranger is the enemy." The stranger may be seen (along the lines of Sartrean psychology) as that *Other* with whom one is always in essential conflict. Here, as theorized by a subject, "The stranger represents in its purest form other-personness. [And the subject then] . . . responds on essential and primordial levels. He can do this because he is unaffected by all of those additional factors that come into play when he is interacting with someone whom he knows."

In general, when the predominant emotional response is anxiety, strangers will be seen as menacing; when hostility is the predominant response, a kind of patronizing view may be assumed, with the unknown others perceived as being absurdly grotesque, ridiculous, or pathetic. These responses are not invariable since, for example, a subject may cope with his anxiety by developing a solipsistic pattern in which other persons cannot harm him for the reason that they are his own mental constructs. Then he may visually perceive others from the same patronizing vantage point as one in whom anxiety is not the predominant response.

One of the most common varieties of negative perception among subjects who take the "patronizing" view of other persons is the perceiving of others as animals. S-2, a twenty-seven-year-old male (LSD), first saw his wife, who he usually thought of as being quite attractive, as having "the head of a snouty hippopotamus on the body of a weasel." For a time he found this view rather funny, but later he found it disturbing and refused to look at her. S would not explore the significance of the distortion, but there was considerable conflict between the couple at the time.

This animalizing or theriomorphizing of others was a constant in S's experience. Standing on a balcony, he saw almost everyone on the street below in terms of some animal correlate. At one point he looked down at the street and began to giggle uncontrollably. He pointed to a fat and gaudily dressed lady who was walking a fat and gaudy Pekingese. He explained that he had visually "switched them" so that he saw "a big, fat Pekingese leading a little fat lady on a leash."

Similarly, S-3, a thirty-year-old physician (LSD), was taken by friends to a large department store where he wanted to experience the variety of "colors and movements." There, in the section selling ladies' dresses, he became convulsed with laughter and had to be taken to a less stimulating floor. S had seen the women around him as "a lot of broken down peacocks trailing bedraggled feathers"; as "clucking, complacent hens"; and, in the Tall Girls' division, as a bunch of "stringy, scrawny, beady-eyed ostriches." He was led out of the store proclaiming amidst guffaws that "Bloomingdale's is a turned-on barnyard."

S-4, a writer in his late thirties, had predominantly hostile perceptions of almost everyone but the guide, who was simultaneously seen by him as an attractive, friendly figure. At the end of his session he visited a restaurant with the guide and describes his visual impressions as follows:

"Seated in a restaurant where I have been many times before: ordinarily, this is a dimly lighted place; but tonight, it seems to me, many additional lights are burning; or the same lights are burning, but much more brightly . . . My pupils, dilated, are drinking in light to an abnormal degree . . . Always in the past this has seemed to me a pleasant and cheerful place; but now, seeing everything much too clearly, I no longer find it so. The waiters, I remark, all seem to be pimps, thieves, cutthroats—in a film they surely would be pirates; the tablecloth appears to be worn, dirty and stained; and, across from us, I see great ugly red blotches on the face of a man who is drinking yellow wine and who frequently pauses to lick fat wet lips that are drooling. Another man, sitting at a nearby table, is partially paralyzed, so that bringing each forkful to his mouth seems an awkward, agonizing labor; and a small gray creature, reeking of death and resembling a gargoyle, scurries past the stools lining the bar and is swallowed by a night that has pointed teeth and is yawning . . . *In the room the waiters come and go/speaking of Antonin Artaud . . .*"

Here, the subject's perceptions combine elements of hostility and anxiety; while at the same time, as previously noted, his peception of the guide was very positive and included a slight distortion of appearance "in favor" of the guide. Also, in this case most of the distortions are not, with respect to vision, so drastic as in the examples just cited. Most of the same perceptions might have been possible without the drug; but they are lopsided in their emphasis.

The distorted visual perceptions of the psychedelic drug subject sometimes have been equated with caricatures; but while this appears to be a fairly plausible observation in some cases, it is not so in others. Among the possible resemblances to caricature, in some of the subjects' perceptions a single aspect of the physical appearance or apparent character of a person may be seized upon, overemphasized, and then employed to sum up, as it were, the one perceived. We find here the mental economy or minimized expenditure of thought associated with caricature. However, unlike caricature, there need be no conscious hostility or aggressive intent. Nor is it necessarily some *defect* of the one "caricatured" that is exaggerated. And while the facial expression may be distorted into a grimace, it would seem that the same mental process as regards method may be utilized to transform the countenance in the direction of enhanced beauty, serenity, strength or some other positive attribute.

It is true that every visual distortion of the other is to some extent gratuitous and a violation of the other that transmutes him into something "not himself." It is also true that the majority of distortions, whether in the direction of the beautiful or of the grotesque, involve a reduction and oversimplification. If we wish, when the other is rendered ugly, grotesque or ridiculous, we may regard the process and its product as caricature. But what then shall we call the same process when the end-product exhalts or enhances in some way the person thus perceived?[1]

Apart from the guide, most *positive* distortions are of individuals well known to the subject and towards whom he is very favorably disposed. In general, love, strong friendship, and desire are productive of visual distortions that may suffuse another with extraordinary beauty or some other much-valued attribute. Some of these positive distortions, subjects say, involve not a reduction but rather a "complexification" of the other, a "symbolization" of the other's now-known complexity with all of the richness of the other visible in the perceptual distortion at the same time it is conceptually apprehended.

These "rich" and "complexified" perceptions of the other often are described by subjects as being not distortions, but valid perceptions. The distorted perception was the old one that denied the other her due and derived from habit, conditioned response, accumulation of grievances, and so on. This phenomenon of perceiving, in the drug session, the other as she "really is" has been likened to a kind of *deja vu*. "Suddenly one turns the corner and sees the other in terms of a richness once seen, but lost through over-familiarity. With this perception, closed circuits are reopened and the persons communicate in ways and on levels long inaccessible to them. Also, new circuits may be opened and new ways of communication become possible." (Subject's description.) Or the subject may feel he is seeing the other in all her richness and complexity for the first time.

Ambivalence with regard to the other may yield a particularly rich variety of perceptions, with the other seen alternately as ugly, drab, beautiful, or whatever, often in terms of the specific relation in which the two persons temporarily find themselves. For example, a woman may perceive her husband as extremely handsome in his role as intellectual companion; and then, should he attempt to exert his authority as "head of the household," perceive him as a shrunken, ridiculous, and inept figure. Such perceptions may, but do not always, point to specific areas of conflict of which the subjects were unaware.

In another type of common visual distortion, the other person is perceived as surrounded by or extruding intricate patterns of wires, loops, electrical and color wave emanations. In a typical case of this kind S-5, a male in his early thirties (LSD), first looked into a mirror and saw himself as the source of great circular loops of neon wires that entirely surrounded him. The loops were many—"hundreds of thousands"—and consisted of his attachments to himself and to every aspect of his life—"memory loops, love loops, hate loops, eating loops, mental block loops." Upon re-entering the living room he saw his wife and immediately became absorbed in studying her since she, too, appeared to him to be surrounded by her loops. He had always thought of her as being "a rather simple person" and was "altogether amazed to discover that she is every bit as complicated as I am." Subsequent to his session, and for about a week, the subject claimed to be able to see dimly a tangle of loops surrounding himself, his wife, and almost everyone with whom he came in contact. These were not, he emphasized, "meaningless hallucinations," but revealed to him something important about the character of the other person.

S said that this experience was especially helpful to him in understanding his wife and coming to know her as the "subtle and complex being she really is." This recognition, he felt, had enabled him to "react to her on many more levels" than was possible in the past. As he considered the phenomenon he decided that in large measure he was recapturing a view of his wife that he had had at the time of their marriage. "Habit had withered and custom staled the infinite variety of her ways," at least for him. But, in his session, he had "reappropriated her complexity" and now took it into account in his relationship with her.

Of 25 LSD subjects who experienced this perceptual and ideational recognition of the richness and complexity of the other, 19 were of the opinion that the recognition was of actual values residing in the other, not just a projection produced by wishful thinking, a momentary upsurge of affection, or whatever. The subjects generally felt that with the passage of time they had conditioned themselves not only to simplify their perception of the other, but also to place the emphasis on her poverty. For the most part, it was the guide's opinion that these subjects were in fact recognizing real, not just illusory, values in the other person.

In another fairly common departure from normal perception, the other is seen in terms of his "potential." In a very simple case of this kind, S-6, a housewife (LSD), perceived her rather corpulent husband as "basically thin." After the session she continued to insist to the husband that his personality really belonged with a much more slender body. Whatever his reasons, the husband agreed that the wife's perception was of an easily fulfilled potential and that his personality would be better suited to a slender body. In only six months he had dropped 30 pounds and it was generally agreed that his "new" body was much better suited to his personality than the former fat body had been.

As a final example of visual change, some subjects, for periods of varying duration, experience feelings of "universal love," "fellow-feeling," or "love for all mankind." This state results in most cases in positive visual distortions with other persons being seen as all very beautiful, loving, friendly, and good. These eruptions of universal love will be discussed at some length later on in this chapter.

There are, of course, many implications present in this perceptual material. Here we will remark that if, as we believe, the drug-state distortions are magnifications of tendencies found also in "normal" perception, then they afford unique opportunities for studying the perceptual process.

Communication. Another often strikingly unusual aspect of interpersonal relations in the psychedelic drug state is *communication*. Factors of especial importance in producing the peculiarly "psychedelic" varieties of communication include the following: the much-increased tempo of thought; feelings of empathy; heightened sensitivity to nuances of language and to non-verbal cues; greater use of gestures and shifts of posture and facial expression as means of communicating; the sense that communication is multileveled and much more meaningful than at other times; the sense that words are useless because the experience is "ineffable"; the feeling that communication by telepathic and other "extrasensory" means is possible; and the illusion that one is communicating when one is not—particularly, that one has given voice to a message when actually nothing was said.

Subjects may range from the garrulous to the taciturn, depending upon a great variety of factors apart from the usual behavioral pattern. In general, the peyote subject is more talkative than the person taking LSD; and the larger doses of LSD are most productive of speech economy, the subject variously preferring nonverbal methods, feeling that fewer words are needed to convey his message, or developing the mentioned illusion that he has said a great deal when in fact the message has remained on the level of thought. Since in general LSD, particularly in doses of 200 micrograms and upwards, yields the more interesting phenomena, the examples to be found in this section will be of LSD subject communication.

To expand a bit upon the foregoing, it is common for a drug subject to feel that because of the rapidity with which his thoughts unfold, it is impossible to communicate by ordinary means and so he must abandon the effort or develop new means more adequate to the situation. He may also feel that speech is largely superfluous since the high degree of empathic communion has made him very communicative on even the most subliminal levels—from one spoken word conveying a bookful of ideas and associations, on to total telepathic communication. Also, he may feel that gestures, postures, and subtle shifts of facial expression, on the part of both himself and the other(s), can communicate volumes of material otherwise verbally inexpressible. Subjects thus may think that they are doing a highly effective job of communicating with one another even though very little in the way of speech passes between them. Nor is it possible to say with certainty that they are always wrong, or that communication by other, still less orthodox means does not occur. Subjects repeatedly insist with some vehemence that they are able to "tune in" directly on the moods and thoughts of the guide and other persons, especially other persons who also are taking the drug. They sometimes seem to do so, and any assertion that they always are actually picking up ordinary sensory cues cannot be based on the guide's visual observations and has to be based on the assumption that the subject is alert to cues the guide has missed. Underlying such an assumption, of course, usually will be a theoretically grounded rejection of the possibility that such phenomena as telepathy can exist.

The conveying and receiving of complicated messages, without the normal amount of verbalization, is made possible also by the subject's alertness to nuances of language. Double meanings and other word plays may be picked up instantly. Apparently simple statements and even single words yield manifold meanings and implications that all seem simultaneously accessible. Much speech that ordinarily would be needed now seems pruned away and the result is a terse and cryptic spoken "shorthand" that may be entirely satisfactory to the subject but is likely to be enigmatic to others.

For example, two subjects, S-7 and S-8, were participants in a group session. Previous to the session these two men had only a nodding acquaintance. But during the session they sat across a table from one another and communicated "psychedelically," later feeling that many thousands of words had been interchanged (although aware that *spoken* words had been few). They considered this "conversation" the most meaningful, interesting and important of their lives. The interchange, although brief when written down, consumed one-half to three-quarters of an hour and went approximately as follows:

S-7: Smiles at S-8

S-8: Nods vigorously in response.

S-7: Slowly scratches his head.

S-8: Waves one finger before his nose.

S-7: "Tides."

S-8: "Of course."

S-7: Points a finger at S-8.

S-8: Touches a finger to his temple.

S-7: "And the way?"

S-8: "We try."

S-7: "Holy waters."

S-8: Makes some strange apparent sign of benediction over his own head and then makes the same sign toward S-7.

S-7: "Amen."

S-8: "Amen."

These subjects said that they had initially become aware of a deep bond of mutually shared feelings and ideas that united them. Their "conversation" had ranged over "the human condition" and such subjects as cosmology, theology, and ethics, to a shared exploration of the significance of each to the other and, finally, of their personal relationship to the Infinite. They had felt themselves at all times to be in a rare state of accord and understanding. Much had been conveyed, they added, by slight gestures and changes of facial expression that had escaped the guide's attention.

Apparently successful complex communication, effected mainly by extra-verbal means, can be intensely interesting, instructive and also disturbing to a person with preconceived ideas about what is possible in this area.

S-9. Male. Graduate student in philosophy. At the time of his session S was largely committed to logical positivism and was writing a dissertation dealing mainly with Wittgenstein and A.J. Ayer. S's interpretation of positivism tended to put the whole burden of the world's meaning on the interrelationships of words. He was ordinarily an incessant talker who would, however, speak for hours without making a single gesture and with virtually no change in his facial expression.

In the drug state, S almost totally reversed his behavioral pattern in this respect. He lapsed into lengthy periods of silence broken from time to time by a "loaded" single word or brief phrase or by gestures aimed at the guide or at various objects in the room. Surprisingly, the guide found these occasional words and gestures to be quite meaningful and often very rich in content. Subsequent reconstruction of the session indicated that S had managed to convey a great deal of what he had intended to communicate.

During the post-session talk S said that while in the drug state he had felt that his thought processes, although extremely complex and subtle, still were largely pre-logical and therefore pre-verbal. He thus had found it necessary to communicate his feelings by the use of an occasional "*ur*-word" or by means of gestures and facial expressions.

S said that he recognized very clearly the "somewhat mystical implications" of this statement and felt that he should be "extremely skeptical" about what he had said. Yet, at the same time, he had the feeling that his experience and analysis of it were valid and cast serious doubt on many of his previous philosophical certainties. His doubt deepened as he began to suspect that the experience which at first he had interpreted as a regressive preverbal one also could be seen, "because of its complexity, as a kind of evolutionary preview into future post-verbal modes of communication."

Whether this subject is to be regarded as helped or harmed by his drug experience will depend upon how one evaluates the merits of his subsequent actions and ideas. Continuing to grapple with the insights he had gained, he became increasingly dissatisfied with his dissertation and finally abandoned it altogether. With much additional expenditure of time and energy he wrote a new dissertation, switching his allegiance to a philosopher about as opposed to Wittgenstein as could be.

While LSD inhibits or seems to minimize the need for speech in some cases, in other instances the subjects become more verbose than usual and sometimes much more eloquent. The loquacious subject may talk a great deal because he finds that he has many important ideas he wants to share and has also the capacity to express them. Or, he may talk a great deal because he is anxious or confused and talking helps him preserve his sense of identity and his contact with some supportive figure. It is not always easy for the guide to determine which of these motives is operative.

A few subjects seem to achieve a previously unparalleled lucidity while in the drug-state. Individuals who normally limit their conversation to routine small talk may speak with some brilliance of a great variety of matters or make extensive analyses of their own mental processes as affected by the drug. These are not always persons who are "starved for good conversation." Those who know them may be astonished at the comparative erudition and talent for conversation they display. Two such subjects have continued to be more effective conversationalists after their sessions; but most at once relapse into their former chitchat and declare themselves baffled by the temporary verbal facility and regretful at its loss. These are not, it ought to be added, uneducated persons or persons of low intelligence. They are inarticulate persons who presumably drew upon information always accessible but rarely put to use in conversation and, in some cases, rarely thought about.

The varieties of *illusory* communication encountered in the sessions are also of considerable interest. In the first example we have the case of an LSD subject, S-10, whose wife was on hand for a portion of his session but did not take the drug. As reconstructed and substantially condensed, the following brief interchange between S and his wife W was heard and respectively assimilated by them about like this:

S says: "You are looking very beautiful." With these words *S means to convey, and thinks he has conveyed*: "I have just recognized to what extent I have lost sight of all your good qualities. I used to see them, but somehow I developed a sort of blindness. Now, however, I am seeing you as the beautiful person you truly are, and I intend to maintain this recognition after my session so that we will be able to recapture all the happiness we once had."

W says: "It may be just the drug, but I appreciate the compliment." *W means to convey, and thinks she has conveyed*: just what she said, although her enthusiasm for the compliment is not great.

S understands W to have meant: "I am going to accept this statement of your good intentions for the time being, but will wait and see whether you still feel the same way after you are out of it. You have done a good many things I didn't like, but I can still forgive you if you will change. I do love you and I understand that you want to do better."

S says: "You're smiling. Are you happy?" S *means and thinks he has conveyed*: "I can see by your smile that you are very pleased with what I have been saying. You may still have a few doubts, and so may not yet be completely happy, but I see that you are much happier than before and things are going to get even better. You are very understanding and seem somehow to sense what I know to be true, that I am a greatly changed person who means every word that he says and who is going to treat you much better from now on. Just seeing you so happy is reward enough for me. Now that we have arrived at a real understanding . . ."

W says: "Oh, yes." W *means*: Nothing very much. She is just being agreeable. W *is thinking*: "Naturally I smiled. He looks pretty funny all stretched out on the floor there. Well, at least he doesn't seem too crazy and nothing else bad has happened either. He has several more hours to go, but everything seems okay so I can leave pretty soon and spend the rest of the afternoon shopping with my mother."

S *understands* W *to have meant*: "Oh! Yes! I am very, very happy! I can see now that you really mean what you have been saying and really are changed. We are communicating so fully, understanding each other as we never did before. We are not talking much, but who needs words? You are revealing yourself to me and I am revealing myself to you in many, many ways all at once. Oh! Yes! Now that we have broken through all the barriers that used to separate us, we love one another as never before and will go on loving one another like that. I am so happy!"

In the above example of illusory drug-state communication, S first supposes that W has understood all that he meant and thought that he had conveyed by his words. In addition to this, S believes that he has received from W answers never given to messages never sent, much less received by W. In the following example, S-11[2] was visited during his session by a girl he was in love with but had never found the courage to tell about his feelings. He believed at the time of the session and also afterwards that he had spent several hours telling this girl how much he loved her. In fact, his "long declaration of love" was never made at all and the few words he spoke to her over a period of several hours were innocuous when not almost meaningless. (He had taken a large, 350 microgram dose of LSD and in spite of having had much previous

psychedelic drug experience became confused and sometimes inco-
herent.) What S actually said during a portion of her visit, and his
account of what he thought he had said, are as follows:

S looks with eyes closed at images and remarks: "I see a big jeweled
butterfly." Opens his eyes and looks at his beloved (B) through some
pussy willows standing in a Japanese vase: "How beautiful. Oriental.
No, now you look Greek." Closes his eyes and observes more images.
"Greek again. A forest. I hear music. Now it seems to be Aztec." Long
pause. "So many places. So many times." Long pause. "Computers.
We're just computers. It is very bad. No, I don't know why." Lies on a
couch with eyes closed for a long time, then looks over at B. "I am so
sorry. I mean, you must be bored . . ."

Occasionally, during this period, B made brief inquiries as to what S
was seeing or asked him to elaborate on something he had said. However, B admitted later that she was preoccupied at the time and had
paid only minimal attention to S. She had been present at psychedelic
drug sessions before and found this one comparatively dull. B says that
she had no idea at the time that S loved her, much less that he was
proclaiming his love to her. S, for his part, seemed to ignore or gave
very terse responses to B's few attempts at conversation.

Later, however, S wrote a report more than 50 pages long detailing
what he thought he had communicated to B. We here quote a few
excerpts from the passages corresponding to his actual words as re-
produced above:

"From above me, many-hued, its giant wings fluttering, the great
jeweled moth descends and alights upon the table and the wings, as I
open my eyes, have become translucent, brilliant, incredibly fragile fans
that you are holding and that pass for an instant across your face, then,
unmoving, become its frame. Between the silken fans—which I know to
be flowers, but which are fans still—your face is oriental: very white, as
if heavily powdered or painted, but unbelievably, exotically beautiful.
And now, between the brown branches, studded with their small soft
buds, it is equally beautiful but classically Grecian. Forgive me if I fail
to understand you when you speak. It is my apprehension of your
beauty that destroys my capacity to focus upon your words.

"Standing, in another time and place where I observe you only from
a distance, you are Rhea: yawning black mouths of caverns at your
back and panthers and lions at your side. The green depths of the forest
ring with the cries of your worshipers, the night descends slowly, and
the torches borne by the procession of your priests illumine—what

again is this room, where you are standing and seeming to listen to what
I, too, am hearing . . . For even at this moment, in this room, from far
off, as if echoing across time from the depths of a torch-illumined
forest, there lingers the sound of horn and pipe, of drum and castanet.
But we are Aztecs now, and you are my queen, and your hair frames a
beauty turned barbaric and cruel as the eyes of a tiger. Before us
assembled multitudes cry out as you raise an arm heavy with flat golden
bracelets and rings of unparalleled brilliance glow in a moonlight that
encircles and suffuses the sacred enclosure where we stand.

"Atop a pyramid, studded with what seem great buttons of ivory,
inlaid with sapphires, rubies and emeralds, again we are standing side
by side. My arms are bare, bronzed and heavily muscled, and in my
hand is a sword around which a living, writhing serpent is entwined. . . .

"In all of those times, in all of those places, but now I seem so old
and you—you are always, unchangingly just as you were then.

"It seems to me that I think only of love, speak only of love, and
that you are telling me: 'Go on. Go on. Go on.' . . .

"Floods of images: the mind's interior—we are computers, feeding
one another, incessantly feeding one another, and linked by tapes that
emerge from one metallic surface to vanish into the other. My flesh is
crawling and my heart is made of brass. How dismal to be computers,
and how terrible to be linked to you only by tapes. . . .

"Always, again and again, I come back to the single theme of my
love for you. I would like to change the subject—free *you* from *my*
monomania. I have forced myself to fall silent; to think a thousand
thoughts, about different times, places, things; yet my ideas, however
remote they seem at first, invariably refer back, as I see all too quickly,
to the single, inescapable source of my obsession.

"I send my mind floating down swift streams and over waterfalls;
roll my self up in a ball that is fired at targets distant as stars; strive to
thrust my thoughts into an orbit that will circle and center upon anything, anyplace, anyone *else*—and cannot avoid or renounce the rejoic-
ing that accompanies the succession of my failures.

"The walls dance, the ceiling shimmers, tiny red wisps of light go
darting, sometimes to collide and explode or unite, through the spaces
above me. My awareness—fragmented—focuses with what seems equal
intensity upon a dozen or more objects: vase, ashtray, pillow, painting,
window, the arm of a chair, the leg of a table, sounds, smells (for these
are to me at the moment as much objects as the rest), a radiator, my
own hands and feet—I apprehend them all, my thoughts circle around

them, envelop them, take them in from every perspective—but as satellites of you!

"All of this, I feel—I know—is unjust, unfair, an unwarranted taking advantage of our present situation. You have come here because I told you I might need you, yet I use this occasion almost wholly as a means of furthering my relentless efforts to possess you. I am ashamed of what seems an exploitation, and is surely ingratitude; yet my love for you is so great I no longer am able to contain it. . . ."

Such examples of illusory communication as the foregoing should not be isolated and then used as weapons against the psychedelic drug experience. Important authentic communication also takes place as numerous instances cited in this book repeatedly demonstrate. Here, as in many other areas of the drug experience, we encounter a curious blending of the valuable with the bizarre. Also, even the bizarre or ludicrous experience may be of value in terms of long-range consequences. For example, S-10 did in fact change his thinking about his wife and their relationship improved as a result. Much of life's happiness, after all, flows out of one illusion or another.

Empathy.   About ninety per cent of our psychedelic drug subjects have experienced at least once some state of mind that many term "empathy." These experiences, while to some extent similar, are not identical and in particular cases subjects seem to be talking about sympathy, accord, concord, rapport, affinity, psychological correspondence, understanding, likemindedness, union, communion, or some combination of these. We will discuss these various states under the heading of "empathy"—indicating our reservations by placing the term in quotation marks.[3]

In the more common varieties of "empathy," the subject identifies with another person much as an actor may identify with his role, then feels he has gained a high degree of understanding of that other; by a kind of "reverse empathy" the subject assimilates an other into himself, rather than "feeling" himself into the other; or his experience resembles *sympathy*, defined as "a similar relation between persons whereby the condition of one induces a responsive condition in another." Or, here, we may take a definition from physics—"the relation between two bodies whereby vibrations in one produce responsive vibrations in the other"—and substitute *psyche* or *self* for *body*.

At the extremes of the "empathic" experience, are solipsism on the one hand, and mystical union on the other hand. Typically, the solipsistic subject appropriates the other person, the other being drawn into oneself and regarded as a part or extension of oneself, or even as nothing more than a product of one's imagination. In the mystical union, with its sense of "I am You—We are One," the self is described as being finally extinguished altogether. The solipsistic experience, because it denies the separate independent reality of the other, yields little of value and when described as "empathy" is only an illusion of empathy. Distinctions between the mystical and empathic experiences will be made in our discussion of mysticism.

There is also a variety or type of drug-state "empathy" that should be regarded as one of the most important experiences available to psychedelic subjects. The condition referred to might be imperfectly described as one in which distinctions between I and You, or I and It, become blurred and the subject-object relation between persons seems to yield to a sense of mutual intermingling with openness to and knowledge of the other. In this seemingly most genuine, and definitely most transformative, of "empathic" states there remains an awareness of the respective identities of the self and of the other. At the same time, individuation no longer imposes the usual insularity. Among the following cases, Subjects 14, 15 and 16 are of this type.

Since a subject's claim that he has experienced "empathy" has to be mainly assessed in terms of his description of his own subjective state, the content and validity of the experience elude exact evaluation. However, certain phenomena sometimes occurring within the "empathic" context tend to support the claim of a breaking through the normal boundaries separating persons. The simultaneous sharing of images and visual patterns and apparent telepathic communication are examples of experiences supporting the claim. Instances of the latter, with accounts of experiments, are given in the section to follow.

S-12, a musician, and his wife, S-13, first had separate LSD sessions and then had a session together. The husband was having an affair with another woman at the time and this had given rise to conflict between him and his wife.

During their joint session the subjects repeatedly claimed to experience identical or almost identical eyes-closed images and also ideas. This remarkable phenomenon both astonished and delighted the couple. They declared themselves "LSD twins" and embarked on a lengthy mutual exploration of the meaning and implications of what they had experienced. Particularly impressive to these two was the "fact" that they many times found themselves simultaneously seeing (imaging) themselves together in various ancient cultures.

One cannot rule out in this case the possibility of a well-intentioned dishonesty. One of the subjects may have claimed to be experiencing what the other was experiencing, and then the two of them jointly played the game from there. However that may be, the couple said that they felt themselves "reborn" to a new sense of unity and harmony. Six months later, the husband had gotten rid of his mistress and the marriage was prospering as a consequence. One year later, he had the mistress back—but the marriage was prospering in spite of it. Rightly or wrongly, the definite and still-lasting improvement in their relationship was attributed by the couple to their "empathic" LSD experience and subsequent analysis and reinforcement of it.

A still more unusual case of this sort occurred in a session in which two of the five participating subjects were twin sisters. These twins, S-14 and S-15, achieved a degree of what they called "empathy" that bordered on the eerie.

During their childhood the mother of these girls had done everything she could to make one sister literally indistinguishable from the other. The twin sisters were given identical clothing, identical haircuts, and compelled to engage in all of the same activities together. So successful was the mother that she herself often could not tell one child from the other one.

By the time the two girls were thirteen years old, each deeply resented the other. Each wanted to be "a real individual, not just one half of a Siamese-twin team." The effect of this resentment, as the two grew older, was for each to differentiate herself as totally as possible from the other. In their teens, one sister decided on a science career, the other decided on the arts. They dressed in opposite styles and if one sister was wearing her hair long, the other wore it short. By the time they were thirty, one sister had become a physician and the other was an avant-garde painter. They were still strongly antagonistic, quarreled heatedly over the most trivial matters, and continued to dress and to wear their hair in very different styles. Even so, and although both denied it, the resemblance between them was considerable.

Despite their apparent mutual hostility the twins saw one another fairly often and one sister arranged for the other to be a co-subject at the group session. For the first hour or two of the session, the pair kept up their customary bickering. Then they became absorbed in their altered sense perceptions and images and soon began comparing notes. To their astonishment each was experiencing almost the same changes of perception and the same images experienced by the other. They repeatedly inquired of the three other subjects in the room what those subjects were experiencing; and found, somewhat to their dismay, that the others were having quite different and highly individualized experiences.

The twins also discovered that they were reacting almost identically to ideas and people, finding the same things funny or sad for the same reasons, and drawing similar conclusions about their co-subjects. They went on comparing notes for some time, beginning to enjoy their "inexplicable mutuality," until a man in the room complained that they should keep their "Gemini perceptions" to themselves and asked, "Christ, don't either of you exist apart from the other one?" He added that the twins looked to him "like one person with two heads and four legs."

These remarks had a strong effect on the twins, who reacted by intensely contemplating one another for a long time. At first they giggled at one another nervously, but then became pensive and finally appeared to be in a profound and almost trancelike sort of communion. It was while in this "empathic" state, they said later, that they had discovered themselves to be "essentially the same person." Each woman proclaimed herself to be "variations on my twin," but declared that the "overlapping of identities" no longer was a source of discomfort.

The effect of this experience was to make the sisters "great friends" —and so they have remained for more than two years. At a time when one sister was going on a trip, she solicitously urged a family friend to "take care of my other self"—something she "could never possibly have said" previous to the LSD session.

It might be added that among the most unusual examples of shared experience in this case were several involving a shared synesthesia. Both women claimed to react to the same piece of music by "seeing the sounds"; and later, looking at the painting, they both said that they were able to "taste the color red." Again, in this case, we have the possibility of deception; but here it seems unlikely.

A fairly common component of the "empathic" experience is the illusion on the part of one subject or both of an interconnectedness of the bodies of the two persons. S-16, an LSD subject, described an "empathy process" in which he gradually became aware of "neural and dermal fibers of communication" extending from himself toward the other and from the other toward himself. Gradually these fibers "grew together and meshed into a total tapestry" containing his "life and the life of the other." S felt during this experience that he "knew" the other as he had never known her before, and had discovered and even literally "felt" values in her of which he previously had been unaware. These values were first experienced by him as "colored threads, color tones of the mutual tapestry," before they became "cerebrated as specific values."

In another, somewhat similar case the subject, S-17, first experienced his "empathy" in terms of the "physically felt rhythms" of the other person. Whether these rhythms were bodily processes, heart beats, humming nerves, S could never decide to his own satisfaction. But he "felt" and later "heard" the other person as a "symphonic complex with a great range of percussive beats." He expressed his "empathy" by "entering into the music and rhythms" of the other, swaying and snapping his fingers to the other's "orchestration." The person with whom S was "empathizing" responded with delight to this "musical rapprochement" and swayed and snapped along with him.

Drug-state "empathy" often begins with a feeling of great looseness, unknitting, and relaxation on the part of the subject. This feeling then may pass over into one of liquefying, flowing or becoming oceanic. At this point the body boundaries may be experienced as melting and indefinite, so that the subject may find himself uncertain as to where his "body leaves off and its surroundings begin." Finally, the psyche or self may seem permeable, transcendent and "empathic."

Subjects experiencing this unknitting and dissolving of boundaries, self-transendence and receptivity are likely to attribute a similar condition to the person with whom they enter into an "empathic" relationship. But such an attribution may be only a projection, and then the subject may experience a genuine feeling of "empathy" on his own part while erroneously believing that the other is also "empathizing" with him.

For example, during a group LSD session, a male subject, S-18, told a female friend: "Walls are falling away from me. My walls are crumbling down." He then observed her closely for a while and added: "And your walls are falling away, too. You're not so damned enigmatic as you usually are. I feel for the first time that I really know you." S told the guide later in the session that he had felt an intense communion with his friend, "a communion much closer than any sexual communion."

On the other hand his friend, also taking LSD, told the guide that throughout her session she had felt "no empathy whatsoever" with S. On the contrary, she had mostly felt that the two were "different island universes drifting in space and not at all related to one another. His contemplating me so intensely merely annoyed me and I thought: 'How dare you try to encroach upon my universe!' I felt that his contemplation of me was a terrible invasion of my privacy." Had his friend been less honest, perhaps "just to be agreeable," S today might be extolling LSD "empathy" instead of proclaiming his "skepticism" with regard to it.

Finally, it might be added that "empathy" with objects or with music is much more common than "empathy" with persons. It is also easier and for most more enjoyable, subjects frequently explaining that "things" do not resist one's effort to "empathize" with them as persons often do. Also, the "empathizing" subject may be extremely sensitive to feelings of indifference or hostility on the part of others and his "empathic" forays into the other thus may meet with painful psychic snubs.

Successful "empathy" with things may enable the subject to move on to successful "empathy" with persons. Here, as in some other experiences to be examined, the nonhuman world is often the gateway to the world of the human. And the Thing-World is one that some subjects must traverse and come to terms with before they are able to accept and find acceptance in the World of Other Persons.

"Telepathic" and Other "ESP" Phenomena. We have mentioned on a number of occasions the claims by psychedelic drug subjects that they are able to communicate "telepathically," particularly that they are able to "read the minds" of other persons. This alleged capacity seems to function at its best within the context of an "empathic" relationship; but it is said to function in other contexts as well.

In addition to this claim of a drug-induced or "drug-liberated" telepathic capacity, subjects from time to time report experiences that they feel involve other varieties of extra-sensory perception (ESP). For example, they may claim to be able to see or otherwise know what is taking place outside their own environment (clairvoyance); to be able to obtain from an object something of its past history ("psychometry"); or to be able to see or know future events.

Should the psychedelic drugs in fact be a means whereby certain

ESP faculties in man could be made operational and effective, then the significance of these drugs for interpersonal relations would of course be enormous.

Since very remote times there has existed a lore associating psychedelic and hallucinogenic drugs with a broad range of ESP and occult phenomena. Some of this lore undoubtedly refers to actual occurrences, but ones which may be understood without appealing to ESP. For example, the use of various *Solanaceae* derivatives by witches appears to make intelligible to us on a scientific level many phenomena formerly seen as involving elements of the supernatural.

On the other hand, there are legends and writings by old historians describing events that do not easily lend themselves to explanations acceptable to most present-day scientists. To take a very early example, it often has been suggested that the priestesses of some of the Greek oracles made use of hallucinogenic drugs to activate clairvoyant and other paranormal faculties. Descriptions of the behavior of the pythian priestesses of the oracle at Delphi lead the authors of this book to conclude that again one or more plants containing the *Solanaceae* drugs was employed.

Some of the most impressive of the more recent reports of "telepathic" (or clairvoyant) phenomena associated with psychedelic drugs involve a psychochemical found in the western Amazon region and first discovered in 1850. The narcotic derivative or group of closely related derivatives is known variously as *ayahuasca*, *caapi*, *yage* and *telepathine*. The principal alkaloid producing the psychedelic effects is probably *harmine*, but some other chemicals also seem to be involved in the production. Despite various studies over the years, *caapi*, etc., remains but poorly understood.

In 1927, Dr. William McGovern, assistant curator of South American Ethnology, Field Museum of Natural History, provided one of a number of reports attributing apparent "telepathic" powers to the individual ingesting a drink prepared from the *Banisteriopsis caapi*.[4]

Describing some of the effects of *caapi*, which he took with the natives of an Amazon village, McGovern wrote:

"Curiously enough, certain of the Indians fell into a particularly deep state of trance, in which they possessed what appeared to be telepathic powers. Two or three of the men described in great detail what was going on in *malokas* hundreds of miles away, many of which they had never visited, and the inhabitants of which they had never seen, but which seemed to tally exactly with what I knew of the places

and peoples concerned. More extraordinary still, on this particular evening, the local medicine-man told me that the chief of a certain tribe on
the faraway Pira Parana had suddenly died. I entered this statement in
my diary and many weeks later, when we came to the tribe in question,
I found that the witch doctor's statement had been true in every detail.
Possibly all these cases were mere coincidences."

Similarly, in 1932, a Brazilian colonel named Morales experienced
for himself the seeming telepathic or clairvoyant properties of *yage*.[5]

Colonel Morales "was on a military mission far up the headwaters
territory of the Amazon, toward the borders with Eastern Peru, when
he heard from an old Indian about this queer plant. Morales, by way of
an experiment, drank a decoction of it. It produced on him an amazing,
hyperesthetic effect which seemed to dilate the normal consciousness.
He asserts that he heard the music of an orchestra playing in what was
apparently American surroundings. He says he also became conscious
of the death of his sister in a house far away from where he was located.
The house was in Rio de Janeiro some 2,900 miles distant, as the crow
flies, from the remote village where he then was. A month later, a
runner brought him a letter . . . telling him that his sister had died about
the time Morales had drunk the infusion of the *yage* plant. . . ."

Since LSD is of rather recent vintage (psychedelic properties discovered in April, 1943), it has no ancient history and lore of strange
events; only a monumental recent lore. Peyote, however, has a history
of use for the purpose of inducing telepathic, clairvoyant, prophetic,
necromantic and other capacities going back well beyond the fifteenth
century. Several decades ago the principal peyote alkaloid, mescaline,
was already being tested to determine the validity of claims that telepathic communication was possible in the drug-state. Dr. Félix Martí-
Ibáñez writes[6] that "Even as a medical student, I had heard about
mescaline experiments. A renowned Spanish pharmacologist, Dr.
Bascompte Lakanal, had told me of the work being done at the Pasteur
Institute in Paris using mescaline. An alkaloid from the Mexican cactus
peyote, mescaline caused a 'luminous drunkenness' in which the world
turned into an orgy of color, a bacchanal of swirling lights, a rainbow
symphony. The most extraordinary result was that, when telepathic
experiments were carried out with the mescalinized volunteers, they
could reproduce words, sketches, and musical notes, pronounced, sung,
or drawn by other people in a distant room of the same institute. Some
physicians then began to wonder whether the pharmacologic arsenal
had not become enriched by its first 'telepathic drug!' "

Concerning these few instances we have mentioned, and many others of which we have knowledge, we maintain a position of open-minded skepticism. They are cited only as fairly typical examples of the lore of ESP phenomena as it has been associated with the psychedelic drugs.

Attempts of the last decade or so to demonstrate ESP-enhancing properties of LSD, mescaline and similar chemicals have been inconclusive—when not plainly abortive—in experiments with both "sensitives" and persons not aware of possessing any ESP capacities. A number of instances of apparent telepathy, precognition, clairvoyance, and clairaudience have been reported, but seemingly they occurred with no greater frequency than in experiments where no drug is administered. Psychedelic drugs are said to have worsened the performances of some experimental subjects. In other cases, the plus deviation from the usual performance was less than noted when tranquilizers and amphetamines were given.

The theory often underlying such use of the psycho-chemicals is that ESP is a natural faculty of mind that is inhibited or kept inoperative by the production of body chemicals developed in the course of human evolution to serve just that inhibitory purpose. The inhibiting chemicals, that is, served to prevent man from perceiving a "larger reality" that would be too distracting and so interfere with his survival and progress in the world. The "medium" or "sensitive," then, is a person whose body does not produce these chemicals in the normal amount and whose mind, therefore, is not normally inhibited. If, as has been argued, psychedelic drugs "inhibit the inhibitors," then the drug subject might be able to experience what the medium experiences.[7]

As noted, however, experimental ESP results do not seem sufficiently impressive to compel our acceptance of this theory. But the theory is not thereby discredited, since parapsychologists have noted a variety of factors that might have a detrimental effect upon ESP performance even where the potential for improved performance has been activated by the drug.

The present authors, as noted, are skeptics with regard to parapsychology and the phenomena with which it is concerned; but, at the same time, we are not closed-minded or antagonistic. Some testing of LSD subjects has been done and we will present the results without making any claims of having conclusively proved anything.

Our efforts at demonstrating a drug-induced capacity for clairvoyance have yielded very little. Some subjects have reported themselves able to visit distant places and have "brought back" reports of what they "saw"; but all of these reports have tended to be vague and the more impressive instances still might be put down as "lucky guesses." A subject might be told, for example, to "go" to a house or apartment at a certain address where the occupant and general contents were known to the guide but not to the subject. A few subjects then gave fairly accurate information, describing persons and objects in the house. This is not, as some will note, a good test of "traveling clairvoyance" since the possibility of telepathy or the subject's "reading the mind" of the guide has not been excluded.

S-19, a housewife in her mid-thirties, complained in the course of a LSD session that she could "see" her little girl in the kitchen of their home and that the daughter was taking advantage of her mother's absence to go looking for the cookie jar. S then further reported that the daughter was standing on a chair and rummaging through the kitchen cabinets. She "saw" the child knock a glass sugar bowl from a shelf and remarked that the bowl had shattered on the floor, spilling sugar all around.[8]

S forgot this episode, but when she returned home, after her session, she decided to make herself some coffee and then was unable to find the sugar bowl. She asked her husband where it was and he told her that while she was away their daughter had "made a mess," knocking the sugar bowl from the shelf and smashing it. The child had done this "while looking for the cookies."

Since the child often went looking for the cookies, and had almost smashed the sugar bowl before, it is easy to "explain away" this particular incident. Apparently more baffling is a somewhat similar case involving a subject of another guide.

In this second case, a friend guiding a session phoned us to say that an LSD subject had reported seeing "a ship caught in ice floes, somewhere in the northern seas." She could read the name of the ship on its bow: it was the *France*. Two days after the phone call (and three days after the session), there appeared in the newspapers an item relating that a ship had been freed after being trapped in ice, somewhere near Greenland. The ship was the *France*, which had gotten into trouble at about the time of the subject's session. There would seem to have been no earlier news items concerning the incident.

We have nothing of value to say concerning this type of phenomenon, which is heard of often enough where no psychedelic drug is involved.

Much more relevant to the present chapter are controlled experiments conducted by one of the authors (J. H.) in an effort to examine the validity of claims by subjects of "telepathic communication." The initial aim was to study various aspects of the "empathic" experience. However, testing is likely to disrupt the "empathic" state; and most subjects therefore had to be tested for "telepathic" capacity in the drug-state but outside the empathy context.

In an experiment involving 27 subjects, the guide used a standard 25-card Zehner ESP pack to test for possible changes in extra-sensory awareness on the part of the subjects. The guide's method was to sit across the room from the subject, running through the pack ten times (250 cards) and shuffling upon the completion of each 25-card run. She would lift up the top card, look at it and ask the subject to tell her what it was—circle, square, cross, star, or waves. She would put the card down, and make a note of the subject's response, and then go on to the next card.

Most of the subjects very quickly became bored with this process, regarding it as a waste of valuable psychedelic time. This subject resistance or indifference may have affected the results, especially in 23 cases where the subjects performed on the levels of chance or below chance, dropping to levels of two and three correct guesses out of a possible 25 toward the end of the testing.

The average test run (based on the ten runs) was as follows:

4 - 5 - 5 - 6 - 4 - 2 - 2 - 3 -1 - 3 (Score 3.5, or 1.5 below chance).

On the last five runs, where the scores fall off sharply, the subject was usually especially bored with the test and his resistance was increased accordingly. Some were apparently throwing out guesses with no attempt at all at telepathy. There remains, however, the possibility that the consistently below-chance scores on the last five runs might be an example of a kind of "negative telepathy," the resisting subject expressing his opposition to the process by misreading the cards. No subject, however, consciously tried to make mistakes as far as could be learned.

In the case of the remaining four subjects—a female (F) and three males (M)—the results were considerably and consistently above chance. It might be of significance here that each of the four subjects was a good friend of the guide and thus better motivated than the others to help her with the experiment. Also, a factor of greater claimed feelings of "empathy" on the part of these four should be noted. Their scores (averaged for the ten runs) were as follows:

M-1: 9 - 8 - 9 - 10 - 12 - 13 - 9 - 5 - 4 - 4
F-1: 8 - 13 - 10 - 11 - 8 - 11 - 9 - 10 - 6 - 5
M-2: 11 - 9 - 8 - 8 - 11 - 13 - 10 - 10 - 7 - 4
M-3: 8 - 7 - 10 - 12 - 9 - 11 - 4 - 6 - 4 - 3

Tested in a comparable non-LSD situation, only one of these sub-jects scored significantly above chance; and his performance remained well below that achieved with the LSD factor added. Even with these high scorers, one notes, performance tends to decline rather sharply for the last three runs. In an LSD context it does not seem feasible to try to inflict a series of more than ten runs on an experimental subject.

Of some other researchers with whose work we are acquainted, one sponsored a very large number of similar tests under psychedelic drug conditions with dismal results. On the other hand, another researcher, Andrija Puharich, reports that his testing demonstrates significant im-provement of the telepathic performance early in the drug (*Amanita muscaria*) experience. His data may be found in his book, *Beyond Telepathy*.[9]

Testing the hypothesis that the card test may be a poor one for the particular circumstances—or that card testing may be, as a subject charged, "psychedelically immoral"—an attempt was made to devise another test that would be more compatible with the subject's mental state and therefore more congenial to him. The guide had noticed that her subjects often seemed to pick up random images that crossed her mind; and the subjects seemed most adept at this in the case of images that had for the guide some emotogenic force—i.e., images that were esthetically, historically or otherwise personally potent or emotionally charged.

It was thus decided to write down ten such images and to place them in ten envelopes. The subject would sit across the room from the guide (G-1) or in an adjoining room with another guide (G-2). G-1 would pick up an envelope and image the scene described on the paper inside the envelope. The subject would relay what he had "picked up" to G-2, who would record the subject's words. G-1 would then say "Now!" and think of the scene described in the second envelope, and so on. After "sending" the contents of the ten envelopes, the image sent by G-1 would be compared with the description given by the subject. The number of approximations occurring with this test seemed significant. Out of 62 subjects tested, 48 approximated the guide's image two or more times out of ten. Five subjects approximated the guide's image seven and eight times out of ten.

By "approximation" is meant the following: The scene would be described on the paper in the envelope as "a Viking ship tossed in a storm." A subject would be considered to have approximated this if he reported, for example, "a snake with an arched head swimming in tossed seas." The paper in the envelope might read: "An arab on camelback passing pyramid." An approximation then might be "a mummy lying in a gilded sarcophagus."

In a number of cases an official error was attributed to the subject although the guide was unable to image the scene described in the envelope, but imaged something else. Or the guide might "lose" the initial image, and find it replaced by another. In some such cases the subject would accurately pick up the guide's "accidental image" instead of the written image she intended to transmit, but still would be charged with an error. The sealed envelope procedure was used as an additional control.

Of the 14 subjects who received less than two out of ten of the images, almost all were persons not well known to the guide or persons either experiencing anxiety or primarily interested in eliciting personal psychological material. The data on subject performance appear as in the following record of an especially high scoring subject:

PAPER IN ENVELOPE READS	SUBJECT PICKS UP	G-I WAS IMAGING
1. Viking ship tossed in storm.	Snake with arched head swimming in tossed seas.	Same as in envelope.
2. A rain forest in the Amazon.	Lush vegetation, exotic flowers, startling greens —all seen through watery mist.	Same as in envelope with some exotic flowers growing.
3. Atlas holding up the world.	Hercules tossing a ball up and down in his hand.	Same as in envelope.
4. Greek island with small white houses built on terraced hills.	A circus.	Same as in envelope, but with an earthquake, houses falling down.

5. A sailboat off a rocky coast.	Sailboat sailing around a cliff.	Same as in envelope.
6. Ski slope in New England — white, with skiers sliding down.	A forest fire.	A forest fire. Guide was unable to image the ski scene.
7. New York City traffic scene.	Geisha girl in full oriental regalia.	Same as in envelope, but very brilliant colors.
8. A plantation in the Old South.	A Negro picking cotton in a field.	Many images relating to pre-Civil War plantation life, including a Negro picking cotton.
9. An arab on a camel passing a pyramid.	Camel passing through the inside of a vast labyrinthian tomb.	Same as in envelope.
10. The Himalayas— snow-capped peaks.	A climbing expedition in the Alps.	Same as in envelope.

Whatever else might be said of this test, there can be no doubt that the subjects greatly preferred it to the ESP-card testing. They felt that it grew more naturally out of the psychedelic drug experience; that it took advantage of the subject's much-increased ability to image; and that it was certainly more entertaining, or at least less productive of boredom and irritation.

In another experiment, the subject would be asked to "get into the head of" (or "identify with") some historical or contemporary personage concerning whom the guide, it was believed, had much more knowledge and "inside information" than did the subject. The subject was told to "incarnate" himself in that person, to "be" that person and think and behave accordingly.

In some of these cases the results were remarkable, the subject changing his voice, way of speaking, posture and even, it seemed, his appearance and way of thinking. The subject would not, however, lose his awareness of his own identity. He would, rather, "be two people," and would talk about his "new" and "second self" with a plausibility that sometimes verged on the uncanny.

Of such a "test," it must be said that it is never possible for the guide to be certain of the extent of the subject's knowledge of the person with whom he "identifies." Asking the subject to "get into" a person totally unknown to him is not productive. At the very least, however, this game has elicited some outstanding performances from persons not previously aware of any acting ability. Some of the performances also would necessitate the subject's calling upon reservoirs of information, or memories, not consciously in his possession. Further, there seems to be demonstrated here a heightened capacity for empathy.

Instant Love and Galloping Agape. Twentieth-century man in the Western World has come to be almost obsessively concerned with the difficulties of the interpersonal relationship and with the "necessity" for tearing down the walls that separate one human individual from another. Confronted by the possibilities of nuclear self-destruction, an imminent population crisis and the emergence of Red-Fascist and other tyrannies, we seek ever more frantically after means by which men and nations may be able to coexist in harmony. With the contemporary supremacy of physics over metaphysics, the most urgent need of man seems no longer to be to find the meaning of his place in the cosmic scheme of things. Defining his position *vis à vis* God has ceased to be man's central quest. Instead, with mounting despair and desperation, he attempts to define and improve his position *vis à vis* the Other Person.[10]

Such intricate analyses of the interpersonal relationship as Buber's *I and Thou* and Sartre's *Being and Nothingness* reflect Western man's concern and also serve to deepen and complicate the problem even while shedding some light upon it. Psychoanalytic, phenomenological, and other psychologies produce, even as they instruct us, a sense of confusion and frustration in the face of the revealed complexities of the human psyche. Man's isolation, opaqueness, estrangement, and the consequent imperfections of communication with and knowledge of other minds emerges as the most pressing and seemingly insoluble problem he confronts.

The psychedelic subject, while rarely a philosopher, psychologist or even a good student of those arts, is nonetheless affected by the *Zeitgeist* and gropes toward a solution of problems dimly or clearly sensed. And a good many subjects seem strongly affected by one of the most influential and popular notions of our time: that "love" is the means whereby man will find himself able to transcend his own singularity and also be able to break through the wall of separateness that encloses the other and makes the other inscrutable and inaccessible to him. Given social direction, this idea emerges as the belief that a universal or brotherly love is possible and constitutes man's best if not only hope. Not bothering to define "love" too closely, it exerts its most powerful impact on the young, the young student, or recent graduate in particular. An easy shortcut to authentic lovingness is strenuously desired; and the psychedelic Drug Movement has gained a good many converts and peripheral adherents on the basis of published data indicating that people become more loving, more tolerant, etc., as a consequence of their drug experiences.

We, too, in the course of our research, and especially as the literature and lore of drug-love proliferate, have encountered numerous claims from our subjects and others to the effect that they have become more loving, more "outgoing," more "related" to their fellow men, more altruistic (with diminished egoism), and so on. Unfortunately, we find these claims—the ones made with respect to other-persons-in-general—among the most dubious and self-delusive obtained from our subjects and those others we have interviewed. Yet, since the claims are so prevalent, and since the *desire* to love seems sincere as well as urgent, we have felt it necessary to discuss the drugs in their relation to "lovingness."

In the 1950's, when psychedelic drug research in this country was in its first phases, and when many persons taking the psycho-chemicals had read no drug literature at all, the psychedelic experience rarely ever yielded claims of a drug-induced or -awakened sense of brotherhood. It is only more recently, with the emergence of a "love"-oriented drug literature, and also as brotherhood has grown very fashionable, that subjects with an ever-increasing frequency have decided that to partake of the peyote or LSD is to quaff at the fountain of universal agape. That many proclaimed conversions of this type thus appear to derive from the wishes, public postures, and expectations of guide and/or subject does not of itself negate the validity of what the subject says he has experienced. But these elements, combined with various others, lead us to require something more in the way of evidence than the subject's willingness to check off "more loving" on a questionnaire soliciting his description of the in- and post-session effects of his peyote or LSD consumption.

Claims of altered emotional and ideational responses to "the world," to "humanity," and also to such large and controversial human groups as Negroes, Jews, Germans, and Puerto Ricans, are very predominantly positive and usually take on a euphoric, euphuistic tone. "Now I am able to love everybody!" and "At last I have learned the true meaning of tolerance!" are, in essence, typical expressions of the upwelling of benevolence as perfervidly avowed in the psychedelic drug state. Should the dispensation persist beyond the session, it may be described in slightly more austere but no less stereotyped terms.

The authors are not, should it need to be said, opposed to anyone's becoming genuinely imbued with love and tolerance and brotherhood. But experience has taught us the need for assessing the extent to which universal love proclamations are hypocritical, based on neurotic need and wishful thinking, or involve self-deceit and self-delusion with consequent damage to the individual. The delusion that one loves when one does not, but only wishes to, can lead as it sometimes does among those in the Drug Movement to mere indiscriminate associations offered up as proof of loving everyone.

S-20, a teacher with an M.A. degree, first was interviewed a little over two years ago. At that time he had recently been a participant in several LSD sessions with friends who had obtained their drugs from blackmarket sources. Then twenty-eight, he was neatly dressed and well-groomed and gave an impression of alertness and efficiency. He wanted to discuss his drug experiences, saying that while he now seemed to be more tranquil, more "extroverted" and more interested in life generally, he had some reservations and wondered whether long-term use of LSD might be dangerous. It was obvious that he wished to be told there were no dangers and that he resented the failure of one of the authors to give him this response.

S emphasized that his drug experiences had made him more loving, more tolerant, and better able to relate to others. He stated, by way of illustration, that previous to these experiences he had avoided looking into the eyes of other persons on the street because he saw there only indifference, hostility, or sexual interest. Also, most persons he encountered appeared to him to be ugly or drab so that he avoided looking too closely at others for that reason. Now, however, he was spending much time walking, looking into people's eyes, "relating to them and noticing how really warm and beautiful they are." He was learning, with the aid of LSD, to love everyone and others were either responding to his love or he was no longer "poisoning" his perceptions with a negative, unloving attitude.

About a year and a half later S was seen again, this time by both of us. Thereafter, he was seen on several occasions, spread over a period of about six months. He had changed considerably, in appearance and otherwise, and not in our estimation for the better. At the first meeting, he was willing to admit that "externally" his new way of life might seem to "warrant criticism." Again, however, his real wish was for a reassurance that could not be given; and at subsequent meetings he increasingly closed his mind to the possibility that his drug use might be doing him harm and that his life did not look to others anything like the beautiful, chock-full-of-love existence he proclaimed it to be.

S was now a full-fledged member of the Drug Movement, a leading participant in the doings of a psychedelic drug-taking group. His experience with drugs now included, in addition to LSD, peyote, mescaline, psilocybin, DMT, and "Heavenly Blue" and "Pearly Gates" morning-glory seeds. The drugs were often taken in various combinations, with amphetamines, marijuana, hashish, and cocaine sometimes added to make the turn-on even more transcendental.

Having given up his regular job, S now was living on his savings and what he was able to earn from occasional part-time work. His attire was somewhat eccentric and he seemed to have lost considerable weight. He spoke for the most part in a "cool" Drug Movement jargon, some of it borrowed from the Beats, and his whole life now seemed to revolve around the group of drug users to which he had attached himself.

Although now "completely tolerant and loving," S became, at the final interview, very agitated, defensive, and hostile when one of the authors inquired about some of the more dubious activities of his group and mildly ventured the opinion that perhaps he should try to devote his life less exclusively to drug experiences with his friends. S obviously felt he was dealing with a frightful "square" who had failed to glimpse salvation at the end of the psychedelic pilgrimage. Later, when it was suggested to him that he and his friends were headed for trouble, and that activities like theirs might result in eventual police action, he changed his diagnosis to "paranoia."

That S, through his use of psychedelic drugs, became able to feel himself "warm and loving" was certainly a factor of some importance in determining the course of subsequent, seemingly self-destructive behavior. However, the main point we wish to make is that this love of others-in-general was transparently illusory and delusional. "Loving everybody," S soon managed to demonstrate his rapport with humanity by cutting himself off almost wholly from the world and withdrawing into a tight little microcosm of fellow true believers. Here he was assured of approval and of being told that his "love" was returned. This yearned-for approval and love he had not received when earlier he had attempted to put into practice his indiscriminate love-of-all-persons.

S, more fervently than ever, claims to "love everyone"; but this love quickly turns into something quite different when one withholds unconditional approval of all his activities and those of his group, or of various Drug Movement prophets and sacred cows. This does not appear to be normal loyalty, which even though misplaced is to some extent praiseworthy. It is, instead, fanaticism, with all the defensiveness and closed-mindedness that fanaticism breeds. And fanatics immersed in small cults never "love all mankind."

The claim of universal love and tolerance is not persuasive unless supported by appropriate actions. Since most often it is based upon some form of self-deception; and since the need to experience a cosmic benevolence seems satisfied by words without deeds, we do not encounter the appropriate actions very often. In the case of the drug subject this particular self-deception rather often arises out of a kind of narcissistic solipsism in which the person regards the world as existing in-himself or for-himself. Then, what the subject loves, in fact, is himself. The following case, while more than usually comical, is not too atypical.

S-21. Female. Age about fifty. Widowed. LSD.

This subject, among other things a theosophist and the author of countless verses about daisies and meadow larks, is a scatter-brained but happy and friendly individual who nonetheless had never quite achieved the "Christ-like love of all beings" she so passionately craved. During her session, however, she announced that she had at long last reached her goal.

Several hours into the session S fell into a kind of solipsistic reverie in which it seemed to her that nothing existed but herself. She reported that, at the start of this experience, the room became misty and persons and objects in the room were seen merely as "thicknesses of mist" —that is, she got rid of them. She then extended her arms in Christ-like imitation and performed a reverent genuflection to herself. After that, she murmured, "I am the universe. I am Love. Love. Love. Love. Love." Asked to expand a little upon her rapture, she spoke at some length, cataloguing the range and various beneficiaries of her cornucopic feelings. While lamentably this lady's exact words were not preserved, the oration went pretty much like this:

"Negroes and little fishes, lampshades and vinegar. These I love. Coats and hats and three-ring pretzels. Radios and Russians, bobolinks and tree sap, medicine chests and Freud and the green line down the center of the street on St. Patrick's Day, these I love. These I cherish. My old blue sweater and the Cherokees. Pots and pans and cold cream and books and stores and the dear little moron on——Street who sells the comic books. Hair spray and Buddha and Krishna Menon. My love overfloweth to all. My nephew——and mushrooms. Red cars, red caps, porters, Martin Luther King, Armenians, Jews, Incas, and John O'Hara. Love. Love. Love. Love. Big yellow Chrysanthemums and the sun and pancakes and Disneyland and Vermont and cinnamon and Alexander the Great. The UN and aluminum foil and apple cider and cigars. Clark Gable, Tony Curtis and salamanders, crochet, the aurora borealis and dimples, mustard plasters and even Mayor Wagner. I am just bursting with joy, with love. I want to give . . . Give to all . . . Give . . . My Love . . . To . . . All . . ."

And so on. And on. And on. And on.

No joke or leg pull here, rather—"An effluvium of joy, an efflux of love/wisdom effulgent, effused from Above"—i.e., an efflation so emphatic it mobilized her Muse.

In reviewing her session on the following day, S remained enthusiastic and declared that henceforth she would lavish love, charity, and tolerance upon anyone who got within her range. There was, however, no subsequent observable change in her behavior to make the alleged love credible; and when seen for the last time, about six months later, the subject's galloping agape seemed to have subsided to the usual trot with occasional prances. It had been an illusion based on wishful thinking and, as mentioned, seemed also the product of a kind of narcissistic solipsism.

We might add that those persons experiencing the solipsistic and related states have been, among our subjects, preponderantly individuals who are somewhat fearful and inhibited in their everyday interaction with the world and especially with other persons. During the psychedelic experience such people often find themselves able as well as willing to swallow up the world and its details and so make everything and everyone their own. Their declared sense of "love" and "harmony" with-the-world and for-the-world then is really a psychological and semantic mask behind which they take their narcissistic, egoistic holiday.

There seems to be no good reason to cite further cases or otherwise extend our discussion in this particular area. Additional cases, although illustrating various other mental processes, would finally serve only to make the point once again that "instant love" is probably more than humanity can hope for even with the aid of potent psycho-chemicals. Some drug subjects do eventually, and apparently as an outgrowth of their sessions, improve their relations with others-in-general or with groups of others. But they do so by first resolving conflicts and achieving harmony with particular others—with "key" or "problem" persons in their lives, with whom they must come to terms *before* they are able to "branch out" and experience genuine good will and fellow-feeling for others-in-general. There are also some subjects who, after their sessions, appear to be less hostile and anxious than before; and diminished hostility and anxiety, while not "love," can also make it much easier to live and move among one's fellow men.

Five:
The Guide

Up to this point it has seemed to us sufficient to define the guide only as one who conducts a psychedelic drug session, leading or assisting the subject over the unfamiliar terrain of his expanded or altered consciousness. Now, as a preliminary to the more complex chapters to follow, the qualifications and functions of the guide must be considered in some detail.

First of all, the work of the guide with a particular subject neither begins nor ends with that subject's psychedelic experience. There are also important pre- and post-session duties to be carried out. With regard to the former, the guide prepares the subject for the session, giving him whatever information he requires, clearing away any misconceptions, and establishing himself as a figure the subject will be able to trust and with whom the subject will feel at ease. Subsequent to a session, the guide continues for some time to keep in touch with the subject, answering any questions the subject may have, observing him to see that all is going well, and also gathering additional research data.

The term *guide* is appropriate since the subject so often conceives of his psychedelic experience as a kind of journey. Also, the term leaves open the question of the purpose of the session. Thus, the guide may be

a therapist who directs the subject along certain paths of self-exploration intended to lead to a specific therapeutic goal. But a guide also may
accompany a subject on journeys intended to have other destinations;
and the term leaves the choice of the destination free and up to subject
and guide to determine.

The role of the psychedelic guide is new in our society, but the
newness of the role should not blind us to the antiquity of its precedents. Priest and shaman, after all, were the first purveyors of its techniques. Seer and sibyl mapped the cosmography of its domain. Perhaps
the finest of its precedents is to be found in the figure of Virgil in
Dante's *Divine Comedy*.

In the first canto of the *Divine Comedy* we find Dante lost in the
dark woods, haunted by strange sounds and shapes. But then, when his
confusion is at its greatest, he is met by the figure of the master poet
Virgil, who says to him: "I shall be your guide to lead you hence
through that eternal place. . . ." It is then that Virgil proceeds to lead
Dante through the ethics, the cosmogonies, and the historico-political
order of the medieval universe. With time suspended, and all of life at
hand, Virgil can lead Dante through all imaginable spheres of reality:
through past and present, grandeur and corruption, history and legend,
tragedy and comedy, man and nature. He can introduce the *dramatis
personae* of extended reality: figures from antique mythology, fantastic
demons, gods and godlings, symbolic animals, allegorical personifications, mighty archetypes, the whole hierarchy of Christianity. He can
lead Dante through the vast tapestry that is the medieval universe,
evoking divinity, beauty, and meaning. And so, in the *Divine Comedy*,
we are led by Virgil through an enhanced *reality* wherein everything is
bound up with everything else in a pattern which is absolute for the
whole universe. The social hierarchy reflects the psychological hierarchy, the cosmological hierarchy and the celestial hierarchy. And the
final point of the masterful guidance is to reveal how all these interre-
lated orders reflect and are basic to the life and being of Dante the
man.

Virgil guides Dante to a realm of changeless eternity and there
shows him the manifold aspects of reality. Furthermore, all this reality
does not unfold upon a single level or within a single event, but involves
instead a great variety of events and several levels and these are displayed within a near-infinite spectrum of tone and feeling.

It is thus with the psychedelic experience. Once the threshold of
altered consciousness has been crossed, we are flooded with a kaleido-

scopic vision of extended perceptual fields and psychological insights; a visionary torrent of cultures and contexts, myths and symbols, remnants of what may seem to be racial or transpersonal memory—that near-infinity of components that appears to constitute our being. Like Dante in the dark woods we can easily lose our way in the labyrinth of strange byways and unknown paths: an all-too-frequent episode in the unguided psychedelic experience. It therefore should be one of the chief duties of the guide to lead the subject through this newly exposed terrain and elicit its varied contents to lead finally to their interrelationship in the experiencing subject—much in the same way as Virgil led Dante through the medieval hierarchical cosmogony so that its parts became integral to Dante the man. It should be one of the chief tasks of the guide to assume the role of Virgil in this chemically-induced Divine Comedy and to help the subject select out of the wealth of phenomena among which he finds himself some of the more promising opportunities for heightened insight, awareness and integral understanding that the guide knows to be available in the psychedelic experience.

Background and Training of the Guide.   In the absence of large numbers of Virgilian paragons, able to do all we say the guide should do, it is necessary to settle for less; and probably the master guide will never be much more common than is the master poet. But the guide, even now, should have certain minimum qualifications; and, as our knowledge increases, psychedelic guide training should become far more thorough and effective and the personal qualities and talents desirable in the guide much better understood than is possible at this time.

Apart from his specialty as therapist or whatever, the guide should have a broad educational background including a good practical knowledge of human psychology. He should be mentally and emotionally stable and possess the capacity to stimulate feelings of security and trust in the subjects. And his experience as a guide should be sufficient to enable him to cope with emergencies and to manipulate the subject when need be without, at the same time, dominating or otherwise unduly interfering with the subject. This last, of course, implies that the guide have received some training in this specialty. It implies as well that the guide has himself been a subject, preferably on several occasions—that is, that the guide has experienced the drugs and so is able to understand the experience of the subject.

Several of these stipulations require that we elaborate upon them and some of the more important points will be enumerated as follows:

Educational background: Ideally, the psychedelic guide will have two (if not more) specialties. First, he will be a psychotherapist, educator, anthropologist, or whatever. Second, he will be a psychedelic guide, and his training will be both in general guiding and in guiding for his own special purposes—in the management of a psychedelic session for therapy, for education, for explorations of primitivistic belief and ideation, or whatever. Presumably a guide-psychotherapist rarely is qualified to function also as a guide-educator, and vice versa. Mature, intelligent individuals with widely divergent interests and talents as well as different specific professional training will be needed if the psychedelic experience is ever to yield up all of the treasures it promises.

Moreover, in addition to his specialties, it is highly desirable that each guide possess a broad background especially including knowledge of history, literature, philosophy, mythology, art, and religion. Materials from all of these fields, and from others, emerge in many of the sessions and the guide must recognize the materials if he is to be of maximum effectiveness.

Mental Health: There exist, so far as we know, no psychiatric or other screening procedures for determining who will make an effective guide—or who will make a poor or dangerous one. Ordinary psychiatric interviews and diagnostic tests, even when expertly applied, may not "catch" the individual likely to succumb to the temptations and threats peculiar to the guiding situation. Since inept or exploitative management of a session may make it a painful and possibly damaging experience for the subject, it would be very desirable to have *effective* tests of this type. However, to date there has been much more interest in disputing the matter of which profession or professional specialty is to control the use of the drugs than in screening out individuals who should not be permitted to guide drug sessions. Among other things this has resulted in guiding by psychiatrists and others who were eminently unsuited to the task and who inflicted some appalling experiences on their subjects.

Guide should have been subject: It is agreed by most persons who have worked with the psychedelic substances that the guide, to be effective, must himself have taken at least one of the drugs, preferably on several occasions. We see neither the need for nor possibility of a satisfactory alternative to this, and would add that the psychedelic experience of the guide-to-be should include at least two guided sessions in which he is a subject.

Since the psychedelic experience includes so many elements not a part of nondrug-state experience, the guide never will be able to understand the subject or communicate with him adequately unless the guide himself has first-hand knowledge of the drug-state and its phenomena. This point has become controversial, but we see no sound reason why it should be. Persons not capable of coping with a drug experience of their own are not likely to be able to cope with the experience of a subject either; and thus the sessions of the guide-to-be may serve the additional purpose of helping to eliminate from a training program candidates too disturbed or anxious about the psychedelic state. On the other hand, this should not be taken to mean that anyone who has a "good" experience is thereby in any way qualified to be a guide. Neither does it mean that a single "bad" experience will in every case demonstrate a person's incapacity to function effectively as a guide. Subsequent sessions, for example, may be handled very well by that person; and the initial "bad" one may turn out to have been the result of faulty guiding or of the intrusion of some other element to which the subject should not have been exposed.

The argument that the person who has taken the psychedelic drugs thereby disqualifies himself as a person able to objectively view and evaluate the experience, must strike most seasoned researchers as simply ludicrous. It is also unanswerable, since all who might reply to it on the basis of real knowledge are declared in advance to be unfit to deal with the question. Work done by those who refused to take the drugs does not demonstrate greater objectivity than that of persons who have had the drug experience; and doubtless refusal to experience the psychedelic state is a product, in some cases, of anxiety about the person's ability to cope with that state. On the other hand, the charge of diminished objectivity gains force when applied to certain persons who have scores and even hundreds of times dosed themselves with psychochemicals over a period of a few years. Even in these latter cases, however, it is not possible to say just why the repeated experience has resulted in apparently diminished objectivity.

Here we will note that there also has arisen in connection with this work the question of whether the guide should take the drug *with* the subject. At one extreme of this debate we have encountered individuals who insist that the guide, and especially the guide-psycho-therapist, must always or usually take the drug with the subject or patient. This is regarded as an essential aid to subject-guide communication and to the guide's understanding of the content of the subject's experience.

In our view, there may be some genuine advantages to this procedure. However, should a guide take the drug with the subject, it then would be required that a second guide who is not taking the drug also be present for the session. This alone will be sufficient to override the advantages in most cases. But more importantly, any guide working regularly with psychedelic subjects would have to expose himself repeatedly to substantial dosages of a chemical, let us say LSD, when the long-range effects of repeated dosages of that chemical upon brain and psyche remain to be determined. That no physiological damage has been shown does not, we think, warrant taking the risk; and, with respect to psychical damage, our own observation of the aforementioned persons who, scores and even hundreds of times, have exposed themselves to LSD and other synthetics suggests the possibility of some mental deterioration. Whether, in these cases, mental disturbance has resulted from or rather was causal to such behavior we are unable to say. But, given the paucity of knowledge in this area, repeated exposure to LSD seems too risky and this risk should deter the guide from regular LSD self-exposure whatever the possible advantage in terms of therapeutic gains.

Training of guides: In general, a training program for psychedelic guides should cover the whole broad area that constitutes the subject matter of this book. This area would be covered by means of lectures, reading, films, observation of sessions, and by practical first-hand experience as both subject and (supervised) guide. In addition to the general training, the guide would be trained in specific methods of applying his own specialized knowledge to the drug experience.

One of the authors (J. H.) served for a time as instructor in a specialized training program for guides and a few of her experiences may be of interest. This program, terminated several years ago, had as its object the instruction of psychiatrists and clinical psychologists in ways of adapting their own disciplines and methods to the peculiar requirements of the psychedelic session. The therapist, that is to say, retained his particular therapeutic approach, but was shown how that approach might best be applied within the psychedelic context. As we have remarked, no specific psychedelic psychotherapy yet has been developed; and thus there exists no alternative to the rarely satisfactory imposition of standard therapeutic procedures upon the psychedelic experience.

In this author's experience the psychiatrists and psychologists proved flexible and willing to adjust to the novel possibilities of the drug-state. An initial tendency, as subjects, to plunge directly into analysis and psychodynamic self-exploration was easily dealt with in most cases. A brief exposure to the range of the psychedelic phenomena was usually sufficient to persuade the trainee that special methods were called for and would be well worth the learning.

Instead of yielding to the subject-therapist's wish to immediately deal with psychodynamic aspects, the guide found it most effective to insist upon an extended exploration of the subject's enhanced sensory awareness. She would help the subject to become involved in the experiencing of color and light, of form and structure, of sound, smell, touch and music. The subject would be presented with stones, shells, fruit and objects of art and encouraged to contemplate these. He would be led into the experiencing of synesthesias—the hearing of color, the tasting of sound, and so on. Subjects responded to such guidance by becoming deeply absorbed in this "new world" of altered perceptions—often to the point of forgetting altogether their early concern with psychological categories and labeling phenomena in terms of pathologies.

Eventually, however the contemplation of objects would lead into discussion of psychological insights, usually of a personal nature. For example, a piece of delicately filigreed coral would finally become for the subject "the pattern of my life," which he found himself able to "read in the swirling hieroglyphics of a stone," and upon which he would elaborate in terms of the object. A sliced pomegranate became "the seeds of anguish, the wounds of discontent," which the subject then discussed in terms of a patient whose case he said was similar to his own.

Once the subject had established such a "working liaison" between the sensory and psychological realms, he was invited to explore the specifics of a detailed psychological case history—either his own or that of some one of his patients. These explorations, however, were not permitted to become either high-speed analytic exercises or emotional hurricanes (two poles of the psychedelic centrifugal field). Rather, the subject was directed to investigate the problems of the case by taking advantage of peculiarly psychedelic phenomena. For example, he might be urged to examine a problem in terms of his eidetic images, or perhaps from the vantage point of archaic mythological materials which often emerge into consciousness during a psychedelic experience. It would then be suggested that he analyze and compare the insights achieved through this type of exploration with the understanding previously gained through utilization of more orthodox techniques. In this way the subject was provided with a means to discover a synthesis of

methodologies employing both his usual procedures and those techniques of guidance which develop naturally out of the phenomenology
of the psychedelic experience.

Subsequent to his session(s) and the post-session follow-up the
psychotherapist would observe the instructor's handling of several other
sessions. During the first of these observed sessions he would be permitted to offer suggestions; and, during the later sessions, he would function as a second but subordinate guide. Still later, the psychotherapist-
trainee would guide a session of his own with a volunteer subject, the
instructor standing by as observer and in order that she be able to
take over the handling of the session should the need arise. Finally, the
trainee's performance would be evaluated and suggestions made concerning possible ways to improve it.

Setting of the Psychedelic Experience.   An important function of the
guide is to arrange for a comfortable, pleasant setting in which the
subject's experience will be favorably, and certainly not negatively, influenced by his environment. Such a major role does the physical environment play in determining the course of a subject's experience that it
would be difficult to overemphasize the need for this objective climate
to be favorable.

One of the more clear-cut lessons taught us by scientific psychedelic
drug research to date is that the hospital and other clinical settings
should be avoided. When such a setting is offered in combination with
the subject's expectation of a psychotic or psychotomimetic experience
something along these lines will probably eventuate. And a very large
amount of research now indicates that while such experiences are terribly distressing to the subject, they are not of compensatory value to
the researcher.

The lesson of this early research may, however, have some value
apart from psychedelic work. For it teaches in stark and dramatic form
that a hospital setting gives rise to all sorts of traditional fears of illness,
death, and the mysterious and threatening practices of doctors. Science,
the laboratory—these are alien and menacing areas for many persons.
When, moreover, the setting is drab and antiseptic, and when the authority figures are coldly clinical, then anxiety is greatly increased and
the subject's experience becomes even more disturbing and distasteful.
One wonders to what extent these same reactions in less apparent form
occur with all or most patients outside of the drug context and work to

the patient's detriment? If setting is so extremely important to the drug subject, then it is probably also of very great importance to the ordinary patient. We are aware that a substantial amount of attention already has been paid to this point, but few hospitals have been changed sufficiently as a result and the experience of the subjects may serve to emphasize the need for more action.

The pleasant homelike setting has proved to be the indoors one most conducive to feelings of security and a good experience for the subject. It is also advantageous if the subject can be made familiar with this supportive setting in advance of his session. A good way to do this is to conduct the preliminary interviews in the session room. The subject should at that time be encouraged to wander through the room, sit or lie on chair or couch, and handle the various objects. In short, he should familiarize himself with the environment in which his drug experience will take place. He also should be made to feel thoroughly relaxed and at ease in this environment, so that when he re-enters it later he will more easily fall back into a state of relaxation and security.

The session room should be equipped with a variety of objects experience has shown to be useful in extending the subject's awareness and enhancing his enjoyment of his session. These will include an array of paintings, art books, flowers, stones, sea shells, a large and varied record collection, and so on. Based upon what is learned during his interview, the subject will be urged to bring with him additional objects, recordings, or whatever is likely to prove especially meaningful and pleasurable to him.

In addition to the supportive indoor environment just described, the ideal psychedelic setting will further provide the subject with an opportunity to experience attractive out-of-doors surroundings. Natural settings such as forests and gardens, lakes and beaches are especially desirable and evocative of a sense of the world's beauty and of the subject's harmonious place in the overall "scheme of things." Few subjects would ever want to forget what one has described as the experience of "lying on the soft rustling grass at night and seeing the pure white loveliness of stars streaming down from the incredible magnificence of the heavens."

Selection and Preparation of Subjects. Because of the enormous amount of publicity given the psychedelic drugs by the various communications media, a great many persons are always eager to have the drug experience. Not all of these persons are acceptable as subjects and some must be rejected on the ground that their well-being might be endangered by the experience. Others will be unacceptable in terms of the specific needs of a particular research program.

Speaking only of research, as distinguished from therapy, the minimal requirements that must be met by the would-be volunteer will almost always include the following: his physical condition must be such that no damage is likely to result. For example, a serious cardiac condition would be a basis for rejection. With respect to mental health, a volunteer subject should not have a past history of illness and he should not be presently psychotic or otherwise severely disturbed. In general, he should be functioning successfully in his day-to-day life and should not be involved in major overt conflicts at the time of his session. Such conflict need not eliminate a subject but should be regarded as a temporary disability warranting postponement of the session. Undue anxiety concerning the session is another basis for postponement as might be, for example, the menstrual period in women if depression or some other emotional or mental distress is experienced in connection with the period. Of course, some subjects will manage to conceal facts which, if known, would be grounds for postponement.

In our own work, for reasons peculiar to it, we have found it advisable to establish certain other requirements. With regard to age, we have with few exceptions limited our research to persons between the ages of twenty-five and sixty. However, age is not always best measured in chronological terms and we have sometimes permitted considerations of biological age and mental and emotional maturity to override the twenty-five to sixty years' rule. We also soon learned that for our purposes a minimum I.Q. of 105 should be required, and most of the subjects have had I.Q.s substantially higher than that. We also required, although not inflexibly, an educational level of two years of college or more, or what could be regarded as the equivalent. Most of the subjects have been college graduates and many of these have had graduate degrees. Depending upon their purposes, other researchers might adopt considerably more "liberal" policies with respect to age, intelligence, and level of education.

One other basis for the rejection of a subject by a guide should be mentioned. In cases where the guide feels that he has failed to gain the subject's confidence, the guide should not go ahead with the session. Instead, when possible, a session with another guide towards whom the subject is better disposed should be arranged. If no other guide is available it will be better to call off the session.

Obviously, the physical and mental condition of the subject should be determined by medical and psychiatric examination whenever there are grounds for suspecting that something may be wrong or when the subject is not well known to the guide. Most of our subjects have been so screened.

Following the volunteer's initial acceptance, he begins a series of exploratory conversations with the guide. These talks usually will be spread over a period of several weeks and will serve several purposes. The guide will be able to explore the psychology of the subject and will help the subject to determine the intended goals of his session. The guide will try to learn what methods will be most effective in giving the particular subject the most rewarding and challenging kind of experience. A decision will be made as to the most promising general experiential context—aesthetic, philosophical, psychological, religious, or whatever. The subject's ideas about the psychedelic experience will be discussed with the aim of clearing away misconceptions, providing information, suggesting background readings, and so on. Rapport between subject and guide will be developed along with positive expectations concerning the session.

In addition to such obvious points the subject is made to understand that the value of his experience will depend in large measure on his willingness to suspend or abandon his ordinary, everyday ways of thinking and "looking at things." During the weeks remaining before his session the subject is encouraged to practice the suspension of his usual world-view. This involves not only the suspension of the subject's routine value-judgments, ways of apprehending form and color, and so on, but also the temporary surrender of his usual self-image. These practices serve as an excellent preparation for a psychedelic experience wherein the subject will benefit most if he quickly and easily relinquishes many of his usual controls and *a priori* constructs, and permits the possible new modes of experiencing to have a free rein.

Structuring the Session.   Although it is neither possible nor desirable to impose a rigid schedule or any type of inflexible structuring upon the psychedelic session, it still is desirable for the guide to have definite goals and to have some advance idea of the guiding techniques he is going to use with the particular subject. That the goals will to some extent determine the choice of techniques is obvious; but, at the same time, the techniques will be geared to the needs and personality of the subject.

Among the goals of the session will be examination of those areas the guide thinks worthy of emphasis and which he investigates when possible with each of his subjects. These areas might, for example, include alterations in visual perception of persons, certain kinds of eidetic imagery, varieties of drug-state communication, and so on. Here, the guide, while exploring these areas, must attempt not to influence the content or ways of the subject's experiencing. In this effort he never will be completely successful—any more than, say, the Freudian analyst will be successful in eliciting from his patient dreams and fantasies that are not to some extent colored by the beliefs and methods of the analyst. Each guide, then, will necessarily elicit phenomena partially determined by himself, and must try to find means to keep his influence at a minimum when that is desirable.

Also of primary importance among the goals of the session will be such objectives as the subject may have. The subject may wish, for example, to explore the meaning that the work he is doing has for him or why his marriage has "gone stale"; or, he might want to have a "mystical experience." At the same time he pursues his own goals, the guide attempts to assist the subject to reach those goals of the subject that the two have discussed, defined and agreed upon during their pre-session interviews. Needless to say, the subject may also have other goals which he has not revealed to the guide and which will become apparent only in the course of the session. These two basic decisions, concerning the goals to be sought and techniques to be employed in the session, largely constitute the possible structuring of the session as it is planned ahead of time and—hopefully—adhered to during the subject's psychedelic experience. More particular components of the predetermined structure will include decisions as to the musical recordings to be played, the object-stimuli to be presented, and possibly the tests to be administered. A few of these points should be expanded upon briefly.

Although structured in greater or lesser detail, the session always should appear to the subject to be conducted mainly in terms of *his* personality and both long-range and immediate interests rather than the orientation and research goals of the guide. Succinctly, the subject should never be made to feel like a guinea pig. And, in line with this, the subject always should be given ample time to pursue his goals and to go into those areas he decides *during* the session he particularly wishes to explore.

Thus, while the session should be to some extent structured, the program should be very flexible and, importantly, should give the impression of some spontaneity. The majority of subjects, we have found, will develop resistances if they feel they are being too much dominated or led. On the other hand, as exceptions to the rule, a few subjects prefer to participate in sessions that appear to them to be strictly programmed. This illusion (for it is always that) of adhering to a detailed schedule and experiencing only what was planned produces in these subjects feeling of security. "Nothing is left to chance," the guide is firmly in control, and the subject feels he need not fear the occurrence of unexpected—that is, unpleasant—developments. In most cases the pre-session interviews and the subject's reactions early in the session will sufficiently indicate to the guide the amounts of real and apparent autonomy required by the subject.

With regard to his structuring of sessions generally, the guide will profit from careful planning; but he must also have the capacity to quickly and intelligently restructure the session should the subject prove unwilling or unable to adhere to the pre-planned agenda and methodology. However, only in very rare cases will the guide entirely abandon his program and altogether "play it by ear" or permit the subject to determine the course of his own session in all of its details. Thus, versatility, adaptability, and an agile intelligence are characteristics of the successful guide.

If testing is to be included within the framework of a session, the tests should not be inflexibly scheduled as to time but should be administered during some period when the subject is ready and able to co-operate and when some experience of importance to subject or guide will not have to be interrupted (and probably terminated) to that end. To force a testing situation upon a reluctant or otherwise resisting subject may be to mobilize feelings of hostility and/or anxiety. Subjects forced into testing situations usually either prove unco-operative or do considerably less well than they might if ready to be tested. Then, what we test is how the subject is able to perform under duress; and this is usually a less valid measure of how a psychedelic drug affects test performance than are tests administered to a more co-operative subject. Naturally this scheduling in terms of a subject's readiness will involve some difficulties and inconvenience when the tests must be administered by persons other than the guide who have their own schedule to adhere to. But whenever possible testing should be carried out when the subject is ready and not when it happens to fit in with the plans of the person administering the test.

It is not possible for us or for anyone else to speak at this time of some single "best" or invariably most effective method of guiding. As regards specific procedures to be employed, much will depend upon such factors as the purpose of the session, the dosage, and the respective personalities of subject and guide. As we have noted, it is possible to work more or less effectively within a variety of conceptual frameworks. Psychotherapists, for instance, have drawn *faute de mieux* upon their respective therapeutic backgrounds, endeavoring with varying degrees of success to apply the Freudian, Jungian, existential-analytic or other concepts to the psychedelic session. Directive and non-directive counseling methods have been used; but the former, with its authoritarian approach to the subject, smacks of "brainwashing" and should certainly be avoided by non-therapists and probably by therapists as well. Techniques employed by hypnotherapists are particularly useful in some drug-state situations, as will be evident to anyone acquainted with these procedures. Canadian therapists working with alcoholics use very massive doses of psychedelic drugs to break down the ego defenses and induce a "transcendental experience," which seems to be almost always religious in nature. Timothy Leary and his associates make use of a manual they have adapted from the Tibetan *Book of the Dead*. When a religious experience is aimed for, guides may use music, symbolic objects and other stimuli appropriate to that objective.

The approach to the psychedelic experience and ways of guiding it to be described in the remaining portions of this book evolved for the most part out of the efforts by one of the authors (J. H.) to take "depth soundings" of the psyche. This led to a method of guiding based upon an observed pattern of "descent" with four levels of the drug experience hypothesized as corresponding to major levels of the psyche. This approach, since refined, enabled us to structure a more sophisticated functional model of the drug-state psyche and to develop techniques permitting easier access to those deeper levels where the more rewarding and transformative experiences occur. The four levels and stages of the psychedelic experience have been termed by us: the *sensory*, the *recollective-analytic*, the *symbolic*, and the *integral*. Supportive data along with discussion of some of the psychological and philosophical implications of this work will be provided in the later chapters.

In the remainder of the present chapter, we will give a preliminary view of this schema, and also describe very briefly a few of the guiding techniques and procedures utilized in the "depth sounding" approach.

Psychedelic Guiding: The Sensory Realm. In the earlier stages of the psychedelic drug-state, and in later stages too if deeper levels are not reached, the subject's awareness is primarily of sensory experiencing. Altered awarenesses of body and body image, spatial distortions, and a wide range of perceptual changes ordinarily occur. Temporal orientation is also very greatly altered and the subject, closing his eyes, may be confronted with a succession of vivid eidetic images brilliantly colored and intricately detailed.

For many subjects the emergence or eruption of this wealth of primarily sensory phenomena may constitute the first experience of the "dark woods." If the subject here attempts to maintain his normative structures of time and relationship, if he attempts to play Procrustes and fit the psychedelic flood tides to the old predrug-state frame of reference, he may be in for some unpleasant moments. A sense of confusion and chaos are the usual results of the subject's insistence on trying to preserve his normal categorical orientation. When such an effort is made, it is up to the guide to divert him.

Beginning with this initial apprehension of a world of altered perceptions the guide must steer the subject along the course of gradual intensification and expansion of consciousness. The first directions should be simple and familiar, geared to focus the subject's attention on the heightening of color and form perception of well-known objects. Pictures and flowers, music and such objects as stones and sea shells—these should be the things first "discovered" as the subject acclimatizes himself to the psychedelic environment.

The guide may, for example, invite the subject to consider the enigma of a peach. He may cut a door in a green pepper and direct the subject to open it and look inside at the glorious cathedral now revealed. He may propose that the subject observe the quivering life of a flower, or even of a stone. A variety of sensory stimuli may be orchestrated together with profound effect.

One of the authors, for instance, has frequently created a sense of wonder and "revelation" in her subjects by what will seem a very simple technique. Placing before the subject various vegetables and flowers she instructs him to "enter into friendly or harmonious relationship" with them. As the subject reports he has begun to achieve this she puts Beethoven's *Pastoral* symphony on the record player. The surging notes of this hymn to nature combine with the subject's botanical empathy to produce a euphoric intermingling of sight, touch, smell and sound. And then, when the climactic symphonic moment arrives, the guide slowly peels back the husks of an ear of corn—and the subject *knows* that he has witnessed a mystery. To the psychedelic non-initiate this is likely to sound funny, if not ridiculous, but it repeatedly has proved to be an effective evocation of one of the more ancient human rituals.

While the subject, left to his own devices, may continue to enjoy his sensory experiencing as an end in itself, the guide's task should be to utilize the responses to sensory stimuli as a vehicle for leading the subject beyond this comparatively trivial activity. Sensory experiencing may, for example, lead the subject on to meaningful consideration of his place in the world; and this, in its turn, may be the means of his "descent" to a "deeper" drug-state level.

The Recollective-Analytic Stage.   Possibly several hours into his session, and usually after he has spent some time in the sensory realm with its altered perceptions, the subject will pass on to a stage of his experience in which the content is predominantly introspective and especially recollective-analytic. Personal problems, particularly problem relationships and life-goals are examined. Significant past experiences are recalled and may be revivified ("lived through") with much accompanying emotion. A more charactistically "psychedelic" ideation appears as materials not normally accessible to consciousness surge up and determine the thought content and patterns. The materials are sifted, analyzed, and ordered, and the unfolding self-knowledge may be accompanied by eidetic memory images and images tending to illustrate and clarify the ideational materials. With such a wealth of helpful phenomena at his disposal, the subject now may be in a position to clearly recognize and formulate many of the problems confronting him and may "see what needs to be done" as he has "never seen it before."

These and certain other phenomena we will mention are usually the predominant and subjectively most important ones at this stage. However, at any stage of the experience, phenomena more characteristic of and predominant at another stage also may be present.

During this psychic eruption and unfolding the guide often will remain silent for long periods, so as not to interrupt and possibly cut off the process. Only if the subject clearly needs help will the guide, in most such cases, interject himself and offer techniques and suggestions for "changing the course" or making the most of the sudden insights and startling revelations. On occasion, for example, it will happen that the subject may get into a kind of circular rut wherein some insignificant or no longer useful theme will repeat itself over and over. Then the guide will interrupt and begin to direct the subject, assisting him out of his rutted quagmire of warmed-over sins and damaging self-images toward some new perspective on the problem.

In discussing these and some other aspects of guiding, the question arises as to whether the guide is a therapist. It is our belief that although some of the activities of the guide may be in effect therapeutic, this no more makes him a therapist than the therapeutic by-products of education, religion, and philosophy make therapists of teachers, clergymen, and philosophers. Virgil is not Dante's psychiatrist although he effects considerable therapeutic change in the poet. And the main responsibility of the guide toward the subject, as we tend to see it, is that of helping the subject to enlarge his philosophical world-view by way of general consciousness expansion and such particular means as re-examination of values and purposes, enhanced aesthetic appreciation and gaining a new perspective on a variety of other basic and universal human problems. When one considers the enormously rich and varied range of experience open to the psychedelic subject, as to Dante, it can only seem wasteful if not destructive to limit the drug-state explorations to psychodynamic factors. Rather, the guide should be one who travels with the subject (again, we do not speak of *patients*) through the vast panoramic continuum of the psychedelic world; and his work then should be to point out a new dimension of experience here, a possible new interpretation there, while helping the subject toward a greater understanding of himself and his world. This journey may prove to be also therapeutic, including the remission of some symptom or symptoms, but such a result is incidental and not the aim of the guide as distinguished from the therapeutic worker.

Returning to this *recollective-analytic* stage of the psychedelic experience, the guide here feels that he is something of an "open book" to many of his subjects. It has been our experience that even vague stirrings in the mind of the guide often cause immediate interest and concern on the part of the subject who then may go on to identify with surprising accuracy the specific and often esoteric feeling or thought that had just occurred to the guide. When the guide has inquired of the subject as to the source of her information the usual response has been that she was not telepathically reading his thoughts but rather "reading" his face. And the subject might then inquire of the guide: "Why do you react so much to your thoughts?" Thus it appeared that even slight and subtle shifts of facial expression were as meaningful to the subject as if the guide were an actor conveying his message by means of theatrical pyrotechnics. Moods may be conveyed in similar fashion, and thus a transient depressing thought or moment of anxiety on the part of the guide has been observed to trigger much stronger feelings of depression or anxiety in the subject. Because of this non-verbal potency of the guide, it is up to him to try to maintain a state of positive awareness and calm and to try to avoid any gestures, sounds, and facial expressions that might be interpreted in a negative way by the subject.

Communication between subject and guide is also affected by other peculiarly "psychedelic" factors. For example, many subjects will tend to assume that the guide is equally as "sensitized" as they, and go on from this to decide that verbal communication is not at all necessary. Some subjects, as we have seen, feel certain that telepathic and even spoken communications of considerable length have taken place; and only the playback of a tape, if that, will convince the subject that no such conversation ever was held.

On the verbal level the "psychedelic" conversation may include a mutual awareness of nuances rarely encountered in ordinary conversation. There is often, for example, a simultaneous grasping by subject and guide of multiple meanings and shades of meanings all attached to a single word or brief phrase. It can be of very great importance if the guide, in pre-session interviews, is able to learn some of the "key" or "pivotal" words of the subject. These personal key words together with recurrent words employed by the subject in the session may be employed with great success to lead the subject into deeper levels of awareness.

The "loaded" psychedelic conversation, in which a few words suffice to "speak volumes," sometimes yields in a minute or two insights capable of effecting a valuable shift of perspective in the subject. We will reproduce such a brief conversation, including a rather typical "psychedelic pun," that the subject felt served to "illumine" his "whole view of matter and attitude towards it."

S: (to G) "You smile."

G: "The earth smiles."

S: (Accepts a stone G hands him and examines it) "The smile in the heart of matter. But does it matter? Does anything . . . matter?"

G: "Go into the stone and find out."

S: (Studies the stone for several seconds and speaks without taking his eyes away from it) "Yes, I matter . . . Deeply, I matter . . . In the very heart of creation I . . . matter."

G: "And your 'nothingness' that you were complaining about a while ago? Where is it now?"

S: (Looking up and weeping tears of joy) "*When Being begins, Nothing* matters."

Some extremely valuable insights may be had on this *recollective-analytic* level and these may be sufficient to enable the subject to revise his thinking and self-image and to alter his behavior in desirable ways. However, much greater gains are possible when the subject uses this level to effectively formulate his problems and goals and then "carries" this material "down" with him to the experimental level and stage of descent we have termed the *symbolic*.

The Symbolic Level.   On the symbolic level of the psychedelic experience profound self-understanding and a high degree of self-transformation may reward the subject who is properly prepared. Since our later discussion of this level, reached by some forty percent of the subjects, is extensive, here we will be brief. We will also be very brief as concerns the integral level to which an even more extensive chapter is devoted.

The eidetic images become of major importance on this *symbolic* level as does the capacity of the subject to feel that he is participating with his body as well as his mind in the events he is imaging. Here, the symbolic images are predominantly historical, legendary, mythical, ritualistic, and "archetypal." The subject may experience a profound and rewarding sense of continuity with evolutionary and historic process. He may act out myths and legends and pass through initiations and ritual observances often seemingly structured precisely in terms of his own most urgent needs.

If the subject before reaching this *symbolic* level has been able to see his life in terms of some universal myth or legend, or if he has recognized his readiness and need to pass through a certain rite, then the mythic acting out or ritual passage will be powerfully experienced by him. He will image and feel himself totally into the rite or into a myth involving a figure with whom he is able to identify because he has come to see his life in its broad outlines or even in many particulars as repeating the life of the legendary figure. In this latter case, should the myth be one that ends in some unfortunate way, the subject is helped to restructure it along more positive lines or else to go beyond the myth to a new one or drop the mythic identification completely.

Since our society offers so little in the way of the important rites of passage and initiations provided by other civilizations, these experiences provide in many cases means for growth and maturation apparently not possible for some persons when no rite is provided. That our society suffers from the lack of these means of growth has been noted by others, but the psychedelic experience affords some important documentation in behalf of this belief.

When the subject does not become a participant in a symbolic drama of myth or ritual, he still may achieve the aforementioned sense of continuity with historical and evolutionary process, and this may be of considerable value. He may *feel* in his body his continuity with these processes and may witness by means of the eidetic images many of what he believes to be the details of evolutionary and historical unfolding. But unless he is able to participate directly in and respond emotionally to the mythic and ritualistic re-enactments he will be unable to descend to the deepest level of the psychedelic drug-state. Neither will he reap the very great benefits already possible on the level he has reached.

The Integral Level. Only eleven of our 206 psychedelic subjects have reached the deep integral level where the experience is one of psychological integration, "illumination," and a sense of fundamental and positive self-transformation.[1] In each of these cases the experience of the *integral* level has been regarded by the subject as a religious one; even so, we see no reason why this level and its effects could not be experienced in other than religious terms.

On this level, ideation, images, body sensation (if any) and emotion are fused in what is felt as an absolutely purposive process culminating in a sense of total self-understanding, self-transformation, religious enlightenment and, possibly, mystical union. The subject here experiences what he regards as a confrontation with the Ground of Being, God, Mysterium, Noumenon, Essence, or Fundamental Reality. The content of the experience is self-validating and *known* with absolute certainty to be true. Further a kind of *post facto* validation is forthcoming in the form of the after-effects: the behavioral and other changes.

The climate on this level is intensely emotional. It is felt that this intense affect serves to synthesize the experimental components and to effect a lasting, positive integration of the restructured psychical organization. Many of what the subject regarded as ineffectual and self-damaging behavioral patterns seem to have been effaced, cut through or overlaid in a kind of imprinting or reimprinting process. The subject knows with perfect conviction that he will in the future respond in terms of the new insights and new orientation instead of making the old, painful and non-productive responses he has made in the past.

The subjects who achieve this kind of experience are always very well prepared for the psychedelic drug-state. They have exceptional self-understanding, usually achieved after long hard effort, although the ways of arriving at this self-understanding have been various. Some have achieved it mainly through psychedelic drug experiences. Some have worked with techniques of self-development including yoga and mysticism. One had largely conquered a severe anxiety neurosis through self-analysis alone. Several had been analysands. All at the time of their sessions were comparatively very mature, developed personalities who, at least in their public lives, would be generally regarded as functioning in a superior way in the world.

The after-effects of these "transforming experiences" are remarkable in those cases where the subject is not already so well-adjusted and so far advanced toward his personal goals that "great leaps forward" no longer are possible for him. The subject may be strengthened, energized, made more serene, creative, and spontaneous. There is a much-heightened sense of being in harmonious relation with other persons and with things—with the world generally. Sense perceptions may be sharpened with a consequent enhancement of aesthetic response to a wide variety of stimuli. The mirror image and also the *felt* body image may seem to have undergone changes for the better; and, along with this, the person may feel lighter and better co-ordinated, generally more "fit."

Following such an experience the subject usually expresses himself as having no need or wish for another psychedelic experience in any near future. He feels that enough has been achieved and that the experience was a fulfillment, taking him as far as he is able to go by this means at this time and at the present stage of his development.

While the effects we are describing resemble, for example, the effects described by A. H. Maslow as resulting from varieties of the (nondrug) "peak experience," we believe that the change is more profound and fundamental in the case of the psychedelic subject. If this is true, then the reason for it probably lies in the much greater duration of the experience on the integral level as compared to the duration of the usual "peak" experience which, whether mystical, religious, aesthetic or whatever, is almost always very brief—rarely more than a minute or so at the most. The psychedelic subject, as distinguished from the person having the nondrug-state "peak experience," ordinarily remains in the intensely affect-charged climate of the integral level for from fifteen minutes to two hours—and on two occasions, for as long as four hours. The integration of the eidetic imagery into a purposive ideation-image-sensation-affect complex also is of great importance in achieving the transformation of the person. But the extended duration of the experience of the integral level's powerful affective climate is probably the final and "clinching" factor producing a deeper, more permanent "imprinting" than usually occurs in the more familiar "peak" and "conversion" experiences of a very brief duration.

Before closing this discussion we would add that our criteria for determining whether the subject has reached this integral level and undergone profound transformation are strict. Thus, while some ninety-five percent of the subjects claim to have been benefited and changed in some positive way by their sessions, and while about forty percent have declared themselves profoundly and positively transformed, we evaluate only slightly more than five percent of the cases as involving radical transformation of the person on the *integral* level. As remarked, this percentage would be doubled if we limited consideration to the last 60 cases—cases handled after our *schema* had been considerably refined and elaborated. Probably it would go higher still with further work; but, even so, we doubt that the very high percentages of profound transformation reported by some other workers in this field ever could be achieved in terms of our criteria, even if the criteria were considerably loosened.

Finally, we would like to say that we are about as uneasy with such terms as "transformation," "self-understanding," "illumination," "realization of potentials," and so on, as some of our professional readers will be. We, too, would "feel much better about all this" if a more scientific terminology could be effectively employed. Unfortunately, however, we deal here, and especially when discussing the integral level, with areas psychology has tended to ignore and with which neither science nor philosophy has done much better.

As concerns participation by the guide, his activity stops at the threshold of the *integral* level and the subject experiences the final integration unassisted and alone. Somewhat as Virgil had to leave Dante at the portals of the "realms of bliss," so must the guide withdraw and do no more than bear witness to the culmination of the process he has launched and directed to this point. The state of being we call *integral*, like Dante's Paradise, is an intensely subjective and private one and there the guide may not follow.

Six:

The World of
the Non-Human

In preceding chapters we have dealt with the psychedelic subject's consciousness of his own body and with his consciousness of other persons and of himself in relation to others. In the present chapter, we will deal with the subject's sensory level experiencing of the world of non-human phenomena. We will also discuss the eidetic images and the transition from the sensory level to a "deeper" one.

Most of the experiences described in the earlier chapters are fairly typical of psychedelic sessions and their occurrence has little to do with how the session is structured or even with whether the session is structured at all. Our purpose in presenting these more or less random experiences was to further familiarize the reader with the drug-state phenomena and also to give him some notion of what the psychedelic experience may look like when considered outside the context of any particular system of guiding or overview of the essential nature of the experience. Hereafter, we will deal with the drug-state in terms of our own discovery of its phenomenological pattern and of our methods for bringing about, or preventing blockage of, the unfolding of that pattern. Our intention will be to demonstrate possibilities always latent in the drug experience but which up to now have been too seldom realized for the reason that the pattern was unrecognized. Thus, goals and procedures were imposed that were alien to and disruptive of the *natural* psychedelic process.

It should be kept in mind that the sensory level is the subject's first experience of the new "psychedelic consciousness." The subject is thrust into a new world, makes his adjustment to it and then is able to delight in and profit by its wonders. His now useless "real world" categories fall away before a novelty first of percept and then of concept. If all goes well, his non-categorical experiencing of the psychedelic "world's" phenomena prepares him to later, on deeper levels, confront the contents of his life and psyche with equally fresh and novel perspectives.

Thus the sensory level should have as a major function the *deconditioning* of the subject. By presenting a wealth of hitherto unknown perceptual possibilities it can dissolve or temporarily suspend the effectiveness of those psychical mechanisms whose functions would appear to be to inhibit emergence of certain processes and contents of the mind. Once these inhibitions are dissolved, the ground has been prepared for the free psyche to function in such a way as to result in the beneficial transformation and self-realization of the individual. As we will see, this transformative process would seem to be entelechical and, when the conditions for unfolding are met, will move in strange but effective ways to provide the subject with that measure of fulfillment for which his past life has readied him.

The Perceptual Feast. Havelock Ellis once described the psychedelic (peyote) experience as "a saturnalia of the specific senses, and, above all, an orgy of vision." This emphasis on vision is especially appropriate when discussing the onset of the drug-state and sensory level phenomena. Later, the subject may go on to some almost equally exciting tactile experiences; and none of the senses need be denied its portion of novel and pleasurable stimulation.

The drug-state consciousness sometimes erupts with a spectacular hypersensate fanfare. "All at once" colors are bright and glowing, the outlines of objects are defined as they never have been before, spatial relationships are drastically altered, several or all of the senses are enormously heightened—"all at once" the world has shed its old, everyday façade and stands revealed as a wonderland.

When a period of fairly gradual transition ushers in this change, the subject may notice first of all a pulsing, vibratory excitation of the atmosphere and remark small, curved, flickering and sparkling particles of light that appear to dart to and fro, dance briefly in place, then dart away again, and disappear. This phenomenon of flickering light and atmospheric excitation is like that seen in the work of the impressionist painters and was theorized about by Seurat, who believed that all objects are precisely a coalescence of these (energy) particles.

Then, as the phenomena swiftly multiply and greatly gain in richness, fluid colors stream and mingle at the edges of things and colored objects stand revealed in all their characteristic drug-state vividness. When the phenomena progressively accumulate, rather than making simultaneous appearance, these color perceptions quickly may be followed by a host of other phenomena including objects shrinking and growing, leaning and displaying in bold delineation the sharpness of their angles, dissolving into whirling particles, melting, undulating, expanding and contracting, and so on. The attempt to banish from consciousness this new world of stimuli yields only fear and confusion, and the same result is forthcoming when a desperate effort is made to at once impose some rigid order upon it. If, however, the subject is willing to lay aside his everyday assumptions and categorizations, then the drug-state environment becomes increasingly stable, although on its own "psychedelic" terms. A kind of order is discernible and the bombardment of stimuli slackens with things "presenting themselves" singly and in such a manner as to enable the subject to fully perceive, think about, and even empathize with the particular object of his attenton.

When the psychedelic experience is had out-of-doors the heightened and distorted perceptions may be somewhat different from those just described. Fairly typical of responses to the out-of-doors setting is the following peyote experience of a young woman. This subject, S-1, a recent university graduate, writes:

"I walked in the light of a full moon across a great meadow. . . . I became aware of almost electrical surroundings . . . (and) there was also the sense of the body's biochemical processes, rhythmically throbbing . . . My senses became extremely acute. I could see an ant upon a tree at a great distance away. I could hear the whispering of my companion, with whom I had shared the peyote, far off from me. Biting into an apple, I felt the granular surface of the chunk intensely magnified. I could rarely close my eyes because of my fascination with the external stimuli, and so probably missed a number of 'visions' [i.e., eidetic images].

". . . As dawn came, my heightened ability to organize caused each cloud to take on recognizable shape. I felt a great peace. The pink sky was hyper-pink. A myriad of multicolored telephone wires hummed as they wriggled like serpents . . . When I closed my eyes there was an endless flow of dancing geometrical forms in the most magnificent combinations of color. I could not help thinking at this time how a man in advertising might make his fortune were he able to capture just a bit of this. . . .

"As I watched a wooded section I was surprised to find the branches of the trees flapping as a bird does, only in harmonious slow motion. Distant scenery waved gently so as almost to resemble a tapestry gently swaying. I was amused to see the brick walls of a house tirelessly undulating. Fascinated, I drew near trees whose trunks heaved, and whose bark from afar flowed and pulsated in a manner suggesting organic growth. Close observation of the bark was astounding. I reminded myself of the mental patient one sees in films, on the lawn of the institution, drawn next to the inanimate in watchfulness. And here I was, leaning against the brick house, bound by concentration on the microcosmic growth and flow of the particles. A dandelion I glanced down at grew two feet high. Everything was magnified. As I strolled, my attention was wholly grasped by a small dewdrop on the grass. It was utterly captivating."

From such aesthetic appreciation S, as is common with the psychedelic subjects, moved on to some philosophical reflections—in this case, a type of thinking made popular by some Eastern-oriented writers whose works have been influential with students and with the Drug Movement. She writes:

"Emotionally there is a profound feeling of oneness. . . . I was joyful to understand the concept 'all things are animate.' It is true for one who witnesses the supposed inanimate fibres of her dress, breathing and undulating . . . The proposition presenting matter as the interaction of light energy is something I feel as though I could confirm. I beheld the One and the Many emphasized in Eastern philosophy. It seemed true—the tree, my companion, and I—we were all the same thing— dying in and out. Status and classification appeared as mere superficial differentiation, in the light of the harmony I saw among all beings."

In the foregoing description we find accounts of the two major types of perceptual change encountered in the psychedelic experience—the heightening of perception and the distortion of perception. Impairment (diminished acuity) of perception also may occur, but usually is mild and has little significance for the overall experience.

That sense perceptions are heightened at all has been denied by some investigators who, administering standard tests, have found that in terms of the test there was no such heightening. But this would be a difficult finding to "sell" to most psychedelic subjects and certainly to the subject whose experience just has been described.

It is our own belief that *for consciousness* a heightening of sense perception definitely occurs; but it may not occur in such a way as to be measurable by the tests now in use. We do doubt that the eye is absolutely seeing more (some effects of pupillary dilation possibly excepted), or that the nose is smelling more. Rather, it seems likely that more of what the eye sees and more of what the nose smells is getting into consciousness. Some of this MORE doubtless results from the subject's paying greater and prolonged attention to the stimulus than he usually does; but deinhibiting factors also may be involved. That the subject firmly believes his perceptions are much more acute is not to be doubted.

That the subject is seeing "better" or "more clearly" the colors, lines, and other specific properties and parts of things appears to be often explained by the fact that the object in such cases no longer is being apperceived in terms of function, symbolism or label categorizations of the object not accessible to sense perception alone and which usually work to dilute the immediacy of the perception.

In most cases, on this sensory level, the classification of the thing as box, jar, or whatever is noted but seems then to be dismissed as irrelevant and so has little or no effect upon the perception. Occasionally, however, a subject will bypass categorical recognition altogether. Then a scrap of wallpaper may be perceived with such immediacy, such instantaneous and total immersion in the sensory detail, as to oblige the subject to inquire what it is he now is observing. If that question is not answered, the subject soon will be able to find the answer for himself; but it still may take as much as a minute for him to recognize and label the object when he has not done so at the outset.

The distortion of perception yields a much greater range of phenomena and is psychologically much more significant than the heightening of perception which is only a consciousness of seeing, hearing, tasting, smelling, or touching "better" than before. The distortions may serve to impose a symbolism upon the environment, may be an essential component of empathic and mystical experiences, and may be an extremely important aspect of the subject's participation in the transformative symbolic dramas occurring on the deeper drug-state levels. We will return to the varieties of perceptual distortion from time to time in this chapter and also throughout the remainder of the book. They confront us with a highly complex interaction of perception with ideational, emotional and inferred unconscious factors; thus, discussion of some of the specific examples will be required.

Aesthetic Images. Few aspects of the psychedelic experience are so impressive to the average subject, or so well remembered after his session, as the eidetic images—images previously recorded by the brain or, in some cases, possibly a part of the phylogenetic (or "Racial") inheritance, and which emerge into consciousness during the drug experience. These images usually are seen with eyes closed, although they may be seen in a gazing crystal or on some suitable surface, such as a movie screen. They are almost always vividly colored and the colors typically are described as rich, brilliant, glowing, luminous, or "preternatural"— colors exceeding in their beauty anything the subject has ever seen before.

The images are most often of persons, animals, architecture, and landscapes. Strange creatures from legend, folklore, myth, and fairy tale appear in wonderful surroundings. Ancient temples and castles are imaged, and figures and incidents from the historical past. Persons, places, and objects observed in the course of the subject's life may make their appearance, especially on the *recollective-analytic* level where life-historical materials are the main concern. More often, however, the images are not of specific, familiar faces, scenes, or things, but probably are synthetic creations combining elements of several recorded images. In general, whatever the subject knows about, has seen or is able to imagine may, as eidetic image, appear to him somewhat as these might be seen in technicolor still photographs or motion pictures. The unconscious process by which recorded images could be synthesized to result in a new creation is not explained by saying that the images and image sequences represent an unconscious act of creation; but that is about as much of an "explanation" as it is possible to give. Probably the images have a common source with the images of dreams and hypnotic states.

The eidetic images may appear as a sequence of related or unrelated single "pictures," or they may unfold as a continuous movie-like drama in which the subject may or may not play a part. The images may enter into consciousness as meaningless and so have only "entertainment value"; or they may be supremely meaningful, illumining the most important areas of the subject's life.

On the sensory level of the psychedelic experience the images are almost always meaningless, or mean nothing more than what they most obviously are. Thus, an image of a grazing cow is just an image of a grazing cow, and nothing more. The cow has no discernible relevance to the subject's life; it is not a symbol or, if it is, then the symbolism does not become apparent. The image has no function for the subject and, at best, will entertain him. This type of functionless or purposeless image we have termed the *aesthetic* image, so distinguishing it from the highly meaningful and otherwise functional *purposive* images met with on the deeper drug-state levels.

Unless they are especially frightening, little emotional response is made to the aesthetic images. They may give some pleasure and so induce a mild euphoria. Some researchers have reported sexual excitement as a response to images with erotic content; but this is rare and, so far as we know, unimportant on this level of the guided session. Only when the images are especially hideous or in some other way menacing does the subject respond to them strongly on the sensory level. Then he may respond to the hideousness of the image as he might to a similarly hideous art work or photograph; or, he may be disturbed because it is his image.

In a representative example of the usual sort of entertaining or innocuous aesthetic image sequence a male subject, S-3 (peyote), experienced the following:

"A platinum snail about twelve feet high and studded with rubies was pulled along on its wheels by a much smaller and brightly painted dwarf carved from wood. The curious couple was closely followed by a host of metallic, gem-covered insects—grasshoppers and beetles, bumblebees, and mosquitos, all of fabulous size and brilliantly gleaming, gliding or walking or hopping with the precision of wound-up toys. These then were followed by strange creatures from some wildly imaginative bestiary—all converging upon a lush oasis in the golden desert where the foliage seemed to have been created by Rousseau."

As regards the "twelve feet high" snail, very often the subject *knows* the dimensions of the imaged object although, of course, the size of an image cannot be measured. This may be true even when the imaged object occurs alone and cannot be compared with other things in the environment. Also, as in this case, the scene may be such that nothing in it offers any clues concerning the size of the object. Apparently, in the unconscious act of constructing the object certain specifications have been made and these become conscious along with the image.

In some cases of eidetic imaging there is a transition from initial crepuscular imagery to increasingly more vivid images. Usually, there is at least some intensification of the images. But it is by no means unknown that the images appear in full vividness at the beginning or any earlier, vague images pass unnoticed. Also, such complex images as those described in the example are preceded in some cases by simple images—geometric forms, drifting "clouds" of color, clusters of "jewels," and so on.[1] In the following case we are given an excellent description of the transition from simple to complex images. The subject, whose peyote experience remained entirely on the sensory level, also describes a few typical perceptual responses to the environment. More importantly, this account of his experience, including a final assessment of it, is representative of the evaluations likely to be made by a mature and nonmystically inclined individual whose experience has remained on the sensory level. The subject, S-4, a forty-one-year-old journalist and former musician, writes:

"The first impressions began to appear in about an hour. With the eyes closed I saw multicolored lines and streaks, faint at first but growing stronger, in a sort of moving kaleidoscope. The constantly shifting patterns reminded me of Disney's visual interpretation of the Bach-Stokowski orchestral transcription in his *Fantasia*, which I had seen some fifteen years before. These images involving play of light, color and movement, were replaced by a static series of patterns of rich hues and abstract design, somewhat like tapestries. They followed at regular short invervals, changing automatically like a slide projector. There seemed no way of detaining a particularly pleasant one by concentration. . . .

"It seemed more pleasant to keep the eyes closed and enjoy the train of inner visions than to examine the various objects in the room. Though their colors and shapes sharpened, which made an ordinary household object a thing of beauty, I did not have Huxley's feeling of perceiving the Platonic essence or *Ding-an-sich* of the objects in view.

"The objects seen with the eyes closed seemed unrelated to thought or experience. As they gradually became more perceptible, scenes involving human forms and architecture began to emerge accompanied by play of light and color, a 'technicolor' of the mind's eye. As the visions grew more interesting, I could still convey my experiences to the guide, although my engrossment in the sensations was such that I did not wish to interrupt them for too long . . . Most of the scenes were oriental—brilliantly illuminated landscapes, strange towers, pagodas, and temples, furnishing the background to exquisite lovely dancers, often with delicate breasts, who could have been Balinese maidens. The most vivid image appeared in a timeless setting: a Japanese girl, nude, standing motionless before a temple, her skin a lovely amber, her hair a glistening black. The colors seemed to glow with an inner light. It seemed a glimpse of something timeless and primordial, a sort of breakthrough into the realm of the absolute. There were no religious or mystical associations—the vision was there, objective, eternal, and yet ephemeral—in a few seconds I moved on to another. . . .

"We took a little stroll and outside in the warm Louisiana summer night—it then was after ten o'clock—the world was transfigured. The full moon shone so brightly it seemed like a sun, and like the sun, one could not focus one's eyes upon it any longer than an instant. The foliage appeared to be a lush tropical garden, the wax-like leaves and blades of grass taking on a deep olive hue. It seemed as if I could distinguish every leaf, every blade of grass. It was like walking through a fairyland, a tranquil, dreamlike landscape unassociated with anything I had previously known.

"With regard to time, what impressed me most was how heavily each moment weighed in the scheme of things—the incredible amount of experience a few minutes could contain. Yet, in retrospect, each of the ten or twelve hours taken up by the experiment seemed to have lasted only a few minutes. Afterwards, I felt I had gone through a powerful experience, but there was no desire to repeat the experience. In a few months, perhaps, yes; but for the moment I had had enough of such strange and uncontrollable sensations.

"I have read that certain tribes of American Indians use the peyote in religious experience. At no time during the experiment did I associate my sensations with religious or mystical feelings. To be sure, there were visions; but for me they were purely sensations. Sensation is a matter of degree; heightened through peyote or other drugs, it still does nothing for me except perhaps emphasize the mystery involved as regards sensory perception.

"Since the sensation is pleasurable, I suspect that some who experiment with psychedelic drugs for 'religious purposes' are subconsciously rationalizing in an attempt to justify the taking of drugs in a society where drug-taking is taboo. Rationalization enables them to indulge in a pleasant and guilt-free experience; even taking drugs becomes a moral act if identified with the search for the Buddha."

As suggested, very little is known about eidetic images. Even the question of an experiential ground is open to debate. Unknown, too, is why a particular image appears when it does and why it stands in its peculiar sequential relation to other, apparently unrelated images. As we progress in our discussion of the levels of the psychedelic experience, the basic mystery of the eidetic images will not be solved; rather, the mystery will deepen along with the drug-state levels.

Although one cannot explain the eidetic images, there is much that can be said about them. We will say only a little at this point, and will limit discussion to a few immediately relevant items.

First of all, the image has its own space, in which the objects appear and the action unfolds. This resembles the imaginary space of the dream and is the space of an unreal as distinguished from the real world. Also, the image has its own time; or it is timeless. With most eidetic images, time is irrelevant, although in the dramatic sequences there may be experienced transitions from day to night and even from week to week or year to year. Even so, the image has a peculiarly timeless flavor, giving to the dramas of the deeper levels their curious aura of fatality.

This fact that the image has its own space makes it immediately distinguishable from both normal percept and visual hallucination. The visual hallucination occurs in the "real world" environment and may be mistaken for a real object. The eidetic image, with its own environment, is never mistaken for a real object. Even a panic reaction to an image probably never means that the image has been mistaken for an object and event in the "real world."

Whether the eidetic image is related to the hallucination and even may stand on a kind of continuum with it, is a question to which there is no certainly valid answer. Occasionally, in a brief span of time, a subject may experience both hallucinations (apparent perceptions of real objects when no such objects are present) and images. Moreover, the images and hallucinations may seem to be ideationally and/or affectively related—as if both were "working to make the same point." However, we have never heard of an eidetic image evolving or developing into an hallucination; or, rather, when we had heard of such an instance, investigation has tended to disprove or cast serious doubt on the occurrence.

The temporal and spatial difference between image and percept, and other distinguishing factors such as the greater vividness of the image, appear to serve as built-in safeguards against the subject mistaking the imaged for the perceived reality. Yet, as we have noted, the images may frighten the subject and so produce anxiety reactions. Of course, the question arises as to whether the image actually produced the anxiety, or whether, instead, anxiety resulted in the production of an image which then further intensified the anxiety? That the images are, at least in some cases, "clothed affect" seems to us a plausible conclusion; but it seems highly improbable that they always are that.

When frightening images do occur they are likely to make their appearance on the sensory level of the drug experience where the image is not a recognizable symbol but is "only itself." Then, if the response is not wholly emotional, the subject may become ideationally involved in the image and begin to read meanings into it. While proper set and setting should prevent the disturbing image experience, its occurrence is always a possibility. This possibility is increased when the drug effects begin very quickly as happens when administration is by injection. In the following cases the subjects received LSD and DMT, respectively, by intramuscular injection and in both cases the onset of the drug effects was swift and the subject's anxiety wholly or mainly attributable to a lack of time to make any gradual adjustment. Both subjects, whose sessions were with other researchers,[2] were "psychedelic veterans" who had had no trouble in previous sessions when the drugs were taken orally and the effects came on gradually. But on the occasion now to be described, the "hell experiences" came at the very start of the session.

The first case is especially unusual in that the subject's experience was of "simple" eidetic images or even what might be called "pre-images." Also, a rarity early in the session, the subject had a tactile as well as imagistic awareness of the tempestuous chaos of liquid and often amorphous colors which threatened to inundate consciousness. This forty-four-year-old author and scholar, S-5 (LSD: 300 micrograms), writes:

"I am a veteran explorer of those depths and labyrinths that are my own self, but for such an immediate and furious onslaught I was not ready. Surging wildly across the surface of my mind—even, as it seemed, across the surface of my brain, a brain now capable of intense sensations—swirled a purple sea, irresistible, angry, and teeming with clammy, serpentine shapes that I thought tried to fasten and feed, but then were swept brutally away in the seething, terrible, thick liquid. The much too suddenly deluged self reeled and trembled before the force of the tidal wave of whatever atrocious stuff had engulfed it. Unexpectedly assailed by so fierce and monstrous a turbulence, even the most seasoned voyager may come to know a new kind of dread that threatens at any instant to degenerate to panic.

"Purple, but with throbbing, bulging, vein-like masses of green and red and black, I think that sea was; and of the texture of syrup, or of blood that is congealing. Heavy, tumultuous seas, and thickening, rising up to awesome heights—with consciousness tossed as a lifeboat is tossed in a typhoon's onrush. Capsize seemed imminent and I longed to cry out my terror, to beg for an antidote; yet somewhere in the midst of bewilderment and the fear of being swept away altogether, was my pride which insisted I ride out the storm. I hung on to this pride, once I found it, as if it were the shattered mast of the vessel of my self. Then, in the midst of a raging sea of colors I could name, but which were horrible, I saw myself clinging to that mast; and the waters gradually turned black and still; and an eerie silver sun came up; and I knew I was saved."

S's session "after this unpromising beginning, was not unpleasant except that throughout there were moments of confusion and, afterwards, 'blank spots' in the memory of the session"—something that never had happened to him before.

In the second (DMT) case the subject, S-6, a young woman in her mid-twenties, experienced "the most terrifying three minutes" of her life—three minutes that seemed, however, an eternity.[3] She then experienced some other, less frightening images, but only one brief sequence which she regarded as pleasurable. The final "face of God" image seemed to her in retrospect an appropriate, mocking commentary on her "foolishness" in taking, under adverse conditions, this particular drug—she got the God that she deserved! S writes:

"I had been up for three days and two nights working on a manuscript. That was the first mistake. The room where the 'experiment' was to take place was a dirty, dingy, insanely cluttered pesthole. That was the second mistake. I was told that I would see God. That was the third and worst mistake of all.

"The needle jabbed into my arm and the dimethyl-tryptamine oozed into my bloodstream. At the same time the steam came on with a rhythmic metallic clamor and I remember thinking that it would be good to have some heat. Within thirty seconds I noticed a change, or rather I noticed that there had never been any change, that I had been in this dreamy, unworldly state for millions of years. I told this to Dr.——, who said, 'Good, then it is beginning to pass the blood-brain barrier.'

"It was too fast. Much too fast. I looked up at what a minute ago had been doors and cabinets, and all I could see were parallel lines falling away into absurdities. Dimensions were outraged. The geometry of things crashed blindly into one another and crumbled into chaos. I thought to myself, 'But he said that I would see God, that I would know the meaning of the universe.' I closed my eyes. Perhaps God was there, behind my eyeballs.

"Something was there, all right; Something, coming at me from a distant and empty horizon. At first it was a pinpoint, then it was a smudge, and then—a formless growing Shape. A sound accompanied its progress towards me—a rising, rhythmic, metallic whine; a staccato meeyow that was issuing from a diamond larynx. And then, there it loomed before me, a devastating horror, a cosmic diamond cat. It filled the sky, it filled all space. There was nowhere to go. It was all that was. There was no place for me in this—*Its* universe. I felt leveled under the cruel glare of its crystalline brilliance. My mind, my body, my vestige of self-esteem perished in the hard glint of its diamond cells.[4]

"It moved in rhythmic spasms like some demonic toy; and always there was its voice—a steely, shrill monotony that put an end to hope. There should not be such a voice! It ravaged the nerves and passed its spasms into my head to echo insanely from one dark corridor of my mind to another. Me-e-e-e-yow-ow-ow-ow me-e-e-e-yow-ow-ow-ow me-e-e-e-yow-ow-ow-ow—the incessant, insatiable staccato went on. It would not have been so bad if it had just been diabolical noise. The chilling thing was that I knew what it was saying! It told me that I was a wretched, pulpy, flaccid thing; a squishy-squashy worm. I was a thing of soft entrails and slimy fluids and was abhorrent to the calcified God.

"I opened my eyes and jumped up from my chair screaming: 'I will not have you! I will not have such a God! What is the antidote to this? Give me the antidote!' But as I said this I doubted my own question for it seemed to me that this was the only reality I had ever known, the one I was born with and the one I would die with. There was no future beyond this state of mind, there was no state of mind beyond this one.

"'There is no antidote,' said Dr.——. 'Relax, it's only been three minutes. You've got at least twenty-five more minutes still to go.'

"I looked around the room. The seething symmetry had calmed down some. Instead of evoking terror it merely made one seasick now. 'Euclidian nausea,' I thought, and closed my eyes again. I found myself on a small planet of a distant star. A spaceship built like an amoeba reached with long tentacles out to grab me. The center of the space ship was diaphanous like an embryo's head with a network of blue veins, flowing blood, and shifting cellular wastes. It pulsed and pulsed and whirred and cackled. I did not wish to be a part of this protoplasmic blob although it was far cheerier than the first vision, and so, as its tentacles were about to enclose me, I opened my eyes and escaped its interstellar plans for me. By this time I was learning how to manage—or should I say Escape from—the experience. I thought that I would start to call my own shots, find my own planet.

"I closed my eyes again to discover a world of blue horses. The land heaved gently and the necks and heads of stately blue horses rose and fell as waves on the planet's surface. It was a land of perfect peace, a blue equine paradise.

"But still I hadn't seen the face of God! I would make a final effort at ultimate visions. My eyes closed and I found myself looking through one end of an immensely long cylinder. At first, there was nothing at the other end—a trillion miles away. Then God came and peeked in at me. I burst out laughing.

"The face of God staring at me from the other end of the cylinder was the face of a very wise monkey!"

Concerning this case it may be superfluous to remark that the subject should not be told she is going to "see God" or discover "the meaning of the universe." Yet more than one researcher and therapist we know of has done this sort of thing repeatedly, and probably never with benefit to the subject or patient. Medical doctors no less than other kinds of workers with psychedelic drugs have promised visions of God, revelations of Ultimate Truth, and so on. And for the self-anointed psychedelic priest, it seems to be just a small further step to assuming the role of God Himself! Sidney Cohen and others have warned about this danger—the threat that an unaccustomed power will corrupt the guide with resulting damage to the subjects, and possibly even greater damage to the guide himself. This, as we also have observed, is a real danger; but psychiatrists have no immunity to the disease and they go astray when advancing such a hazard as a basis for restricting all work with psycho-chemicals to themselves. There exists not a shred of evidence to indicate that the limiting of guiding to one or a few professions will do anything at all to eliminate abuses of power and corruption by power.

A further point that should be made concerning the eidetic images has to do with their relation to clock-measured or "real" time. Psychedelic subjects may feel that an image sequence has lasted "forever," for "years," or for "many hours," when in fact the sequence has been clocked as lasting only a few minutes or even a few seconds. Sometimes the subject's estimate of the time consumed is based on the imaged events. If the subject has imaged the day-long coronation of a king he may feel that the image sequence has taken all day to unfold. More commonly the estimate of the time a grouping of images has taken to unfold is based on the feeling that *so much* was "seen" that "hours" or "days" or "aeons" must have passed in order for "all that" to have been experienced. This resembles, of course, the similar phenomenon of time distortion in dreams. Such a compression of images and imaginary events also may be induced in the hypnotic trance state. As often has been demonstrated, a hypnotic subject may draw upon the contents of his memory to see again in a few seconds a feature-length motion picture that is experienced as running at just the same speed as it did when first seen in the theater.

Not only images but thoughts as well are enormously compressed in time in the drug-state, although the compression may be greater at some periods than at others. It is this speeding up of the mental processes that is experienced by the subject as a "slowing down of time." The thoughts do not seem to be coming any faster, but a great deal more may be thought in any given amount of clock-measured time. It is of course because of this that "such a lot" seems to happen in the psychedelic session.

Slowed-down time produces many curious experiences. A subject lights a cigarette, smokes it for "hours," looks down and the initial ash is still only a quarter-inch in length. Walking down a flight of stairs "takes forever." The guide leaves the room, immediately returns, and the subject complains about having been left alone for "such a long time." And so on.

There are also other, more baffling experiences where it seems to the subject that events of the session are "known before they happen," so that the actual occurrence seems out of sequence (not a repetition or *déjà-vu* phenomenon). Here, a "second" dissociated consciousness may live through events A-B-C-D-E before these events are experienced by the "first" consciousness which remains with the body, communicates with other persons, and fulfills the usual tasks of the normal consciousness. Then when the events experienced by the "second" consciousness are "later" experienced by the "first," the former knows exactly what will occur because it already has experienced these events. Or the subject may "turn around in time" a series of events so that events A-B-C-D will exist in memory as having occurred in the order D-C-B-A. The processes governing these and some other time-out-of-joint phenomena are not understood.

Tactile Experiences.   Some of the most important and interesting experiences on the sensory level are those involving tactile phenomena and unusual kinds of body feeling. The more pleasurable of these experiences are most likely to occur in a nature setting since subjects almost always prefer the natural out-of-doors environment and have a high degree of sensory and other openness to it. This extraordinary openness especially facilitates certain types of empathic experience rarely encountered under other conditions.

Empathy in the natural setting may differ in several significant respects from that usually experienced indoors. First of all, the subject, almost from the start, already has achieved a kind of empathy with his surroundings as a whole, although not with any particular object. That is to say, nature seems to the subject a whole of which he is an integral part, and from this characteristic feeling of being a part of the organic "body of nature" the subject readily goes on to identify with nature in its physical particulars and processes. No drug subject similarly identifies with a room or other artificial environment, and the empathy with nature seems to be especially abetted by the warming rays of the sun, the playing of the breezes over the subject's body, his contact with the earth below him, and various other types of tactile experiencing of the environment.

This larger empathy or harmony with nature then may become particularized through the physical contact. The subject, at first subconsciously, becomes related in a tactile-empathic way to that stimulus with which he is effectively in contact. Then he gradually becomes aware of some part of his body as partaking of the substance of the earth or stone or grass upon which he stands, or of the air around him, the sunlight, or the wind. The sense of physical separateness increasingly diminishes and may be altogether lost—sometimes moving the subject towards a mystical-type experience. But what is unusual here is that the body-nature empathy or synonymity begins with a preconscious physical merging with the environment so that by the time the subject becomes aware of his "tactile-empathy," of his identity with grass or stone, the empathic state already is *fait accompli.* Then may follow the "psychological empathy"—the psychical at-oneness with the object which is the more commonly occurring type of indoors empathy with objects. In another sort of tactile (partial) identification with the environment, the subject retains his awareness of his body's outlines and separateness from the environment, but feels that his substance now is the same as that of some part of the environment. Thus, he reports that his body or some part of it feels as if it has *become* the stone or clay upon which he stands, or that his hands have become like the water into which they were dipped—these "watery hands," however, retaining their form and a kind of comparative solidity. Two subjects, thrusting their hands into dusty earth, have experienced an instantaneous metamorphosis of substance—"So, it is true! Dust into dust!"

A number of subjects, standing in the wind, have become the wind, experiencing their bodies as an amorphous, weightless movement or "dancing" in the atmosphere. However, the experience of standing *against* a fairly strong breeze has produced a different experience for half a dozen subjects and one that was strikingly similar for all six. Here, while word choice naturally varied, the subjects spoke of having become *permeable to* the wind and of feeling the wind blowing through them. There was no wish to resist this penetration by the wind. On the contrary, it was welcomed or regarded as being "in the nature of things"; and two subjects even went so far as to "molecularize" themselves in order that the passage of the wind might be facilitated. This position with regard to the wind (which ordinarily one senses as "parting" and "breaking around" one's body) represents a capitulation to the phenomenon such as one rarely encounters in or out of the drug-state. Since the wind is experienced as remaining precisely itself, without any blending of its being with the subject's, all alteration is on the part of the subject and the wind is accorded a dominant status not met with when there is empathic merging or union with the phenomenon. Much more than empathy, this goes directly counter to the main tendencies found in the subject's usual encounters with non-human phenomena—encounters wherein he both attempts to negate the otherness of the thing and also imitates the thing or certain of its attributes. The negation is partially effected by a sensory-ideational appropriation of the thing that blurs its otherness and so makes the thing at least to some degree an extension of the subject. The "imitation" of the thing, occurring as if in response to a suggestion by the thing, we see exemplified in the stiffening of the body and some other responses made by the subject when he touches a rigid substance such as metal; and, when not impeded by countersuggestions, it culminates in the tactile empathy with the thing.

Returning to the latter, "submissive" response to the wind, some subjects have said that they felt the wind stands to the person in a kind of ruler-ruled or even God-man relationship. The wind then is experienced as a tangible manifestation of the awesome power of the universe, as "God's breath" or "Nature's exhalations." In the face of this expression of a tremendous force benignly restrained, it is up to the person to make himself "open" to the wind somewhat as one might fall upon one's face in the presence of some Ultimate Sovereign. Such an attitude towards the wind has, of course, very ancient antecedents; and thus the phenomenon may seem in some cases to be yet another of the countless archaisms encountered in the psychedelic experience. That some of the subjects thus "mythicizing" the wind experience feel "cleansed" and "inwardly purified" by the wind's "clean sweep" through them, is consistent with the archaism.

The drug subject's experience of the sun is also of considerable interest and again, in some cases, has a distinctly antique aspect. Again there is the sense of penetration, but here by what has been frequently described by subjects as a direct life-giving principle. Some female subjects have experienced the penetration by the sun as sexual, speaking of the sun as a "cosmic lover," or using other words to that effect. Women much more often than men, it would seem, derive sexual stimulation from lying in the sun; and the male, in or out of the drug-state, is more likely to feel himself sapped by the sun of his sexual vitality while not experiencing any or more than a very transient erotic stimulation.

Experiences such as these with sun and wind very readily lend themselves to creation of rich mythological fantasies by the subject; and increasing involvement in the fantasy may carry the subject along to experiences on "deeper" levels, especially the symbolic. In one elaborate case the subject, S-7, a housewife in her mid-thirties (LSD: 150 micrograms), lay down on the grass in a field beneath a bright sun and soon was living out an epic of creation in which she identified with "the Great Goddess—Mother Earth."

S's experience of this identification began when she first became aware that "for some time" her body had "no longer existed in its usual, limited form" and that now she was "one with the earth" upon which she "had been" lying. As this vast feminine Earth, S then received the penetration of the "great Masculine Father—the Sun God," and so was fertilized by him. The effects of this fertilization were immediate, since S then felt that "out of the conjunction the world is continuously being born." "All of the things of the world" were felt by S to be streaming out of her womb, passing out of her body and into the world.

We will see later how the symbolism of such an experience may take on increasingly personal meanings for the subject; meanwhile already in this experience we see the opening of a gateway through which the subject may pass to go beyond the sensory and on to other, deeper levels. It is, of course, a part of the function of the guide to help make transitional the aesthetic experience in which the potential for transition is present.

In general, to touch a thing or a person is to enter into a closer, more intimate kind of relationship than is possible when one only looks at the object. Thus, since an intimate relation with the object is the one most conducive to going beyond it, the psychedelic subject is repeatedly encouraged to hold things, to enter into a tactile relationship with them. A few types of objects notably excepted—for instance the metallic, which yield negative responses—this intentional touching of the thing soon eliminates any anxiety or hostility towards the thing and, by extension, tends to improve the subject's relation to the whole of his physical environment.

When the subject is especially alienated from things, or when his mood of the moment is negative, he may be expected to respond in a negative way to the object that is offered him. Presented a stone to hold and asked to describe what he is "getting from" the stone, he is likely to mention "hardness," "coldness," "opaqueness," or "deadness"—*not* typical responses under other, more favorable conditions. An effective procedure for the guide is then to take the stone out of the subject's left hand, keep it for a few seconds, and then place it in the subject's right hand. Since, in the psychedelic experience, a few seconds can yield a whole new orientation, while the "attitude" of one hand may be quite different from that of the other, this shifting of the stone from left hand to right makes it possible for the subject to take up a new position with regard to the stone. However, some more help is likely to be needed, and the subject now is told not to look at the stone, but rather to feel it and to become aware of the stone as it becomes softer in his hand. "Make the stone give, press on it so that it changes its shape." When the subject announces that this has been done, he then may be urged to "Go ahead, keep on squeezing. Squeeze the stone until it becomes soft as cotton. It's soft as cotton? Good. Now look at it again and describe how it looks." Frequently, when such a procedure is employed, the stone will appear to have lost its sharp definition and will have taken on a cotton-like or perhaps even gaseous appearance. By this time the subject will be sufficiently caught up in the "game" to comply eagerly with further suggestions concerning the stone. The guide then may induce an empathic relationship, telling the subject to "Let yourself go into the stone, let yourself dissolve into the stone. Be one with the stone, so that you understand it and so that it understands you." By such means, experiences of empathy are made possible for persons who never have had even remotely similar experiences before; and once such a breakdown of subject-object boundaries has been experienced, the drug subject becomes a great deal more accessible and in many cases spontaneously proceeds to an examination of his own life and especially his own human relationships—so opening the way to a movement "down" to the deeper *recollective-analytic* level.

In a great many ways a variety of objects may be used to help the subject break through the barriers he has erected around persons and ideas and feelings; barriers which, moreover, may block him from moving on to deeper drug-state levels where the inhibitions and values structures may be confronted and re-examined. It may happen, for example, that the subject becomes intensely involved with a thing, then the thing becomes a symbol and may be identified with some key person in the subject's life. Then, the intense involvement with the thing becomes an intense involvement with the person, and there is a freedom to think and feel about that person such as the subject never has known in the actual relationship.

For example, a fifty-two-year-old man, S-8 (LSD: 150 micrograms), disclosed in advance of his session that for all his apparent success in industry he usually viewed the world "like somebody looking at goods in a display window." He felt that he very early in his life had decided that "if you don't touch anything, nothing is going to touch you." For himself, he was right about that; but, as a consequence, he lived in a world he recognized to be one of impoverished emotions and even perceptions. He was ready to "smash the window" and take his chances; but he found this was "easier thought of than done" and hoped the LSD session would "help melt the ice"—ice being a term he used interchangeably with glass in describing the barrier between himself and the world.

S, an exceptionally strong-willed individual, proved himself unusually successful at resisting the effects of the drug. He displayed no anxiety, and denied the resistance, but admitted that his "iron self-discipline" was "deeply inbedded and hard to let go of." There was very little perceptual change and he wandered about grumbling over some mildly unpleasant physical sensations and wondering aloud "if this damn stuff (LSD) is just another fraud?" After more than an hour had gone by in this way, S was finally persuaded to choose from among various objects standing on a shelf. He selected, as "the silliest of the lot," a small cork of the kind that is used to cork a bottle of wine. He held it, turned it over, looked at it, and finally sat back with eyes closed and the cork enclosed by a fist. After several minutes of this he announced that the cork was "coming alive" in his hand. He clenched his fist even tighter as if trying to squeeze the "life" out of the cork—what in fact he was trying to do, as he later admitted.

S now appeared to be growing more and more angry. Asked what was the trouble, he said that the cork he was holding had become identified with his son, "a spoiled brat." S then, speaking directly to the cork, launched into a bitter tirade against his son that was phrased as if the cork were his son. Then, he suddenly seemed to wilt and acknowledged that he had "spoiled" his son in an effort to buy from the boy an affection he could not hope to gain otherwise. Unable to "express love," S had only been able to show the love he felt for the boy by showering him with money and presents. With this, S began to experience characteristic *recollective-analytic* level phenomena, regressing to his own boyhood to find there the origins of his "stoicism."

That such an object as a cork may serve this kind of purpose for the drug subject is attributable in part to the tendency of the subjects to play with words, especially to look for double meanings and to seek in the double meaning some veiled reference to self. Thus, S recognized in the cork an appropriate object for "uncorking" all of his "bottled up" emotions. The exercise of only a little imagination will provide the guide with a host of objects useful on a similar basis—and these should be available but no particular object should be presented to the subject; he should have a chance to make his own selection. With considerable frequency the drug subject will select in advance of any conscious recognition of the symbolism just that object which best affords him an analogue or metaphors for his own situation. We think that the object is selected because of its symbolic potential, not yet consciously grasped, and think it unlikely in the majority of cases that the subject simply imposes an arbitrary useful symbolism on whatever object happens to be at hand. He may, of course, do this, but he does it much less often.

Additionally, with reference to this case, we might remark that cork as a *substance* is especially well adapted to the psychedelic experience. Soft and porous, cork as a substance is experienced as nonresistant and even receptive to the attempts at *Einfühlung* by the subject. Also, its surface is such as to easily capture the subject's attention and then draw him into the object through the customary cracks and large pores. The coloring is pleasant and the configuration either highly suggestive or sufficiently innocuous. We might mention here, too, that the large, flat slab of cork, while not so obviously offering the same verbal associations, is an object the drug subject finds especially "friendly" and rewarding to consider, its patterns lending themselves to projective ideation and even imaging. Other kinds of bark as well seem particularly well suited to eliciting desirable ideational and emotional responses.

Symbolizing the Environment. Visual and other perception of things or of the total environment as symbolic is largely a phenomenon of the *sensory* level. On the deeper drug-state levels the symbols are internal—ideas and eidetic images. The symbolizing of some particular thing is common and examples of it have been given; however, the *total* environment or a good many aspects of it may be simultaneously symbolized and, by means of perceptual distortions, be perceived as if the things are the symbols now brought into tangible existence in the world. In this situation, hallucinations also may appear. Then we are likely to have a psychosis-like experience. Again, this ought never to occur and has not occurred in well-guided sessions of which we have knowledge. However, the possibility of such experiences does exist; and the examples to follow warrant inclusion on that basis.

The first case is that of a four-year-old boy, S-9, who was interviewed one week after his LSD (250 micrograms) "session." S's mother, recently separated from his father, was associated with a psychedelic drug-taking (Drug Movement) group in New York City. The boy obtained the drug by taking from the refrigerator an LSD-saturated sugar cube, which he ate. He began to experience almost immediately what, insofar as can be determined, were authentic hallucinations.

Among the first hallucinations to appear were a number of crustaceans, especially (as it could be gathered) crabs and lobsters. This very much impressed S's mother in view of the fact that the child's zodiacal sign is Cancer, represented by the crab, and she felt certain that the boy had no knowledge of this symbolism. Throughout his whole "session," which lasted some twelve hours, with reduced effects in the last several hours (after a tranquilizer had been administered), S continued intermittently to see crabs and lobsters coming out of the walls and crawling across the floor towards him. When first he saw these creatures he "screamed and threw a fit." Later he was reassured when his mother told him the sugar cube was responsible and the effects would wear off. He said he had been afraid "it's going to last and last."

S also hallucinated a whole array of "monsters"—apparently creatures such as elves, dwarfs, and other small, deformed human-like beings. Fearful at first, he gained confidence when his mother encouraged him to "make friends with the monsters"—probably the best suggestion possible and one the boy was able to carry out. After some of his anxieties were disposed of, several of the "monsters" came and sat on S's knees and in the palm of his hand and he talked with them. Others danced around him and made faces. From time to time, S's fears would return; then, with his mother's help, he would overcome his fears again and enjoy playing and talking with the hallucinated beings.

In another frequently recurring hallucination or perceptual distortion, the walls of the apartment would shiver, bulge inward, the ceiling would sag and seem about to collapse, and S would report himself afraid that "my house is going to fall down." This seemed a transparent symbolism, referring to the child's anxieties concerning his parents' separation and previous domestic strife—house falling down = home breaking up. However, suggestion may have played a part in this experience. His mother reported having had the same hallucination or perceptual distortion during one of her recent LSD experiences. She had never discussed this with the child, she said, but it was possible he might have overheard her describing it to someone else. In the mother's case, the walls seemed about to buckle, they were made of wax and were melting, everything was about to crumble away, and so on.

Another of the mother's recurring drug-state perceptions also was experienced repeatedly by S: The floor seemed to be covered with water, about six inches or so deep, and he looked down at his feet as through water—a visual and not a tactile distortion.

There were also, however, tactile hallucinations besides those of touching the "monsters." Sudden "itches" would appear and S would brush away from his skin hallucinatory felt but unseen bugs that would "land on" him and "crawl around" on his bare flesh.

Seen one week after this experience, S did not give any surface indication of having been harmed by it. He is a good-looking, energetic child, apparently in robust health and of better than average intelligence. He said he would not like to have any more LSD; and his mother said he seemed to have lost his appetite for sugar cubes. Four months later, a good friend of S's mother said that the boy still had shown no signs of disturbance resulting from the drug experience. He was "same as always." No psychiatric or other professional examination was made.

It is of interest to compare this child's psychedelic experience with that of a noted philosopher, Jean-Paul Sartre, as described by Simone de Beauvoir in *The Prime of Life*.[5] Sartre, it would seem, could have used someone to persuade him to "make friends with the monsters."

The psychiatrically supervised session in which Sartre was an experimental mescaline subject is described, along with its aftermath, by Simone de Beauvoir in her usual uninhibited way. She relates that Sartre, then engaged in a study of imagery and anomalies of perception, was told going into the session that he would be able to observe his own hallucinations (by which presumably was meant his eidetic images). He further was told that the experience might be "mildly disagreeable" and that he might "behave rather oddly" for a while; but, he was promised, the experience would not involve any dangers.

On the afternoon of the session Simone de Beauvoir called the hospital to find out how Sartre was faring. He answered the phone and told her he was fighting a losing battle with a devil fish and mentioned a number of other disturbing experiences. He reported umbrellas changing into vultures and shoes changing into skeletons, faces that became hideous, and crabs, polyps, and "grimacing things" that he saw from the corner of his eye. He blamed his distressing experiences on the predictions of the psychiatrist.

Sartre apparently recovered from this harrowing experience but, a week or two later, fell into a deep depression that recalled his mood during much of the session. He said he now was hallucinating. Houses had leering faces and gnashed their jaws, and clocks resembled owls. Still later, he described himself as "on the edge of a chronic hallucinatory psychosis." He was being followed by lobsters and crabs (and we do not mind noting an amusing coincidence—that, like S, Sartre's zodiacal sign is the crab); also, by assorted other monsters. The psychiatrists denied that the drug could have provoked the attack and fatigue and tension were blamed. The drug had only furnished Sartre, they said, with "certain hallucinatory patterns"—a rather fine splitting of hairs, it would seem. The abnormal phenomena eventually disappeared and Sartre himself attributed the whole experience to "the physical expression of a deep emotional malaise." In Simone de Beauvoir's account, "Sartre could not resign himself to going on to 'the age of reason,' to full manhood."

We will mention one other case of this psychosis-like type, but one in which there were no hallucinations and the total environment was perceived in a uniformly distorted way.

The (interview) subject, S-10, age thirty, had participated in two previous peyote sessions in which "all went well." A newspaperman, he had been for some time engaged in a frustrating love affair with a girl whose mother disliked him and thus had made many efforts to break up the relationship. On the occasion to be described, S had planned to take peyote with this girl. He consumed his own portion, then sat down in his hotel room to wait for her arrival.

Time went by and the girl did not come. She was an hour, then two hours late. Since he had no telephone in his room, he went down to the hotel lobby to phone her and she told him her mother had refused to let her leave the house. She very much doubted that she would be able to come. S, "bitterly disappointed," went upstairs, lay down on his bed, and became increasingly depressed. The eidetic images were "stupid or drab," so he got up and sat on a chair in the center of a large room. By the moment, he felt more abandoned and lonely.

S became acutely aware of the distortion, the "slowing down" of time. Seconds were hours, and minutes were like days. After another "hour that was ten centuries," he went down to the lobby and called her again. This time she said she definitely would be unable to come before evening, if at all. He told her "Don't bother"—which he instantly regretted—and went back upstairs, feeling that the desk clerk and people in the lobby were looking at him "in a strange way."

S sat down once again in the chair and suddenly felt himself to be a shrunken, withered figure, while around him the room, "a surrealist nightmare," had grown enormous. All of the objects in the room seemed totally alien, as if they, too, had abandoned him. He turned over endlessly in his mind a line from Rilke: "Who loses himself by all things is let go . . ." and felt utterly alone in the world. Now, the walls of the room began to shrink. They were furrowed, somewhat like corduroy, and the previously white walls now seemed an ugly, dirty gray. Gray light of the consistency of glue oozed out of the walls and trickled down them. At the same time the room seemed a kind of cell, its floor space dwindled to perhaps a quarter of its actual size, while the walls towered upward to three times their normal height. And S now felt that his flesh was furrowed like the walls and resembled the skin of a dried prune, or of a mummy.

Whenever he thought of the girl, S was overwhelmed with grief. He had intended, so he now thought, to ask her to marry him; and, since this had been his intention, it was especially cruel of her not to come: How could anyone be so cruel! A minute now was longer than his "whole life up to that point"; his pain, "a thousand times more painful than any known before."

Finally, some five hours into his experience, S played some music, became interested in it, and his mood lightened. The remainder of the experience was "not too unpleasant." However, that night he repeatedly was awakened by terrible nightmares; and, next day, he found himself "definitely insane—the beginning of seventy-two hours of insanity."

Awakening, S found himself immediately pondering the question: "What is permissible?" He felt that he had "lost or forgotten all the rules for behaving in society." He went out, thinking he would try to go to work, but found himself "slinking along the streets like a terrified animal." The sight of a policeman produced "fear and trembling, since perhaps a way of walking in a particular place was a terrible crime." S managed to get home and phoned his office, saying he was ill. For the next three days he went out only at night, then "drifted along like a shadow, trying not to be seen." He constantly watched other people to try to "relearn the rules of living, find out 'what is permissible.' " The "insanity" dissipated gradually, with S gaining confidence in his ability to "behave in such a way as to stay out of trouble." However, he was "unusually fearful for several months afterwards."

In such cases as the three just described the perceptual distortions imposed upon the environment seem very plainly to be clothed affect— anxiety acting upon the visual perceptual process to change the environment which then, as percept, generates still more anxiety and also depression. The hallucinated monsters are the monsters of childhood, the forms fear takes when one regresses to feelings of childlike helplessness. The symbolisms are transparent as in the house falling down = home breaking up, or shriveled walls and shrunken body = depression and feelings of loneliness and deprivation. Yet even such clear-cut symbols will usually escape recognition by the subject. He responds emotionally to what he sees—while what he sees are his own emotions, cast by perceptual distortion in appropriate symbolic form. Intellect here seems deprived by emotion of its capacity effectively to analyze these distortions; and ideation becomes involved in circular, self-pitying and anxious cataloguing of the distortions and the responses made to them. This indeed is psychosis-like behavior; and many psychotics would seem to be responding in a similar way to about the same kind of perceptual distortions as those met with in the drug sessions. The vast majority of psychedelic subjects experience distortions and other phenomena for which the mechanisms seem the same as those of the psychotic experience, but which have a different content because reflecting a different emotional state; or the content is approximately the same, and the type of emotion is the same but does not, for lack of reinforcement by response to the percept, build to the same degree of intensity.

Many factors present in the drug experience ordinarily enable the subject to avoid reinforcing the initial negative emotion by responding in a highly emotional way to the distorted perception. The subject is able to handle the distorted data of his senses by bringing into play mental instrumentalities and knowledge not accessible to or effective for the psychotic. The subject feels himself to have guarantees of his return to the normal world. The distortions he perceives he is able to attribute to the drug. He is malleable and will accept the interpretations or suggestions of the guide. What all of this leaves untouched, of course, is the genesis of the emotional disturbance underlying the perceptual distortions to which the subject (and the psychotic) must react. But it does seem clear that where it is possible for the person to interpret to his own advantage the distorted percept, this interpretation then serves to alter in a positive way or to diminish the force of the negative emotion. That is, the emotion now responds to a conscious instead of an unconscious determinant and thus may be reached and transformed by a calculated manipulation of its effects. Then the even deeper lying psychogenetic factor is disarmed if not transformed.

Transitions. Experiences on the *sensory* level are of shorter duration and tend to be more numerous and more varied than those occurring on the other levels so that it would be possible to engage in an almost endless cataloguing of them. This we will not do, and will only mention a few more varieties of those transitional experiences by which the subject progresses from *sensory* to *recollective-analytic* and, occasionally, to a still deeper level.

In terms of the phenomenological pattern we have outlined the *sensory* level always should be considered a stage along the way to deeper levels where more profound experiences await the psychedelic subject. Its purpose, as we have remarked, is to free the subject from the limitations of his old ways of perceiving, thinking, and feeling. It would seem that only when consciousness has been freed from these limitations is the unconscious free to release (and consciousness able to accept?) those materials and initiate those processes which become conscious and increasingly purposive as the subject moves from one level to the next. Thus it is the task of the guide to stimulate a wide variety of *sensory* level experiences and to continue so doing until the deconditioning has been effected and the gateway to the deeper level swings ajar. Then, when this gateway phenomenon is recognized, the guide, if need be, will assist the subject to pass through it.

How many or what kind of *sensory* level experiences a particular subject will require may be to some extent predictable; more often, at the start of a session, it is not. Thus, the earlier phases of the session are usually to some extent experimental and the variety of experience encouraged serves the dual purpose of enabling the subject to reach deeper levels while it provides the researcher with his best opportunity to explore, without disrupting any purposive moment, those areas compatible with his own research objectives.

One of the experiences most impressive to the subject is synesthesia —the response by one of the senses to a stimulus ordinarily responded to by another of the senses. For example, the subject may find himself able to taste colors or smell sounds. Occasionally the experiencing of synthesias may prove to be a gateway. A subject who had "almost no sense of smell" was invited to try to smell a lemon. Even when he held it up against his nostrils, he reported himself unable to smell anything. The guide then put a recording on the phonograph and placed the lemon on a table several feet away from the subject. He was told to "smell the lemon in the music." At once, the subject declared himself able to "hear the smell." Then he said he could smell the lemon in the music. Then he was able to smell the lemon directly. He took this as evidence that, as he had suspected, his inability to smell was not due to any organic deficiency but rather was due to a functional (psychogenic) blockage. Regarding this fact of a functional sensory inhibition as "proved," the subject began a search for its causes that soon led him "down" to the recollective-analytic level. There, he found that his problem was essentially one of the negative attitude towards matter—a fear and dislike of the physical that was also less strongly manifested in an impaired ability to use his other senses. This antipathy towards matter emerges time and again as a crucial factor disabling the person for a full experience of the phenomenal world. It is also especially likely to affect the capacity for entering without inhibition into sexual relationships. The subject overcomes these blockages by seeking out, if possible, the origins of his condemnation of matter. Then, he re-examines his values and creates for himself a philosophy that does not separate mind or spirit from matter to the detriment of the latter.

We find this negative attitude towards matter illustrated too, and much more dramatically, in the case of S-11, a forty-five year-old minister (LSD: 250 micrograms). This subject was known, in advance of the session, to overreact to spilled liquids and it was proposed that this reaction possibly be taken up at some point.

S was not otherwise especially fastidious. His office, as he had described it, was "a mess," with papers, magazines, books, and other things piled all around. This never troubled him, nor did, with rare exceptions, clothing left strewn around a room or even the stacks of unwashed dishes his wife sometimes left standing in the sink. But any liquid *spilled* anywhere produced in S a very strong need to immediately wipe it up. On numerous occasions he had flown into what he knew was an unwarranted rage on going to the table and finding that water or soup or something of the sort had been spilled on the table top and left there. Even a drop or two could elicit this near-phobic reaction which S never was entirely able to control, although making valiant efforts to do so. Water alone could produce the response, but an even stronger response was made to viscous liquids so long as they were not sufficiently thick to seem to him more nearly solid than fluid.

About an hour into his session, S was led into a dining room where he immediately noticed that some rather slimy looking soup had been spilled on the table top and left there, seemingly by accident. His initial reaction was the usual one, and at once he began to search for something with which he might wipe up the spilled soup. Finding nothing, he pulled out his handkerchief and debated whether he ought to use that. Then, however, he became aware that what he was experiencing was much less anger (as he usually considered his reaction to be) than fear. He looked closely at the droplets and turned noticeably pale. Before his eyes, as he subsequently related, those few tiny drops began to expand, rise up, bubble and seethe, take on a "horribly slimy and gelatinous" appearance, and then surge like a miniature but rapidly growing tidal wave towards the edge of the table. At the same time, he recognized as a cause of his anxiety the fear not only that the room would be flooded with the liquid but also that it would infect whatever it touched, so that everything would be dissolved into the gelatinous slime. He leaped back in horror, wiped away the drops with his handkerchief, and appeared almost ready to faint. But then he approached the table again, picked up the soup bowl, and deliberately poured a good bit of its contents on the table top. He became increasingly calm and described to the guides the visual distortions he had perceived.

S now was urged to "go deeper," to go down into the depths of his own psyche and try to find there some explanation for what he had seen. He fell silent for a minute, then spoke in a voice that sounded as if, in fact, it were coming up from the depths. The phenomenon he had just witnessed, S said, was one that occurred on a level below consciousness whenever he was confronted with spilled liquid. He could tap, from "some deep source," many memories of having repeatedly had such experiences before, although they never had emerged into consciousness. His "fear of inundation," he said, was but one aspect of his "fastidiousness." What the drops of liquid represented was not just "a wetness that might flood over everything." Rather, these liquids he responded to so strongly, were translated by his "unconscious into the most repulsive and terrifying kind of liquid there is—matter in its slimy, oozing, corrupt form," a viscous putrefaction so corrosive as to "rot upon contact whatever it touches." This corrupt matter with its "disintegrative force," S went on, was the material correlative of moral evil in the world; or perhaps, he thought, it was the other way around. Somehow it was "all bound up with death," and he seemed to remember "instantly forgotten dreams" of corpses dissolving into viscous, liquid putrefaction. It was "bound up, too, with sexuality"—a "wet, slimy, and corrupt sexuality," which simultaneously attracted and repelled, setting him in "painful conflict with moral values" which had insisted upon matter as evil with sexual union regarded as a symbolic embracing of the material in its "most corrupt form."

After a lengthy analysis of his values, S touched with his fingertips the spilled soup on the table, then rubbed it around on the table top with the palm of his hand. He licked some of the soup from his fingers and remarked that "Of course, it's just soup after all. It's messy but it's not going anywhere and nothing could be more far-fetched than to think that it could." He then walked around the room, examining objects, and announcing that finally things were "really getting through" to him. He reported that "the insights just keep coming," and that they, too, were "really getting through" and would "stick."

The follow-up on this subject indicated a reorientation of values with an enhancement of aesthetic and sensory reponse to the environment. He felt (and his wife agreed) that his relationship with his family was much improved, mainly as a result of "the loosening of a rigid puritanism." He continued to mop up spilled liquids, "but without getting mad." His reaction had become, he felt, a "reasonable, unemotional response, such as most anyone would make." It is natural, after all, he remarked, to clean up messes and he felt no need to resist what was now "a natural impulse, not an unnatural compulsion."

As a final example of the transition to the recollective-analytic level, we will reproduce a subject-guide interchange showing just how a succession of object-stimuli might be used to lead the subject beyond aesthetic appreciation of the thing to meaningful examination of his own life. When such techniques as the following are used, the transition from an outward to an inward concern occurs smoothly and the subject's feeling of autonomy is carefully preserved. He is enabled to preserve, too, his sense of spontaneity in the development of the session.

The subject, S-12, male, in his mid-twenties, was unsophisticated but intelligent and sensitive. The example is of "key" passages from the dialogue between the guide (G) and the subject (S):

G: (Peeling a purple grape and handing it to the subject) "Here, I have a present for you."

S: (Looking at the grape in amazement as, with perceptual distortion, the grape is translated into something quite different) "What is it?"

G: "What do you think it is?"

S: "It's . . . it's a living brain. . . . My God, I'm holding a living brain in my hand. . . . See . . . there's the fine veins . . . feeding the brain . . . Now it's changing . . . Why, it looks like an embyro . . . a transparent embryo! (Laughs happily) I seem to have all of life in my hand!"

G: (Hands S an orange) "Here, live with this for a while."

S: (After contemplating the orange intensely for several minutes) "Magnificent . . . I never really saw color before . . . It's brighter than a thousand suns. . . . (Feels the whole surface of the orange with palms and fingertips) But this is a pulsing thing . . . a living pulsing thing . . . And all these years I've just taken it for granted . . . (Speaks to the orange) I promise! . . . I'll never take you for granted again. . . . Never! . . . You're a world . . . a whole world in itself. . . ."

G: "Then let me offer you—the world within the world." (Cuts another orange in half and hands it to S.)

S: (Says nothing but silently considers the orange for a long time.)

G: "What are you thinking now?"

S: "I'm thinking that . . . it's a very odd thought . . . that there could be no more perfect death than to drown in an ocean of orange juice . . . I'm thinking . . . that here . . . here in this orange . . . there is design for living . . . the symmetry . . . and the seeds . . . My thoughts are going too fast. . . . I can't explain . . . I start to explain, but before I get to the end of a sentence I've had a hundred new thoughts."

G: (Turns on the phonograph and puts on Tschaikowsky's *Violin Concerto in D*) "Relax now. Put the orange down and let yourself be absorbed into the music."

S: (After listening silently with his eyes closed for about twenty minutes) "Ahhhhhhhhhhhh."

G: "What is it?"

S: "I've never listened to music like this before. . . . I'm hearing so much more intensely with my outer ear . . . and yet . . . at the same time I'm listening with my inner ear . . . I hear melodies . . . and melodies in the melodies. I hear Tschaikowsky himself! And I can see it all too! The melody passes before my (closed) eyes . . . I see . . . I see centuries and all of the glory and the tragedy of man . . . *Everything* is in this music! . . . But especially the tragedy of man."

G: (After the music has ended, hands S a rough piece of tree bark.)

S: "Ah, roughage . . . The tragic side of life. But so beautiful . . . Like flying over the entire earth . . . looking down on all the mountains and valleys. I could look at this for the rest of my life . . . So much detail . . . It's unbelievable."

G: "And the texture?"

S: (Running his hand over the bark) "I feel every rise . . . every crevice. I'm a giant . . . a thousand miles high . . . and I'm running my hand over this little planet."

G: "And the meaning of the bark? Does it tell you anything? Something about yourself perhaps?"

S: "Yes . . . Yes, I see it does. It has so much variation in it . . . so many opportunities. If a piece of bark can have all of these opportunities for differentiation, then what about me? I may have as many possibilities in me as this bark."

G: "Look now at your own hand. Look at the skin texture. You will find that it is just as rough and differentiated as the bark."

S: (Taking a long look at his hand) "Yes, that's so. (Laughs) I'm a planet too . . . and I'm a giant looking down on my own planet-self."

G: "And can you identify with this planetary self? Try now to see yourself as this world of opportunity and differentiation. *Become* your planetary self."

S: (Continues to stare at his hand for some time and then finally begins to smile and nod his head vigorously) "All this possibility that's in me! . . . and all the time I didn't believe that it was there. Christ, what I could do!"

With this, the subject no longer is concerned with externals and exploration moves inward.

Seven:
The Voyage Inward

With the transition to the *recollective-analytic* level the psychedelic subject no longer is concerned with most of those phenomena to which he responded so intensely on the *sensory* level. The external wonder world of heightened and distorted perceptions no longer is of much importance and the perceptions may become, with a few exceptions, normalized. Odd psychical phenomena, such as dissociation, may no longer occur unless serving some specific purpose. This same trend towards elimination of the nonfunctional may be observed in the case of the eidetic images. These images no longer are only aesthetic but become increasingly purposive, serving to illustrate or otherwise illumine the subject's exploration of self. In short, the voyage inward now is under way and will, if fully successful, find the subject traversing his present level to reach the *symbolic* and, finally, the *integral* level—the ultimate drug-state goal of the psychedelic journey.

On the recollective-analytic level there is a readily recognizable and progressive deepening of the emotional tone of the experience. Thinking also is markedly different as it increasingly appears that the usual boundaries between consciousness and the unconscious have been breached and finally in large measure are dissolved. Long "forgotten" memories may become accessible and meaningful in the context of the subject's particular concern. Age regression (similar to that met with in hypnosis) may occur, with the subject "going back in time" to very vividly experience the emotional as well as the other contents of important forgotten or repressed events (while, however, retaining his link with present time). Or there may be a revivification, the subject so totally re-experiencing events from his past as to lose all contact with the present and relive, as child or even infant, the significant occurrences most relevant and crucial to his present (nondrug-state) situation.

What up to now have seemed to the subject to be memories of real events may be disclosed as distortions of real events or as wholly imaginary constructs. The subject may discover that he misinterpreted the real event at the time of its occurrence, so that it has been preserved in memory in its invalid form; or he may find that he subsequently mis-remembered an event and then, after that, remembered the misremembered and not the true version. He may even find that what he has long remembered as an actual occurrence—for instance, sex molestation by some adult—never happened at all but was only a fantasy, based possibly on fear or wishful thinking. Indeed, with regard to the psychical contents generally, there now may be a novel ability to separate the false from the true, the authentic from the inauthentic, and the essential from the mountainous accumulations of superfluities. Association may be exceptionally free and productive, its speed increased, and its scope greatly extended. Abreactive release of unconscious materials frequently occurs, especially if aimed for in a session predefined as therapeutic. Insight is added to insight as the subject typically announces that "The scales are falling away from my eyes and at last I am seeing myself and the world without self-deceit or illusion"—a view that may liberate the subject from guilt, enhance self-esteem, and effect other changes desirable in themselves and prerequisite to still more important experiences of growth and self-fulfillment. Of course, not all of this occurs in every case; but on the recollective-analytic level these are the characteristic phenomena and some or all occur with variations of duration, intensity, and benefit to the normal subject as well as to the neurotic patient.

. What we are dealing with here, then, is a level characterized by phenomena very familiar to the psychoanalyst, the hypnotherapist, and to practitioners of some other psychotherapeutic procedures. As regards these therapists, the very fact that the phenomena are so familiar raises certain problems. For one, the therapist is led to oppose the work of lay researchers with normal subjects on the basis of dangers which may be real in therapy but which have little application to non-therapeutic work. For instance, the therapist may fear that the upsurge of unconscious materials will overwhelm the normal research subject; but this, in our experience, does not happen. Also, it is just because of the familiar nature of the phenomena and their (sometimes more apparent than real) adaptability to existing therapeutic techniques, that psychotherapists have been deterred from evolving more specifically "psychedelic" methods. Especially, they have been deterred from encouraging (or permitting) the subject to go beyond this level into regions where the terrain is unfamiliar but where a much more profound transformation and self-realization is possible.

It would, of course, be the decision of the therapist, made on a patient to patient basis, whether to deal with a neurosis exclusively on this level, then possibly in subsequent sessions encourage the patient to reach the deeper levels. But, where normal subjects are concerned, the deeper levels should be reached whenever possible; and we suspect the neurotic patient also would derive still greater benefits if the deeper levels actively were aimed for (or even, passively, permitted to be reached). That this conclusion will meet with much resistance, we have no doubt. The psychedelic experience provides nothing less than a means of truly going "beyond Freud"—and to venture into these previously inaccessible, or only very rarely accessible, regions of mind where new concepts and methods have to be evolved, learned, and utilized is a challenge to vested personal psychological and emotional as well as economic and ideological interests that many therapists will be reluctant or altogether unable to accept.

The recollection of relevant materials, followed by an analysis of them, is typical of this level and explains our choice of the somewhat burdensome term recollective-analytic. However, equally important should be the subsequent organization of the recollected and analyzed materials into a clear formulation of the subject's objectives, life pattern, or specific conflicts and problems. It is this formulation of the materials which then serves as a basis for the symbolizations and purposive dramas of the next, symbolic level. Given a proper formulation, this symbolization and dramatization will occur spontaneously, may require little or no intervention by the guide, and will unfold in such a way as to best serve the subject's interests and as if in accord with a natural entelechical process of movement towards a unique and specific fulfillment. The way this occurs will be discussed and illustrated later, both in the present chapter and throughout the chapter to follow. Meanwhile, we will exemplify the recollective-analytic level experiences both as they occur when no other level is reached, and as they occur when the subject does make effective transition to the *symbolic* level. Additionally, we will offer some examples of therapeutic results achieved on this level and will suggest some possible further therapeutic applications.

"Instant Psychotherapy." Scores if not hundreds of therapists in many countries, working with the psychedelic drugs, have found it possible in one or a few sessions to eliminate a neurosis that had resisted months and even years of nondrug psychotherapy. In a great many additional cases, presumably there has been removal of the symptom only—often a cure for all practical purposes, since the oft-predicted replacement by another symptom rarely ever occurs. These therapeutic successes have been duly reported at congresses and in the scientific journals, often to be met with nothing more than derisive comments about "claims" of "instant analysis" or "instant psychotherapy." But they merit much more serious consideration than that, and certainly do not deserve to be rejected out of hand by those who arbitrarily announce that results can never be achieved so quickly or so easily. And the fact is that the psychedelic drug results have been consistently played down by psychiatrists and psychologists just because the antagonistic response of colleagues was so readily predictable. Whether this should be called prudence or timidity, the reader will have to decide for himself.

The cure of the neurosis and the removal of the neurotic symptom almost always are products of experiences on the recollective-analytic level. Whether this is because the recollective-analytic is the level best suited to the purpose remains a matter for debate. The writings of some therapists suggest that this may not always be the case; but it does seem to be true that some progress towards dissolving the neurosis must be made on this level if further therapeutic progress is to be made, or even if a deeper level is to be reached at all.

In the two following cases we will provide descriptions of what the follow-ups indicated were authentic examples of so-called drug-state "instant psychotherapy"—a term we do not use in any pejorative way. It perhaps is a further affront to orthodoxy that so very often the therapy is self-initiated and self-directed by the patient or subject with the therapist or guide doing little more than simply standing (or, more often, sitting) by. It should be added that both of these sessions were guided by psychiatrists whose goals, however, were defined as research rather than as therapy.

Although the guide did not know it at the time, S-1, a businessman in his late forties, had "definitely made up my mind to kill myself, and for me LSD was the straw the drowning man clutches at. Although I kept quiet about my intention, for fear I would not be given the drug, this decision to have an LSD experience was the last plaintive outcry for help of a man who was standing on the edge of a precipice and getting ready to jump."

Beginning very early in his session, S dredged up a host of old memories and lived through some calamitous experiences from his early and later childhood with considerable emotion. He then analyzed at length his attitudes and values, claiming to have arrived at some important insights. Yet, none of this occurred in such a way as to suggest that the subject was profoundly involved with his productions. Instead, S gave the impression of someone who is just "going through the motions"—as if this sort of thing were a duty which he felt obliged to carry out. However, after several hours of such behavior, S abruptly regressed to an infantile state, curling himself up into the "foetal position," in which he remained without speaking for perhaps thirty minutes. He then emerged from this state and rather tersely acknowledged the regression. After that, he seemed slightly euphoric but otherwise unchanged. At no time did he discuss his plan to take his own life. Instead, S talked about the drug-state psychology and about philosophical and religious matters. The effects of the drug now diminished rapidly and he was taken to his home.

Only some two weeks later did the subject disclose what had happened to him during his session. He revealed the existence of a long-standing "chronic depression" that had resisted the efforts of several therapists and finally had "helped lead" him to "the very brink of suicide." Since his psychedelic experience, S reported, this depression had been "totally absent." He then went on to say that during his LSD session he had suddenly felt his life "flickering and about to go out, like a burned down candle." He had "died" and then been "reborn," awakening to find himself "all curled up like a foetus in the womb." Once he had "pushed free and unrolled from that position" he had "entered into a new life exactly like someone who has died and been reborn, leaving behind all the torments of the old life."

This experience of "dying" in the psychedelic experience is not a particularly rare one and numerous other writers have made reference to it. And the subsequent "rebirth," as was the case with this subject, often is into a "new life" with "all the old troubles left behind." However, there is another facet to this case which seems of particular interest. The subject remarks that:

"It was absolutely essential that I die. It was not the depression alone that created this urgent need within me. I had lived with the depression for years and while it was extremely painful it was not beyond my ability to endure. No, there was something else that I cannot explain beyond saying how I felt. There was this inescapable and irresistible feeling that I *must* die. I am absolutely certain that had I not 'died' in the LSD session I would have had to die in some other way, and that could only have meant really dying. Committing suicide, destroying myself, as I surely would have done."

These and other statements made by this subject suggest a possibility that seems worthy of serious consideration. The question is posed as to whether in some cases the suicidal individual cannot satisfy his "need to die" by "dying" in a drug session so that he then does not "have to die" by other means and in a final, irretrievable way? Since it is possible in some cases to induce the experience of "dying" it seems to us that therapists should explore the possibility of salvaging suicidal individuals by this method. It should be pointed out, however, that the psychedelic experience is regarded by many as contraindicated where the patient has suicidal tendencies. Thus, at least until many more data are available, such experimental work would probably have to be reserved for those cases where suicide otherwise seems inevitable, so that a radical and possibly risky procedure can be justified.

As concerns the present case, S reported several months later that "the very idea of suicide now seems to me abhorrent on those rare occasions when I think of it at all. The other day I read a magazine article about LSD that warned that this drug might cause people to kill themselves. Let me tell you, LSD can *prevent* people from killing themselves. I know it still is too soon to say with any certainty that I have really been 'reprieved.' I am convinced, though, that it is true, and I cannot imagine ever having been in such a desperate state of mind."

S, for some six months after his session, received weekly encouragement from the guide and then reported himself able to "go it alone." Over one year later, all still seemed to be well with him.

It cannot be emphasized too strongly that the follow-ups must be made and the subject encouraged to hold onto and increase his gains. With the patient, further therapy may be required or simple encouragement may be sufficient. Without the follow-up interviews, gains will be retained in some cases; but they also may be lost, in a few weeks or months, and the follow-ups very often serve to prevent any relapse.

We might also say a word here about the feelings subjects have in the wake of therapeutic or transforming experiences that all of their troubles have been left behind, that they are making a fresh start, or that the old slate has been wiped clean. Of course, this is an exaggeration resulting from enthusiasm over the fact that a or *the* major life problem has been resolved. Naturally, the everyday problems that beset everyone remain. On the other hand, these are usually dealt with better and so actually are minimized in those cases where a major problem has worked also to magnify the painfulness of normal, minor irritations.

In the second case where death also is a factor, although in a quite different way, we find what gives every indication of being another one-session remedy of a long-standing and severe problem. The subject, S-2, a fifty-five-year-old widow (LSD: 200 micrograms), was known in advance of her session to be an alcoholic suffering also from depressions and anxiety.

S had been drinking excessively since shortly after the death of her husband some six years previous to her session. She drank, so she said, to relieve a "deep melancholy" that had been with her "constantly" since her husband's death. But the drinking, with its severe hangover aftermath, served to worsen the depression, also made her "nervous," and then she would "have to drink some more." She lost many friends as a result of her drinking and those she had managed to keep were afraid to invite her to any social occasion where alcoholic beverages would be served. They had "learned the hard way" that S would soon become "maudlin," then "hysterical," would "recover from that and drink some more" until finally she "passed out."

Analyzing in the session her life with her husband, S described a relationship of total dependency in which she had been a willing and happy satellite of a strong, aggressive male figure who had made her decisions, given her abundant affection, and provided for all her material needs and most of her wishes. With his death, although he left her economically secure, she had lost her sense of security in other respects and felt she now was too old to learn to live adequately on her own "undeveloped resources." In part, she had refused to admit her husband's death, keeping his clothing hanging in the closet, leaving his toothbrush and other items in the bathroom, and often referring to him in conversation as if he still were alive. At the same time, however, she always wore black and often spoke at great length and in a self-pitying way of her great loss. This behavior, too, eventually had become too much for some of her friends, who had come more and more to avoid her. Because of this, S felt herself "deserted" and utilized that feeling as another justification for her drinking.

S brought with her to her session a pipe that had been her husband's favorite and which she often looked at and held when she wanted to feel especially close to him. As she recounted the innumerable anecdotes of her thirty years of married life, she held this pipe tightly in her hands. Finally, she closed her eyes and reported that the pipe was "getting warm" and then that she had the feeling of holding not the pipe but instead her husband's hand. She now experienced the first of many vivid memory sequences during which she "relived" with intense emotion a great many past events. Still feeling that her husband's hand was in hers, she walked with him along the beach, attended church, and took an evening stroll. Her husband seemed "real as life" and she wept with joy at his "return from the grave."

S then began to talk to her husband, telling him how much she had missed him since his death, how difficult life had been for her, and how their friends had abandoned her since she had started to drink. To the guide's inquiry, she explained that the sense of her husband's presence was "completely real" and that he listened "very seriously" to her discourse and sympathized with her plight, but managed nonetheless to convey the idea that he "didn't really approve" of the way she had been behaving. She fell silent, and finally reported that the pipe was only a pipe again, that it was growing cold, and the sense of her husband's presence was becoming very faint. Then, however, it returned once again—a presence so powerfully felt that she thought she could "reach out and touch him." She felt that her husband smiled at her lovingly, conveying "whole worlds of encouragement and strength," then slowly turned his back and walked away. Then the sense of presence was extinguished and somehow she knew that he would "come no more." The pipe now was "cold and lifeless" in her hands and had "nothing more to do" with her husband, would "never have anything more to do with him." "At long last," she said, he was "gone. Dead. Really dead. He has made me understand that and I have got to accept it. That is what he would want me to do. That is the meaning of what I just went through."

S did not, it should be emphasized, have any idea that she had been dealing with her late husband's "spirit," or that he had actually "returned" in any way. But she felt that the "sense of presence" and the accompanying ideation had been "so true, so in keeping with what he would do and say if he *could* come back," that she now had received what she would accept as a kind of final "set of orders" from him. These orders were to the effect that she come to healthy terms with the fact of his death, and that she "grow up, create a new life, and no more of this drinking and moping around and living in the past." On the basis of this experience, which she went on to discuss and examine in detail, S later was able to shake off much of her grief, reshape a good many of her attitudes, and begin to live a much richer, happier life. The drinking was discontinued at once and was not resumed. These changes were still in effect about three years after her session.

In the two foregoing cases very serious mental and emotional disturbances were alleviated with what will seem a near-miraculous rapidity and ease in a single psychedelic session in which, moreover, very little therapy of any traditional sort was employed. The extensive psychedelic literature adds hundreds of similar results to the evidence supporting the value of the drug experience for purposes both of therapy and personal growth and fulfillment. We call attention to these results once again in the continuing hope of helping to initiate a public outcry that will force revision of unduly restrictive legislation that has taken psychedelic drugs out of the hands of almost all therapists and researchers in this country. And we will present still more cases which ought to provide further impetus for the protest—while they also serve the purpose of exemplifying the phenomena characteristic of the level with which we now are dealing.

The case to follow includes a good many of these recollective-analytic level phenomena. It also provides a striking example of significant changes in a subject who had no conscious motivation to alter his (homosexual) behavioral pattern and who had no expectation of effecting personal changes of any sort. The case also *may* demonstrate how the drug-state gains can be rather quickly lost when no subsequent effort is made to retain them.

The subject, S-3, age about fifty, was an economist at a southwestern university. He was married, but socially oriented mainly to the homosexual community of the city where he lived. S participated in a group peyote session that included two other male homosexuals, and the guide. All three subjects had some familiarity with the psychedelic drugs and wanted to have the drug experience; but it also was intended that the session be utilized as a kind of seminar to examine various aspects of homosexual psychology and problems of social adjustment peculiar to the invert.

As it turned out, no such seminar was possible. Neither was it possible for the guide to devote very much attention to the other two subjects; and, as a consequence, their experiences were almost wholly aesthetic and remained on the sensory level. This disruption of the plans for the session occurred because S, like many subjects who have been psychoanalyzed, went quickly to the recollective-analytic level, beyond which, however, he could not go. He then monopolized almost the whole of the session and, for various reasons, it seemed to the guide desirable to concentrate upon his productions. The other participants, deferring to S's superior "status," retired to a corner of the room where they conducted their own conversation. After that, for many hours, S recounted many events of his life and occasionally relived with considerable emotion some of the more painful past experiences. His own account of this session and its surprising aftermath follows. He also provides some preliminary personal background material essential to an understanding of his case. S writes:

"At various stages of my life I have conceived of myself in terms of attempting to find an answer to the question: 'What am I?' and in relating this question to my sexual identity. When people are asked 'What are you?' they usually think in two terms: either an ethnic identification, such as 'I am a Catholic' or 'I am a Negro,' or an occupational one, as 'I am a doctor' or 'I am a truck driver.' But with an immediacy that betrays what is uppermost in my mind, I would usually answer such a question—at least silently to myself—with the words: 'I am a homosexual.'

"Yet, at times, there might be some slight wavering. There is this vast area that stands between the one hundred per cent hetero world of people who have never had on a conscious level the least interest or arousal or even curiosity about the gay life, and those at the other end who believe (mistakenly, I think) that they were born homosexual and the image of contact with the other sex leaves them indifferent or repelled. Between these two poles there is that vague field of bisexuality, from those slightly leaning to one side and those almost identified with the other, and the many inbetween. Where was I on this continuum?

"Kinsey and his associates worked out a 7-point scale ranging from

0 to 6. At the 0 point were the completely heterosexual people, and at the 6 point were the opposite extreme. As one went up from 1 to 5, one traveled from being almost entirely hetero, through the midpoint, to almost entirely homo, at 5. When I was interviewed, some years ago, by the late Dr. Kinsey I knew of his rating system and I told him that I was a '5½.'

"What is 5½? Erotic arousal was entirely from men, and gratification largely, but not quite exclusively, from them. Any reasonably attractive male, ranging in age from late teens to my own age (whatever that happened to be at the time), could arouse me. I disdained the extremely effeminate, but other than that the male could be tall or short, intelligent or stupid, and of any race: I was capable of enjoying a relationship and would fantasy one merely by looking at the person for the first time. In my homosexual activities I would take both the active and passive roles in the usual types of contact.

"Then why 5½? Because women are not entirely out of my sex life. In fact, there was a time when my interest was centered more on females than on males. Although my first sexual arousal was toward a male, I was a young boy who at the time wanted a female very strongly, fantasied having one, but didn't know how to go about getting one. At age sixteen, I would fantasy being with a girl, but was expending my energies looking for a man. By eighteen, I had almost forgotten these fantasies: I was homosexual. Yet, I was curious and made the effort, going to a prostitute. When it came time to perform, however, I was totally incapable.

"About six months later, I accomplished with a beautiful young neighbor woman what I couldn't accomplish with the prostitute. I visited this woman a number of times, and apart from my wife, that makes up the whole of my heterosexual experience. Even at that time when I lost my 'virginity' I had already had contact with hundreds of males.

"A few years passed and I had my moments of fun and my moments of remorse. . . Some of my homosexual affairs were one-night stands; occasionally I would be emotionally involved, with deep friendships and even with vows of fidelity, but these would last only a few months at most. Some men need an anchor and perhaps I am one. I wanted sex, but with it a home and something like a family. I finally met an attractive girl and married her, but not before I had gone to bed with her, found it was great, and told her I had had a lot of homosexuality in my life.

"Sex with her was wonderful, but somehow when I left the house I saw only men on the streets, and this continued for many years. And seeing them, I stared, they stared back, and often we ended up in a hotel room, at the man's apartment, or at the home of one of my gay friends. That was what I told Kinsey I meant by 5½ : I could, with some effort, accept sex with my wife, and even get a sense of fulfillment out of it; but I couldn't, even with the greatest effort, resist sex with almost any willing male.

"There were occasional vacillations. When things were just right between my wife and myself, so much love and passion passed from her to me that I drifted over as far as 2 or 3. Then sex with her became frequent and interest in men was only slight. But these periods of high (not heterosexual, but wife-sexual) interest were short-lived, and then I would find myself a complete 6, without even the smallest interest sexually in my wife.

"So it was at the time of the peyote session, when I was deeply involved with Paul (not his real name), another of the participants in the session.

"Before proceeding to the session, another bit of background is required. For all the talk about homosexuality and narcissists I have never been in love with my own body. In fact, I believe that a major emotional problem in my life is that I have always disliked it. Years back, I thought of myself as a rather ugly youth; when I look at photos taken in my teens and twenties I am amazed, not only at the strikingly handsome young man, but even more so at my conception of myself as ugly and repulsive. During my thirties, I developed a strong distaste for mirrors. I use one while shaving, but aside from that deliberately avoid mirrors and rooms containing mirrors. When I go into a restaurant my main and overriding concern in choosing a table and seat is to avoid seeing myself in a mirror. Now for the peyote experience.[1]

"I had never previously taken any hallucinogenic drug, smoked a cigarette, or been even slightly "high" on alcohol or anything else. What I knew of consciousness-expanding drugs was based solely on some reading and conversations with the guide. I arrived at the home of the guide (who was thoroughly familiar with my sex life as well as that of my companions, although himself heterosexual) at 9 P.M. The others, already present, were Paul (with whom I was involved) and Gerald (as I will call him), who at the time was Paul's roommate, and homosexual, but not involved with Paul. Paul is bright, to me relatively masculine, and has a strong aversion to contact with women—a disgust such as some men feel when approached by other males. Gerald has strong manifestations of compulsive overmasculinity: the proud muscular male, the worshiper at the shrine of the cult of supermanliness.

"Some two hours later, we were under the influence of the drug but were reacting to it quite differently. Gerald and Paul experienced strangely vivid colors—tridimensional illusions. But for me, eyes opened or closed, the visual aspect was the same as always. I, on the other hand, felt an irresistible need to talk. I then started a monologue that was to last, with few interruptions, for many hours. More and more it centered around my experiences with my analyst some years earlier, and Gerald and Paul withdrew to be able to enjoy their own experiences.

"As our guide listened, I talked on and on. For hours I free-associated, speaking of things I had never discussed before (although nothing I might not have discussed had the occasion arisen). Free association was especially unusual, because it led me into many seemingly unrelated directions, but I would come back again and pick up the strands where they had been abandoned, and always the central point of the entire discussion was the story of my brief and abruptly terminated analysis. Several features of this free association stand out in my mind:

"The influence of language, words, puns, plays on words, in determing where the monologue would go. I was particularly sharp and sensitive to word play. Any word that had two or three possible meanings, or that would sound similar to another word with another meaning, would jump to mind and lead me off in a new direction, but always to return again.

"I recalled specific incidents and events that I had never 'forgotten,' but that had been out of consciousness for many years, perhaps for thirty years or more, even several I had not recalled during the hours of free association with the analyst.

"I was deeply moved as I relived emotionally and in conversation some of the most painful events of my life: a death in the family, and particularly the abruptness with which I had ended the analysis some years before . . .

"I recalled detail that under ordinary conditions I could not possibly have remembered, including the address on an envelope of a letter that a friend had sent me some years before—an important letter since it had had great significance for me during my analysis. I saw the envelope in front of me, in my mind's eye, recalled the handwriting, and recited the street number and street. (A few days later I went to an attic where I had old letters put away, dug into a dust-laden box, and took out crumpled and yellowing old papers. There, among them, I found the envelope, just as I had recalled it and the details of the address were correct, entirely correct.)

"Thus the night passed. I had lost my sense of time: I might have been in that room for days or years, and yet it was not dragging time. Towards morning, we all sat for a while and watched a flickering candle give off its dying light, held in magnetic fascination by a death agony that seemed to go on endlessly. I saw Paul as I had never seen him before: less than masculine, boyish in a gamin sort of way far too young for his years, and adolescent in that undifferentiated boy-girl way that characterizes some homosexuals and is often confused, mistakenly I think, with effeminacy.

"I was never sleepy, never hungry, and never completely comfortable. I kept having a peculiar feeling of chills that was not shared by the others, and only wanted to talk, talk, talk, which I did.

"Of vivid colors, I finally saw some, but mainly I was seeing gross visual distortions. I put my two hands in front of me and one was much larger than the other; yet, while I saw this, I silently and reassuringly said to myself that this was not so, that it was only an illusion from the peyote, and that my hands were not what they seemed to be. Other distortions I saw included Gerald's face, which seemed scarred and shriveled and aged and ugly. This was an interesting view because only a short time later, the affair with Paul having come to an end, I became deeply involved with Gerald and began to see him as an extraordinarily attractive male. Was I already developing this image, and was I distorting reality because I did not want the complication of this attraction to Paul's roommate, particularly that night when Paul was there?

"As the sun came up, I still was telling everyone else to keep quiet because I had something to say; and I still was saying it, saying it, saying it, over and over and following the threads of association wherever they led, and then always back to where they had started. The young men left around seven and the guide and I went down to a nearby restaurant to have some breakfast; but the sight of the food was disgusting and I said goodby, then went home to try and get some sleep. Now for the aftereffects:

"Arriving home, I made coffee and opened the sugar bowl to put the spoon into it. Suddenly I saw all the different shades of white in the little granules of sugar. Some were dull white, some were lustrous, some shown with an inner glow, and some were like milk. What blindness I had had to color differentiation all my life that I had never seen this before! I had no doubt that the shades and degrees of whiteness really existed, that they were not an illusion produced by the drug, but were real, and that I would see them tomorrow and thereafter. Indeed they were real, and I have often seen them since, although never with quite so intense an awareness as that day. But still I am able to perceive the lovely design of monochromatic whites, posing motionless in an entrancing work of art.

"After coffee, which I enjoyed, although I was a bit too sensitive to the flavor, I walked over to the mirror and put out my tongue, somehow expecting it to be coated with white. But instead of noting color, I saw the size, a huge tongue that surely could never be retracted to fit back into the mouth. I managed somehow to fit it in, stuck it out again, was fascinated, and stood before the mirror, tongue hanging out, marveling and frightened at its size.

"My face was drawn, there were ugly lines under the eyes, and the eyes, although large, looked tired. I wanted to sleep, but found I couldn't. Instead, I still wanted to talk, and in the absence of my wife spent most of the day on the telephone, talking with various people.

"In the afternoon I showered and then went to the mirror to take a shave. The grotesque, enlarged tongue, I discovered, had returned to normal size. I shaved, washed, combed my hair, and took a last look to see if I was in proper condition to go out. What I saw in the mirror was amazing!

"There, staring me in the face, was *a handsome man*, approximately my age! I noted his small mouth and perfectly formed lips, his handsome all-white hair that contrasted with a rather youthful face, his deepset, brown moist eyes. I stared at the man with considerable satisfaction, and then smiled. He returned the smile.

"I met my wife and we went to a restaurant for dinner. When we were shown to a table I took a seat facing a mirror and found myself looking at it more often than at the food or my wife. That night sex with my wife was particularly fulfilling. I felt a strong need and a satisfaction in accomplishment while it was taking place. For about six weeks thereafter we repeated this experience with a greater frequency than ever before and almost always with outstanding success. My eyes strayed to males less frequently and although I had some extracurricular experiences during this time, they were few.

"During this time, too, my love-affair with myself and my mirror image continued. Like the shades of white in the sugar bowl, that had always been there but that I had never seen, so this handsome man of my age had been in front of my eyes countless times before, yet I had always seen him as pretty awful.

"At the end of six weeks or so I noticed the effects were beginning to wear away: I began avoiding mirrors again, and saw my own image as less than attractive. But not entirely so, for at least I could recall what I had seen and then look specifically for those interesting and well-formed features, and then, seeing them in memory, I would find them to be as I had seen them before. 'You look the same to me as you always did,' a psychologist friend said when I told him this story, and I looked at him incredulously. Couldn't he see that I had changed?

"As the attractive image became less attractive, the erotic wife-centered interest also diminished, and somehow they seemed linked to one another, or they were affecting each other. But in each of these two respects I have not been the same since the session as before."

So ends the subject's account of his session, about which some more remarks should be made.

Like most (twelve out of fourteen) of the limited number of overt male homosexuals who have been psychedelic volunteers, there is to be found here a distorted body image—in this case, a much more distorted image than in the other cases. That S's distorted body image preceded and was at least partly causal to his homosexuality is probable but cannot be established beyond doubt. Certainly, the normalizing of the distorted body image produced a marked trend towards heterosexualization; in the same way, the deterioration of the body image later on appears to have preceded and been causal to the resumption of the former homosexual pattern.

After his session, and during the period when the image was most pleasing to him, S went for the first time in several decades beyond his intermittent "wife-sexual" interest to a broader and much less sporadic heterosexual interest. He repeatedly considered "testing" himself by having intercourse with other females; that he did not do so was mainly owing to his lack of knowledge of ways to effect what he desired. In the streets, he consistently saw what he had "never seen before": He noticed the "breasts and bottoms" of women and found them attractive. This was a source of much astonishment to him, since before he always had passed women by without seeing them at all, or noticing them only as if they were objects, "like lampposts or fire hydrants." Moreover, as the self-image began to "slip," S had a (for him unprecedented) brief "involvement" with an effeminate male described by him as "very girlish" —an almost-heterosexual relationship in which the techniques of contact employed were also approximations to the heterosexual.

Over a period of several months, S experienced more frequent than usual revivals of his attraction to his wife. Apparently, she now sometimes appealed to him as a *woman* and not only as a wife.

The "delayed reaction" in which the subject acquired his new image some hours after the session, is not too unusual. Some apparently non-transformative sessions produce significant changes in the subject days, weeks, and (rarely) even several months afterwards. The changes that did occur in this subject are all the more remarkable in view of the fact that he expected no changes at all and had no motivation whatever to relinquish his homosexuality. For reasons unnecessary to discuss here, S had a considerable investment in his homosexuality and this not only prevented the wish to give it up, but also discouraged post-session efforts to consolidate and expand upon the "gains." Thus, one may only speculate as to what would have been possible in this case had the subject been strongly motivated to become heterosexual. What did happen is at least suggestive.

It also should be noted that S fails to mention specifically what was probably the most important single event of his session. He frequently refers to the abrupt termination of his psychoanalysis some years earlier, but does not mention that this analysis was terminated by the death of the analyst. After that death, S had attended the funeral, passed before the open coffin, and looked down upon the analyst's face. During the session he relived this scene emotionally, ideationally, and imagistically. There was no intense reaction, but nonetheless there seems no doubt as to the importance of the experience.

It is also of possible interest to report that apart from S and one other subject, all of the homosexual subjects have had a rather passive demeanor, especially in relation to the guide but also in relation to the other persons generally. Individuals "in authority," including the guide, are approached in a rather apologetic way and the whole manner, including the speech, tends to be diffident. A frequent post-session effect is then a heightened aggressiveness, an impression of greater self-confidence and probably better self-esteem, with a noticeable deepening of the voice in some cases. Also, gestures may become more vigorous, posture more erect, and movements generally more decisive and, in some cases, more "masculine."

The preceding cases illustrate some of the phenomena and therapeutic possibilities of the recollective-analytic level. Cases likely to be of particular interest to the psychotherapist have been selected and should only be taken to mean that the so-called "instant psychotherapy" is in fact a possibility, in the psychedelic experience and on this level. Thus, as so much other evidence also demonstrates, much more—not less!— work with psychedelic drugs is warranted and eventually "psychedelic psychotherapy" may in some cases emerge as a standard therapeutic shortcut resulting in an enormous saving of time and energy for both therapist and patient, and additional benefits of money saved and misery avoided for the latter.

As regards this "psychedelic psychotherapy" of the future, already it is possible to foresee and warn against abuses which surely would limit its effectiveness. For example, any psychedelic psychotherapy must take all possible precautions to avoid the establishment of a dogmatized theory and the other rigidities that in the past have sapped the effectiveness of so many psychotherapeutic methods.

With the psychedelic drugs, especially, the experience of the subject *must not become vicarious*; that is, his experience must not be in terms of the psychodynamic constructs and other ideas of the therapist, but must remain largely his own. The therapist must remain the guide and aide, not the all-knowing, all-powerful leader of the patient.

Present psychedelic subjects display an astonishing ability to direct their own sessions precisely into those areas which will prove most beneficial to them. How long they will continue to do so well may depend upon whether an elaborate and over-systematized, inflexible therapeutic approach evolves. At the same time, it eventually should be possible to construct a more profitable and scientific approach than that of the therapist largely "playing it by ear," as has to be done in the absence of a psychedelic psychotherapy when the therapist does not merely use the drug (so impairing his own effectiveness) as an adjunct to some traditional therapeutic method.

Some notion of the extraordinary array of tools available to the psychedelic drug therapist by now should be available; and the therapist must assist the patient in making the best possible use of all these unique possibilities and capacities. As a veteran observer of psychedelic subjects, the therapist will know what is possible and will have to impart to his patient as much of this knowledge as is in the patient's best interest. But, at the same time, he must display a degree of respect for the patient's autonomy that will not make the patient's experience vicarious or otherwise unduly restrict or deprive him.

If, as considerable evidence would suggest, the psychedelic experience has the potential of initiating the unfolding of an entelechical self-healing and self-realizing process, then more than ever it will be essential that the therapist be able to refrain from interrupting that process by indulging his own authoritarianism or imposing his own ideology on the patient. This will require nothing less than a new kind of therapist who will not receive from the therapeutic experience the same kind of personal power rewards the therapist presently receives. It seems evident that the transition to such a different sort of patient-therapist relationship will not always be easily effected.

Transition—and Transformation. In the final case to be presented in this chapter we will show in detail how the experiencing of the recollective-analytic level may lead the subject "down" to the "deeper" symbolic level. The case will be given in somewhat greater detail than the preceding ones, since it also demonstrates how the effective experiencing of the several levels may culminate in a transforming experience of very great benefit to the subject. As a preliminary to this case we will briefly recapitulate what already has been stated.

Ideally, the subject whose aim is to effect increased self-understanding and other beneficial changes in himself brings to the psychedelic session not only his hopes but also much self-knowledge gained through auto- or hetero-analytic work. If he then, on the recollective-analytic level, re-examines his insights, possibly adds new ones, and so comes to a deepened and more adequate comprehension of his deficiencies and problems, then the chances are good that he will move on to important experiences on the symbolic and possibly the integral level. On the symbolic, if the preliminary work has been done, he may experience a symbolization of the essential psychodynamic and other materials and participate in a symbolic drama leading to a resolution of his conflicts and possibly effecting many of the positive changes that were the subject's goal. In the following case, we observe the unfolding of this process in a subject who provides an almost perfect illustration of how the experiencing of the first three of our levels may be accomplished in those instances where maximum results are forthcoming. The final "descent" to the *integral* level is not accomplished. However, so complete is the symbolic participation, and so appropriate the symbolization, that the transformative effects rival those achieved by some subjects who do "go deeper." And, of course, there is always the possibility of misinterpretation of the phenomenological signs, so that this subject may have achieved the *integral* level even though in our estimation he did not. The case will further demonstrate how much more comprehensive and self-potentiating is this type of transformation than the changes and symptom remissions described as occurring on the previous levels.

The subject, S-5 (LSD: 100 micrograms), is a forty-year-old professor of philosophy at a major West Coast school. He is married and the father of three young children.

S entered his present profession after having spent more than a decade preparing for the Roman Catholic priesthood. During that decade he had been increasingly troubled by "a sense of maladjustment to self and world." As the time of his ordination drew closer, S's "inner tensions and sense of maladjustment were intensified." He then decided he should not be ordained and abandoned his plan to be a priest in the hope that this action "might benefit the inner life." Instead, the action seemed to him, once it had been taken, to be a "social admission" of his "problems," and the effect of this seemed to be to strip away the "mask" he had developed over the years to conceal his "tension and feelings of depression." He "was exposed," his "protective façade" was "torn down," and he was plunged into a deep depression that no longer could be veiled by his customary "mask of serenity." Unlike his previous depression, this present state was one of "general numbness, lack of feeling, lack even of the anxiety" that had been with him for years. So distressing was the lack of feeling, that even the absence of anxiety seemed a painful deprivation.

Shortly after leaving the seminary S entered into a psychoanalysis that lasted for six months. The depression was eased and he terminated the analysis. He again was somewhat anxious, and much less aggressive and involved in life than he wanted to be, but doubted that analysis, unless continuing for many years, could do much more to effect the changes he desired. S then met and married a quiet and rather shy young woman with whom he shares many interests, and who is the only woman with whom he ever has been romantically involved. He embarked upon his academic career, which has been successful if unspectacular.

Shortly after beginning his analysis, S went into a church and there had a "mystical experience" while contemplating a religious object. At first he became conscious of anxiety concerning the nature of his relationship to Christ. This anxiety became specifically a fear of a "homosexual attachment to Christ" (not too uncommon among celibate Roman Catholic priests and seminarians). This was followed by a revelation to the effect that S could "love God without fear of this involving a homosexual love of Christ." After this experience, S felt that his mental-emotional state was significantly improved.

The fear of a homosexual attachment to Christ, S says, was the first time it had ever occurred to him that homosexuality might have any place in his life. He had never experienced any homo-erotic desires or engaged in any homosexual behavior. He discussed the mystical experience with his analyst and was given a Rorschach test with a subsequent diagnosis of "latent homosexuality." Trying to find in his past some indications of an aberrant sexuality, S recalled that at the age of three or four years he had "identified with" a little neighbor girl about his own age and had envied the privileged status of girls—nicer toys, prettier clothing to wear, etc. He specifically had wanted a set of toy dishes (such as that owned by a neighbor girl), but his mother had refused this and told him that such playthings were unsuitable for a boy. During his boyhood S had had several "crushes" on male classmates but never was aware of any sexual interest in the object of the "crush." For a time, he recalled, he was regarded by his classmates as something of a "sissy." But, as he grew older, he no longer was so regarded. Although willing to consider the possibility of a "latent homosexuality," S doubted the accuracy of the diagnosis and felt that, even if true, it had little relevance to his present situation.

S felt that the really important discovery made in the course of his analysis was that of a "castration complex," and with this he had been concerned ever since. He reported frequent awareness of a slight tension at the base of his penis and associated this with his chronic sexual anxiety and also with the unconscious fear of castration turned up in analysis. In discussing what he hoped to achieve through his psychedelic session he remarked that he felt "cut off" not only sexually, but also over the whole range of his sensory experiencing. In every area of his life, he said, he always avoided the concrete for the abstract. He felt that this sense of "being cut off" had been worsened by his seminary training and that he had joined his particular order, in part, because it offered an "abstract, intellectualized approach to life." He also had entered the seminary, he felt, in order to remove himself as much as possible from erotic temptations. Since self-understanding and development, not therapy, was S's aim in volunteering for the session, he did not propose to try to deal directly with the castration anxiety. What he did hope for was that he might become "able to relate to things and others more completely," to establish a better contact with the sensory realm and to become better able "to experience life as a creative process." He also hoped to reorient some of his attitudes and values with regard to sex.

At 10:20 A.M. S was given the 100 micrograms of LSD. At 10:50 he complained of being cold and put on an overcoat which he continued to wear for the next hour. He also mentioned a slight tremor experienced as running through his whole body and a "feeling of constriction just below the abdomen." This later became localized at the base of the penis and was described by S as "the focal point of resistance" to a full participation in the drug experience.

A light, pleasant musical recording was played and S closed his eyes and imaged a series of "richly colored geometrical shapes: green, blue, and possibly red." He opened his eyes and reported that all of his sense perceptions seemed much heightened. Especially, the visual, tactile, and olfactory perceptions were intensified and objects were seen not only with greater clarity but also seemed to be "more meaningful." At 11:10 he reported the impression that his "conditioning" was "cracking and breaking up," that his "categories" were "falling away." There remained, however, a feeling of resisting the drug effects.

At 11:30 the guides played for S a spoken recording that has been used to good effect with a few selected subjects, to overcome resistance and produce a movement toward deeper drug-state levels.[2] S apparently soon was absorbed in the recording and in about ten minutes began to make convulsive lower body movements, most noticeably of the legs— legs jerking out from the body, legs opening and closing—with many twitches and jerks, sometimes as frequent as twenty to thirty per minute. The basic movement then became the spreading and closing of the legs. S appeared to be trying to control this by frequently shifting his position and locking his legs at the ankles, but later said he had no memory of ever trying to control the movements. He also said later that these involuntary movements all seemed to move outward from the point of constriction at the base of the penis. S writes that:

"During the playing of the record I felt myself being swept along by the movement of the words, as if the meaning were coming through directly to me and the meaning itself was a movement, a dynamic flow which carried me along as if on a journey. I did not interpret the words. I simply heard them and they reflected back their individual meaning like sparks . . . I simply gave myself to the movement and to the richness of the voice. All the while I felt my mind being stretched, as if my faculty of abstracting and conceptualizing was being left on the surface, still capable of operating, but not interested in doing so. All the while new dimensions of my mind were coming into being and I was carried along by the sheer movement and rhythm of the voice. Although I felt periodic resistances and the tension of my mind being stretched, I enjoyed the experience of being swept along.

"At the end of the record, I felt that I had been on a long journey and that I had come to my destination. My guides came to me and welcomed me into this 'brave new world.' I felt that I had reached the psychedelic shore and enjoyed the wonderful things around me. I felt joyous and deeply related to everything, as if I were part of a whole. It was a feeling of solidity and yet fluidity, a sense of total relatedness and involvement, bringing with it a sense of joy, peace and wonder. This was the deepest and most sustaining experience of the entire session. It remained throughout, as if it were the base of all other experiences. In my estimation, it was the most valuable dimension of the entire session.

"I explored the room, the flowers, the fruit, and my own hands. My hands seemed wondrously clear. I explored the cauliflower, the flowers, and the grapes. I slowly peeled a grape and enjoyed the intricate patterns of the veins. Throughout the room colors were alive and clear. Outlines were sharp and certain perspectives, especially of depth, were altered from their normal dimensions. In all of this, I felt closely related to the room and the objects and persons in the room."

At 1:00 P.M. S, having shown no tendency to deal with recollective-analytic level materials, was encouraged to experience phenomena characteristic of the symbolic level. He attempted to image scenes from ancient Greece, but met with only very slight success. S now initiated an experience of regression along evolutionary lines, as he describes:

"Then I said, 'I don't want to go to Athens; I want to go to the beginning.' I felt good at this statement and felt myself going back and down into a dark substance. Then I began to move my body—my arms and shoulders, as if I were trying to bring something to life. I felt that I was the earth and I was trying to bring something to life—growing, working, growing, with great effort and struggle and yet driven by a powerful force. I worked and worked and life came forth. It was difficult and I felt the life force within me toiling and striving to come to fulfillment. Then I moved to the floor of the room, where I became the ocean. I was in the ocean and I was the ocean. I moved and rolled like the ocean. Finally I was asked if I saw any animals. I said 'Yes, tigers,' and when asked 'What, no dinosaurs?' I said that maybe I had by-passed them. Then I felt myself slowly becoming an animal. I tried to resist this, but finally accepted it. I found that I had become a panther and writhed about, stretching my limbs as if I were a panther."

S now reported that he no longer was a panther and was back in his own body. Lying on the floor, he reported himself "very relaxed" while, at the same time, locking his legs together at the ankles and apparently exerting much effort to control the leg movements. He finally gave up on this effort and there followed more spasmodic movements of the lower body, accompanied by many sighs, groans, grunts, and snorts. All activity continued to be in the lower body, with little or no movement above the waist. S said he was finding in his movements "a sense of release" and of "relatedness to things" and, thereby, of "relatedness to the world."

At 2:00 P.M. S abruptly entered into the recollective-analytic phase of his experience and continued on this level for two and one-half hours. Without any apparent associational linkage to his preceding ideation he re-experienced with great accompanying emotion the death of his grandmother when he was not quite four years old. He describes the onset of this experience:

"Suddenly I felt as if some obstacle were coming up to me—something large, dark, and vague, but very powerful—as if it were knocking on the walls of consciousness. I said that some block was coming up. Then I said, 'It's Granny's death! I must examine Granny's death!' At once I felt ill and dashed to the bathroom and vomited—not food, since I had not eaten. This vomiting, and all the vomiting to follow, was more a kind of ritual emission of negative emotion than a physical vomiting of food, but I did go through the physical motions of vomiting and spit up liquid."

Returning to the session room, S said he believed at the time of her death that he had killed his grandmother by a magical act—by smashing the head of a doll he had identified with her. This doll he also had identified with himself and with the previously mentioned neighbor girl. He thus, in destroying the doll, effected "the destruction of my world, the concrete world of affection and real persons."

S re-experienced with great emotion the incident that had caused him to destroy the doll. Soon afterwards, his grandmother fell ill and finally died. During the period of her illness his guilt was so great he would not enter her room. After her death, too, he would not enter the room where her body was laid out. And, when the grandmother was buried, S had felt that "a part of myself was being buried with her."

This incident had left him cut off from "the concrete world" and also had been a "symbolic autocastration." Moreover, he now felt, he had never liberated himself from the identification with the neighbor girl. Thus, in a variety of ways, he was blocked from reaching full manhood and from direct, uninhibited experiencing of the world around him. These formulations yielded more affective discharge and vomiting. He later wrote that "In the state of deep relatedness of the psychedelic experience, I was able to experience these negative emotions in a way I had never been able to do before. There was a sense of totality in the experience, as if I had actually entered in to the mythic framework of the world I had destroyed by my magical act."

Memories and regressions continued, accompanied by the recurring nausea, and S was taken into another room where he would be closer to the bathroom. He there lay down on a couch, closed his eyes, and considered further his need to achieve full manhood by overcoming the old guilt, the effects of the autocastration and the feminine identification. Then began his *symbolic* level experiences, image sequences consisting of a series of rites. These were:

A fertility rite. This consisted mostly of white-skinned savages dancing and singing around a fire, "trying to bring something to life." S was emotionally, and through body sensations, a participant in this imaged rite, but his involvement was not great and the rite lasted only a few minutes. It seemed to him to be a preliminary to something more important still to come.

A puberty rite. Here, S was one of a number of youths dancing around an older woman. There was a sense of identification with this woman, who represented "the feminine principle." The youths had coitus with this woman and so shed their identification with the feminine, becoming wholly male. S was totally involved in this rite— experienced on the levels of image, emotion, ideation, physical sensation, and appropriate body movements. At the end he leaped up, dashed into the bathroom to vomit several times, and emerged to say that he had vomited up the whole of his feminine identification. In fact, his appearance seemed to be more strongly masculine than before.

A warrior initiation rite. This rite also began with dancing, which became increasingly faster and more violent. Then the young candidates for initiation participated in the killing of an older man— "the father." They pulled off his genitals and devoured them, thus liberating themselves from paternal influence and so becoming ready to assume their roles as warriors and leaders of the tribe. S also was fully involved in this rite, which precipitated still more strenuous vomiting.

A rite not classified as to purpose. This rite, involving the same white-skinned primitives as the others, again began with dancing. It was a curious combination of primitive and Christian elements and, at the end, passed over wholly into Christian content. It accomplished the salvation of S and made him "whole." Again, participation was on all levels (image, emotion, ideation, physical sensation, kinesthetic). The subject's own account of this ritual series, written next day, provides additional materials of interest:

"I suspended my thoughts for a while and the material simply began to come up. I soon had an image of a group of people dancing. They seemed to be primitive people, but of white skin. They were dancing around something raised, a pole or a platform, and there was a snake associated with this ceremony. They were dancing, dancing, trying to bring something to life. I had a sense of labor and duration. At this point I was lying on the couch and was having periodic spasms of the legs, seeming to come from that point of tension at the base of the penis. These spasms continued through the long sequence of primitive rituals.

"In the next ritual there were boys present and they were having intercourse with an older woman, with the earth mother. Then I saw the image of a huge female figure over me and, at that moment, there was a bursting reaction as of liberation and the figure seemed to move quickly away. I became very ill and dashed to the bathroom to vomit. I retched violently. This was the most intense of the vomiting spells and seemed to involve my whole body. I had the sense of spitting up deep anxiety— from the innermost part of my body, from my very toes. There was a realization that I was vomiting up my identification with the Female—an identification which had led to terrible anxiety about being castrated. As long as I was identified with the Female, I seemed to be castrated, and unless I got to this level and liberated myself, contact with women in my life would ultimately lead to a sense of castration.

"I returned to the couch again and again saw dancing, this time faster and more violent, like a war dance. I think this was the initiation ceremony for new warriors, but I am confused about the sequence here. Then I saw a group of boys killing an older man. This was the father. Then they began eating him. I felt that I was also there mutilating this man. I pulled off his penis and testicles and, at that moment, saw vividly his mutilated body and the wound in his groin. I felt a deep release of tension and, I believe, I vomited again.

"Then I returned to the couch and saw more dancing. This time the people were dancing around a raised platform, on which people were tied by their arms on supports, perhaps two or three males. Then I had the awareness that I was lying down on my back and that someone was placing hot coals in a circle on the lower part of my abdomen near my penis. I was afraid. Then I accepted the situation and entered into the ritual. I ritualistically accepted my own castration. At that moment, a man appeared in front of me, in the same position that the large woman had been in in the first ritual. I knew that he was the Savior. I could not discern his features. His face seemed to be white, without any features, and I could see only his bust. As soon as he appeared I threw over his left shoulder a piece of animal skin; it seemed to have hair and to be a piece of goatskin. At this moment I knew I was saved from castration.

"Then I noticed that the people were on a field and were tearing the Savior to bits and eating his flesh. Then I felt that I was the Savior and was lying on my back being nailed to a cross. Then the cross was lifted up, and at this moment I was a spectator viewing the Savior from a distance as he was being lifted up on the cross on the top of a hill for all the people. From the time the Savior appeared, I had a deep sense of peace and integration. I felt that I was saved and that I was whole."

S now was exhausted and slept briefly, something we have seen in only one other case. At 5:40 P.M. he awakened and thereafter the drug effects appeared to diminish sharply. S described himself as very tranquil and happy. He remained silent for some time and then reported that he had been "integrating" all that had occurred, and that this integration was extremely important. He felt drastically and beneficially transformed. He viewed his image in the mirror and said it was greatly changed. His face now was "much more youthful and relaxed" than it had been for years. He felt "strongly related" to everything around him. His appetite, when a meal was served, proved voracious and he stated he had never felt better or enjoyed food more.

The post-session effects of this session will also be dealt with in more detail than usual, since they convey a good impression of what may occur as the result of a truly transforming psychedelic experience.

In general, at the end of the first week after the session, S felt energized, more masculine, more tranquil, and self-esteem was heightened. His experience of everything around him was more intense and "everything" seemed to be going extremely well. One event of the week was of outstanding importance to the subject.

For almost two years S had been collaborating with another philosopher on a book. Many difficulties had plagued this collaboration, which had reached a virtual standstill. S had long felt that he had the "key to the whole problem—the ideas that would bring the book to a successful conclusion." But, as junior author, he could not insist upon these ideas; and he never had been able, despite strenuous efforts, to get his points across to his collaborator. Now, however, a few days after his session he had a meeting about the book and was able, as never before, to communicate with his co-author. S reported that "This time I found myself letting the issues simply emerge and did not try to look for arguments or tactics. The meeting was extremely pleasant. For some time we ranged over the several issues he had raised. All the while I was trying to move towards a formulation of what I thought was the difference between us: our understanding of metaphysics. Eventually he formulated my basic idea. I said, 'That's it.' For some time then he developed the implications. This was one of the richest moments of communication on a philosophical level I have ever had. I left feeling very much at peace personally and as concerned the future of the book. Professor——was very pleased with the meeting."

Another event of personal importance also occurred. The opportunity presenting itself, S without hesitation accepted leadership of a major departmental project—something he felt he could not have done before. Both of these events he related in a detailed way to materials of his session.

Three weeks after his drug experience, S attended a seminar on Whitehead and found himself understanding and able to explain to others points of Whitehead's philosophy which in the past had always been obscure to him. His other gains were being maintained and he reported, too, that "I continue to experience a deeper relation with my wife. There is less tension and negative affect in the relation. I have a much clearer realization of the significance of her love and understanding to my own personality and invividuality. I have also had a deeper sense of sexual relatedness to her." He mentioned also that "During the last few days I was experiencing a bit of inner tension, which led me to believe that something was working its way to consciousness. Finally it emerged in the context of fantasy images associated with the Attis myth. I experienced anxiety and hostility towards the Earth Mother—Cybele in the myth. The anxiety was over being castrated by her. The hostility was over being subjected to her destructive force. It seemed that I had drunk in the hostility and in its inverted force it became a vehicle of my own castration. I could now hurl it outside and direct it towards Cybele—to turn towards her the knife she directed to my own castration. In this way I felt liberated from her power. This seemed closely associated with the ritual of the puberty rite where I was liberated from identification with the female. The same type of sense of deep affect and physical anxiety was present. Since then I have been able to be aware of a positive dimension of sex as a means of relating to the world."

The subject's progress continued and five months after his session the situation was as follows: For the first time, S was greatly enjoying working with his collaborator on the book. His other work was progressing excellently and he felt that "The sense of integration gained through the session has extended to an integrating vision of my work. Now I am really discovering what scholarship means."

He reported a "continual stream of penetrating insights and deepened philosophical understanding. Common to all this understanding is the new integrated view of the world and the sense of the concrete relations between things." Before his session, all of his relationships "were on an abstract level"; now, however, he had a "continuous sense of immediacy, a sense of existing in the moment, a total commitment to what is being done at the moment." There was a "continuously heightening relatedness to nature—something qualitatively new, a sense of belonging to nature that was not present before. This relatedness to nature has had an important effect upon my relationship with my wife. Before the session, our communication very largely had to do with theoretical intellectual and academic matters; now there is a shared feeling level to the relationship that never existed before. I have also a deepened sense of what it means to be a father and, along with this, a much better relationship with my children. I think, and apparently my students agree, that my teaching never has been better. I communicate feelings as well as cold ideas, and ideas communicated with feeling seem to be communicated much better than when the feeling is lacking. In short, I am happier with myself than I have ever been, and others seem to be happier with me too."

As noted, this is something of an ideal case. The subject came to his session well prepared in terms of self-understanding. The transitions from level to level were smoothly accomplished and the insights and formulations made on the recollective-analytic level laid the basis for a symbolization in terms of rites best suited to enable the subject to move beyond those early experiences which had previously blocked his development. In the chapter to follow, some other varieties of symbolic experience will be exemplified and the phenomena and problems of the symbolic level will be considered and should shed additional light on the present case.

Eight:
Psyche and Symbol

Few of the drug-state phenomena are more perplexing, fascinating and potentially valuable than is the subject's participation in mythic and ritualistic dramas which represent to him in terms both universal and particular the essentials of his own situation in the world. These analogic and symbolic dramas occur most characteristically on the third or *symbolic* level of our functional model of the drug-state psyche. They often are sequentially preceded on this level by the subject's experiencing of historical events and evolutionary processes—usually of less value, but not less likely to perplex and fascinate.

When the historical events are experienced the subject may observe these as spectator only or he may have the sense of being a participant in the event. These battles, coronations, witch trials, crusades, or whatever, enter into consciousness and may be eidetically imaged in intricate and voluminous detail. The historical materials may seem to have no empirical antecedents for the subject, and concerning this apparently groundless knowledge it is only possible to speculate more or less plausibly. Similarly, the subject may observe or feel himself to be a part of evolutionary process, seemingly becoming aware of the whole or a part of the pattern of emerging life on this earth and its progression towards the present point in time. Again, the subject may display a knowledge that remains inexplicable should we insist upon discovering its source in what he is aware of having read, seen, or heard about.

The psychedelic drug "world" of myth and ritual, which is also a world of legendary and fairy tale themes and figures, of archetypes, and of other timeless symbols and essences, is of a more profound and meaningful order than that of the historical and evolutionary sequences. Here, where the symbolic dramas unfold, the individual finds facets of his own existence revealed in the person of Prometheus or Parsifal, Lucifer or Oedipus, Faust or Don Juan, and plays out his personal drama on these allegorical and analogic terms. Or he finds the means of attaining to new levels of maturity through his participation in rites of passage and other ceremonies and initiations.

In the case of the analogic mythical and ritual dramas, these very often are shaped of the stuff of the raw personal-historic data and insights now seemingly viable and plastic to the un- or pre-conscious myth-making process as a result of the subject's evocation and examination of them on the recollective-analytic level. Now, on the level of the symbolic, these memory and psychodynamic materials may emerge restructured in a purposive pattern of undisguised symbols cast in a flowing dramatic form that illumines the subject's life and may even transform it.

As we have noted elsewhere, the eidetic images become of major importance on this level and especially where the symbolic dramas are concerned. Ideally, the subject's participation in these dramas will be total—i.e., a participation by image, ideation, affect, sensation, and kinesthetic involvement, all coalescing as integrated dynamic constituents of the unfolding dramatic experience. The drama, it is true, may unfold on a verbal-ideational plane and without the images, but then the chances of effecting the kinesthetic, affective, and sensory coalescence are diminished; and, in the case of this theater of symbols, the chief purposive function of the eidetic images appears to be the enhancement of imaginary events by drawing into the image-ideation complex the additional factors of affect, sensation, and kinesthetic involvement required to charge the experience with its full richness and transformative potency.

Also of major importance on this level is the work of the guide who here, more than elsewhere, must assume the Virgilian mantle and employ all his art in leading the subject through ever more complex and more personally significant realms of symbolic experience until the subject is able to participate directly and wholly in those dramas that will be most beneficial to him.

While it often occurs that the subject spontaneously reaches the level of possible participation in the personal allegory, it also frequently occurs that he does not participate but only observes, remaining no more than an appreciative spectator as the aesthetic images of curious flora, fauna, and architecture characteristic of this psychical region pass before him, signifying nothing. These are the scenes and figures which Aldous Huxley has told us are not symbolic, "do not stand for something else, do not mean anything except themselves. The significance of each thing is identical with its being. . . . Through these landscapes and among these living architectures wander strange figures, sometimes of human beings (or even of what seem to be superhuman beings), sometimes of animals or fabulous monsters. Giving a straightforward prose description of what he used to see in his spontaneous visions, William Blake reports that he frequently saw beings, to whom he gave the name of Cherubim. These beings were a hundred and twenty feet high and were engaged (this is characteristic of the personages seen in vision) in doing nothing that could be thought of as being symbolic or dramatic. In this respect the inhabitants of the mind's Antipodes differ from the figures inhabiting Jung's archetypal world; for they have nothing to do either with the personal history of the visionary, or even with the age-old problems of the human race. Quite literally, they are the inhabitants of 'the Other World.' "[1]

But what Huxley evidently was unable to tell us is that this "Other World" is one whose surface has been but barely touched by the sort of passive, aesthetic observation he describes without mentioning other possibilities. And these figures "doing nothing symbolic or dramatic" are precisely the unemployed actors who await recruitment as players in the subject's personal drama. The eliciting and formulation of data on the recollective-analytic level increases the likelihood that the players will be recruited and the drama staged; but, as suggested, there is still no guarantee that this will occur, and collaboration of subject and guide yet may be required if archetype and symbol are to arise out of their latency and if the subject is to be participant rather than entertained spectator only.

The historical and evolutionary sequences may be seen as having the function of moving the subject toward increasing dramatic involvement, and thus the guide may fruitfully *induce* the historical and evolutionary experiences. Here, even rather sketchy suggestions may suffice, and the guide need do little more than invite the subject to walk along the Piraeus with Socrates, to witness a battle in the Thirty Years' War, to participate in the bull-leaping at Knossos, or to help with the building of the pyramid of Khufu. The subject may be asked to gaze over the shoulder of that Cro-Magnon man who painted the great bison in the cave at Altamira. He may join in the violent thrust westward of the army of Genghis Kahn. He may have a front row seat at the Battle of Hastings or mingle with those present at the court of Louis XIV.

The subject, whose eyes are closed, then is asked to describe as fully as he can the background, action and *dramatis personae* of the historical events he now is imaging (or perhaps is imagining vividly but without eidetic images). This, as some forthcoming examples soon will demonstrate, he often does with not only a wealth of detail but also, in some cases, with a rather uncanny measure of accuracy not to be explained in terms of the information to which he normally has access or to which he remembers ever having been exposed. Whether one will attribute this rich "reporting," with its impressive note of immediacy, to recall of previously learned but long since forgotten materials or to the subject's having gained access to materials from some other source, will depend upon theoretical commitment to scientific or philosophical postulates. Needless to say, most persons will consider probability to lie with the former attribution; and Freud, for one, has shown us how "completely forgotten" materials may emerge years later as ideas and images which will seem mysterious in origin since apparently lacking the usual empirical ground.

As an effective next step in leading the subject toward symbolization and dramatic engagement, the guide may assist him to "recapture" and participate in evolutionary events. In many cases the subject at this point will begin to discard the spectator role maintained throughout his experiencing of history and will find himself entering into an identification with the evolutionary process that may involve at least some measure of sensory, emotional, and kinesthetic as well as ideational and imagistic participation. For example, the guide may suggest that the subject might want to "become that primordial piece of protoplasm floating in an early ocean"—described by several subjects as a very restful state. Then, perhaps through additional suggestions by the guide, but more often without any further suggestions, the subject may experience a reliving of the evolutionary transitions from gill stage up through "hominization." The experiencing of evolutionary phenomena already has been sufficiently exemplified in the fourth case presented in Chapter One.

Again, the explanation for these vivid experiences probably is to be found in the application of imagination to knowledge collected by the subject during the course of his life and which may or may not be accessible to him under other, non-psychedelic conditions. Alternatively, it might be proposed that what we encounter here is an activation of the phylogenetic inheritance.

The extent to which the factual and directional content of symbolic level and some other drug experiences may have been supplied and determined by the guide, through nonverbal communication as well as spoken hints, is yet another factor to be considered. For it is clear that just as an analyst of Freudian, Jungian, existentialist, or other orientation will elicit from patients dream and other materials appropriate to the analyst's orientation, so does the psychedelic guide elicit materials appropriate to his orientation and interests and to some extent this will occur no matter how stringent and well-planned the precautions taken by the guide. The importance of this factor increases as we move into the area of the potentially transformative symbolic and analogic dramas.

Ritual. Throughout most of the history of man the importance of ritual has been clearly recognized, for it is through the ritual acts that man establishes his identity with the restorative powers of nature or marks and helps effect his passage onto higher stages of personal development and experience. Ritual is the province of renewal and emergence and without its authority man tends to lose sight of purpose and meaning. Man without ritual is man without sanctions, and this, as we know, results in a condition in which the energies of life remain abstractions and man becomes alienated from nature, from other persons, and from himself.

It has been theorized that many of the problems of modern man stem from the fact that he has few if any effective rituals by means of which he is able to experience catharsis and rebirth. Western civilization since the Renaissance is one of the few social orders that does not provide for emotionally powerful rites of renewal and emergence. An anomalous situation thus has been created in which the accumulated ritual requirements of the millennia have been ignored with consequent repression and deflection. It is thus of extreme interest to observe the frequency with which subjects in psychedelic sessions seek relief from tensions and a way out of alienation precisely through participation in ritual dramas.

The most frequently occurring ritual theme experienced on the *symbolic* level is that of the eternal return. The subject usually experiences this theme in terms of the redemption of the vegetation cycle leading to a redemption of human consciousness. In many cases the theme unfolds through a drama replete with such a richness of historical and anthropological detail that again the source of the knowledge displayed arises as a problem confounding both subject and researcher. A striking case in point is the unfolding of interwoven mythic and ritual elements in the experience of a twenty-seven-year-old bookkeeper. This subject, S-1 (100 micrograms LSD), was a high-school graduate whose reading matter rarely extended beyond the daily newspapers and an occasional popular magazine.

The guide initiated the ritual process by suggesting to the subject that he was attending the rites of Dionysus and was carrying a thyrsus in his hand. When he asked for some details the subject was told only that the thyrsus was a staff wreathed with ivy and vine leaves, terminating at the top in a pine cone, and was carried by the priests and attendants of Dionysus, a god of the ancient Greeks. To this S nodded, sat back in his chair with eyes closed, and then remained silent for several minutes. Then he began to stamp the floor, as if obeying some strange internal rhythm. He next proceeded to describe a phantasmagoria consisting of snakes and ivy, streaming hair, dappled fawn skins, and dances going faster and faster to the shrill high notes of the flute and accelerating drums. The frenzy mounted and culminated in the tearing apart of living animals.

The scene changed and S found himself in a large amphitheater witnessing some figures performing a rite or play. This changed into a scene of white-robed figures moving in the night towards an open cavern. In spite of her intention not to give further clues, the guide found herself asking the subject at this point: "Are you at Eleusis?" S seemed to nod "yes," whereupon the guide suggested that he go into the great hall and witness the mystery. He responded: "I can't. It is forbidden. . . . I must confess . . . I must confess . . ." (The candidate at Eleusis was rejected if he came with sinful hands to seek enlightenment. He must first confess, make reparation, and be absolved. Then he received his instruction and then finally had his experience of enlightenment and was allowed to witness the mystery. How it happened that this subject was aware of the stages of the mystery seemed itself to be a mystery.)[2] S then began to go through the motions of kneading and washing his hands and appeared to be in deep conversation with someone. Later, he told the guide that he had seemed to be standing before a priestly figure and had made a confession. The guide now urged the subject to go into the hall and witness the drama. This he did, and described seeing a "story" performed about a mother who looks the world over for her lost daughter and finally finds her in the world of the underground (the Demeter-Kore story which, in all likelihood, was performed at Eleusis).

This sequence dissolved and the subject spoke of seeing a kaleidoscopic pattern of many rites of the death and resurrection of a god who appeared to be bound up in some way with the processes of nature. S described several of the rites he was viewing, and from his descriptions the guide was able to recognize remarkable similarities to rites of Osiris, Attis, and Adonis. S was uncertain as to whether these rites occurred in a rapid succession or all at the same time. The rites disappeared and were replaced by the celebration of the Roman Catholic Mass. Seeking to restore the original setting, the guide again suggested the image of the thyrsus. S imaged the thyrsus, but almost immediately it "turned into" a man on a tree (the Christ archetype). The guide then said: "You are the thyrsus," to which S responded: "I am the thyrsus. . . . I am the thyrsus. . . . I have labored in the vineyard of the world, have suffered, have died, and have been reborn for your sake and shall be exalted forevermore." These are the mystic words that with variations have been ritually spoken by all the great gods of resurrection—the great prototypes who embody in themselves the eternal return of nature and who, in a deeper sense, are identified with the promise of eternal life to righteous man.

The extraordinary aspect of this case lay not so much in the surface details, but rather in the manner, the meaning, and the sequence in which this material was evoked. We notice, for example, how the theme of eternal return, death, and resurrection, moves in the subject's mind from its initial confrontation in primitive rites to highly sophisticated and universal expressions. The sequence began with the Dionysian rites, an early Greek form of the celebration of the vegetation god's struggle, death, and rebirth, linked to the yearly triumph of spring over winter. There next appeared the ancient Greek drama which had in fact evolved out of the form of the Dionysian sacrificial ritual. (In the artistic transformation of this ritual in tragedy the audience no longer consumed the body and blood of the god, but instead experienced a spiritual and psychological ingestion of the body of the tragic hero and, in so doing, found new community and solidarity within itself.) The sequence then found a sublimation in the Eleusinian Mystery, the great ritual of catharsis and spiritual rebirth which itself grew out of the Dionysian rites. After this there followed a proliferation of many myths and rituals bearing upon the themes of the eternal return and culminating in the sophisticated expression of this theme in the Roman Catholic Mass. Finally, the subject himself indentified with the god-thyrsus and invoked the mystic words of renewal. The entire sequence told the same story— the drama of redemption seen on all levels at once; the redemption of the vegetation cycle and the redemption of the human consciousness— each seen through the prism of the tree-man dying to live and yielding, by death and resurrection, life to those of his cult or his cultivators.

Among the ritual materials most frequently encountered in the psychedelic sessions are the rites of initiation and rites of passage. The subject in the following example, S-2, was a twenty-four-year-old Jewish college graduate. At the time of his LSD experience he was working in a law office. (Dose: 100 micrograms)

The guide began the particular sequence by drumming on the table and suggesting that S envision an African rite of initiation—possibly a puberty rite. S then almost immediately began to describe a night scene involving many young boys who appeared to be moving around a fire on hands and knees and who were at the same time being flagellated by older men. The guide asked the subject if he minded the beating, to which the reply was: "No, it is quite necessary if I am to be reborn." He then described himself as being wrapped up in some kind of animal skins. The guide asked him if he knew what kind of skins they were, and was told: "Sheep . . . goat . . . I remain three days and am then reborn . . ." (The foregoing is especially noteworthy in that it confirms the schemas of initiation in which the symbolism of birth is almost always found alongside that of death.) S then discovered himself to be a baby floating in fluid (presumably in amniotic fluid) and moving down the birth canal, pushed along by the contraction of muscles. He next burst into uproarious laughter, for he had not emerged onto a hospital table as expected but, rather, into his own Bar Mitzvah (the Jewish rite of puberty). The guide asked S to attempt an explanation of the entire sequence. S said words to the effect that man is born of woman incomplete. Thus, there must be a second birth of a spiritual character in order for man to pass beyond his prolonged foetal condition. Man becomes completed by engaging in some significant event or rite of passage in which he is obliged to divest himself of his embryonic or prehuman nature and assume that condition in which he becomes fully Man.[3]

As the experience of many drug subjects suggests, and much historical and anthropological evidence demonstrates, the mystery of initiation (whether culturally staged or psychedelically induced) can deliver the young man from shallow adolescent understanding and render his life dimensional. Chastened by the vision of aspects of reality which include the sacred (or extended reality), he must be similarly extended and take upon himself the obligations of the adult state. He must die to his shallow nature and rise to his deepened one. This is a fact of existence about which we still seem to know, even while "officially" regarding it as a tenet properly belonging to archaic societies: that the process by which one attains to spiritual awareness or to a greater sense of reality finds expression in the thematics of death and rebirth. In its psychedelic expression as otherwise, the initiation has a profound and frequently transformative effect upon the participant. At the end of the session we have just described, S declared himself "reborn." Later, he stated that his experience had brought first deliverance and then meaning into his life, linking his personal destiny to that of mankind and liberating him from narrow and selfish purposes.

Specific Symbols. Among the devices employed to facilitate the subject's participation in allegorical dramas are specific, usually traditional symbols, which the subject is encouraged to contemplate, and historic, legendary and mythic figures, with whom the subject is encouraged to identify. The symbols and figures then serve both to trigger and flexibly configure the experience that follows. However, these ensuing experiences do not always take just the form intended, and we will briefly digress to examine several of the forms the deviations may assume.

Here, the guide either verbally suggests a symbol or presents an actual symbolic object—cross, star of David, religious statue—to the subject and proposes that he consider it.[4] In the psychedelic state, however, the symbol does not remain for long in its static configuration, but quickly dissolves and points beyond itself to the dramatic events from which it was condensed, or leads analogically inward to some personal struggle of the subject which it may effectively symbolize. Thus, a traditional symbol like the cross may open outwards upon such historical pageants as those of the crucifixion, the crusades, the inquisition, and so on, or open inward upon some personal drama of guilt and redemption.

S-3, a thirty-one-year-old male (LSD: 100 micrograms), was an attorney and former divinity student who had left the seminary because of religious doubts. For him, to move from religion to law had been to move from chaos to order. Concerning his experience arising out of contemplation of the cross, he writes:

"The guide handed me a heavy cross to hold. At first I didn't want to take it because of bad associations, but finally did so. It was a golden glinting thing, and soon absorbed my entire attention. I found myself observing its every facet with fascination and a kind of awe because every facet, every glinting particle became—when I focused my attention—some historical episode in the story of the cross.

"I saw Jesus crucified and Peter martyred. I watched the early Christians die in the arena while others moved hurriedly through the Roman back streets, spreading Christ's doctrine. I stood by when Constantine gaped at the vision of the cross in the sky. I saw Rome fall and the Dark Ages begin and observed as little crossed twigs were tacked up as the only hope in ten thousand wretched hovels. I watched peasants trample it under their feet in some obscene forest rite, while, across the sea in Byzantium, they glorified it in jeweled mosaics and great domed cathedrals. My hand trembled, the cross glimmered, and history became confused.[5] Martin Luther walked arm in arm with Billy Graham, followed by Thomas Aquinas and the armies of the Crusades. Inquisitorial figures leveled bony fingers at demented witches and a great gout of blood poured forth to congeal in a huge, clotted cross. Pope John XXIII called out "good cheer" to a burning, grinning Joan of Arc, and Savonarola saluted a red-necked hell-fire and brimstone Texas preacher. Bombers flew in cross formation and St. Francis preached to the birds. A hundred thousand episodes erupted from the glinting facets of that cross and I knew that a hundred thousand more were waiting for their turn. But then, and I don't know when or how it happened, I was immersed *in* it; my substance—physical, mental, and spiritual—was totally absorbed in the substance of the cross. *My* life became the glinting, sparkling episodes of the history of the cross, and the hundred thousand remaining events were those of my own life's history. The shame and victory of the cross was endlessly repeated in the minutiae of my own life. *Mine* was the shame and *mine* was the victory. I had been inquisitor and saint, had falsely damned and sublimely reasoned. And, like the cross, I, too, had died, and lived, and died, and lived and died to live again and again. And perhaps once more I would die. But now I knew (and now I know) that redemption is a constant thing and guilt is only transitory.

"Probably the most important thing that happened to me in that session was that I learned that life mirrors its greatest symbols and the cross was the mirror image of mine. That is why I left the seminary and why I had been so antagonistic to the cross. I had expected it to be a thing of constant triumph and had found that its course was as wayward as my own. I am no longer antagonistic. In fact, and I realize this sounds corny (but then, invariably, the corniest things are the truest), I have found that I serve myself best when I serve the cross, when I become, in the words of the old hymn, a Soldier of the Cross. So here I am, back in bondage to an impossible ideal, and damned glad of it!"

Subjects reaching the *symbolic* level of the psychedelic experience do not concern themselves exclusively with traditional or essential symbolisms. In a number of cases symbols hitherto unrecognized as "symbolic" have emerged spontaneously, pregnant with personal meaning, and have provided the subject with a living reality and a directional frame of reference previously unknown. These symbols, novel at least to the subject, would seem to be as effective as their better-known counterparts and like them provide psychic energy for the formation of new attitudes and for the development of more extended and mature states of consciousness. Examples of such emerging symbols have included a personal totemic animal (eagle, tiger, lion), whose idealized symbolic characteristics the subject seeks to realize in himself; geometric configurations (spirals, circles within circles); microcosm-macrocosm analogies; organic growth processes (especially as they occur in trees and flowers); and mandalas.

As an example of another variety of symbolic experience, the subject may wish to feel himself invested with the personality of some archetypal persona famous for sagacity and depth of understanding. Subjects often spontaneously display an inclination to assume the persona of the Wise Old Man in his ideal state or in some of his various historical and mythological disguises—Socrates, Chuang-tzu, Merlin, Winston Churchill. This phenomenon is especially intriguing to the observer in that the face of the subject frequently assumes an antique aspect, his body adjusts to an attitude appropriate to the patriarch, and he intones the weighty sentiments of an ultimate sage. Alas, however, the platitudinous pontifications of such psychedelic pundits rarely attest to any real increment of wisdom. Much more rewarding are the insights which appear to accrue to those few subjects who have succeeded in "putting on the persona" of the Wise Fool or King's Jester. With the assumption of this persona comes the tragicomic revelation into the nature of paradox as the essential construct of reality. The either/or insistence of the Western mind is abandoned in favor of a both/and approach to life and dualistic formulas are seen as an evil which one conquers by satiric laughter. One subject extemporized a verse to describe the understanding he felt he had gained through identification with the persona of the Jester:

> "I see behind the duality blind,
> And for this sight I rise in kind
> To King's own Jester—Fool Sublime,
> Immortal Idiot, Godly Mime."

Mythologies. In the psychedelic drug-state mythologies abound. The guide often may feel that he is bearing witness to a multi-layered complex of mythological systems as they arise out of their latency in the mind of the subject. If they are not produced spontaneously, the guide can elicit a remarkable exfoliation of diverse mythic images and archetypal settings. Lest the subject be inundated by this, the guide must help him to select the most personally meaningful and potentially valuable symbolic possibility out of the dozens that may present themselves, then giving further support and advice as the subject attempts to follow the chosen mythic structure through to its conclusion. As we have noted, the choice of the mythic structure very often will be determined by the preceding recollective-analytic level materials.

One constant of these mythological systems, in both their universal and particular aspects, is that as they emerge in the psychedelic session what they express is something *that never was but is always happening.* They usually relate to occurrences that cannot be specified in space and time but which nevertheless exert a powerful influence on culture and consciousness. The frequency with which they spontaneously appear in the experiences of the psychedelic subjects attests to their continuing potency and relevance to the human condition.

Mythic patterns frequently recurring in the drug-state fall within the following broad areas:

Myths of the Child-Hero
Myths of Creation
Myths of the Eternal Return (Cycles of Nature)
Myths of Paradise and the Fall
Hero Myths
Goddess Myths
Myths of Incest and Parricide (Oedipus, Electra, etc.)

Myths of Polarity (Light and Darkness, Order and Chaos)
Myths of the Androgyne (Male-Female Synthesis)
Myths of the Sacred Quest
Prometheus-Faust Myths[6] (Myths of the Trickster).

The myth of the child-hero is one that occurs in the psychedelic experience with considerable frequency. This motif is often relived in terms of historical and mythological analogues—Jesus, Moses, Heracles —and then is taken up by the subject in a more personal manner to suggest his rebirth experienced in terms of a newborn divine child emerging from the darkness of the womb and undergoing extraordinary dangers in order to begin a life of great promise. The figure of the child-hero becomes for the psychedelic subject a personification of the most profound aspects of his striving towards self-realization.[7] We do not have here, we believe, just a simple regression to an infantile state which presents the subject with an opportunity to "begin all over again." Rather, this appears to be a phenomenon of profound engagement in a potent and potentiating universal drama from which the person emerges with a sense of having been redeemed, transformed, and as some subjects have put it, "transfigured." In the following case we have an example of the child-hero motif as "lived out" during the course of a psychedelic session.

S-4, a businessman in his early forties (LSD: 100 micrograms), came to his session feeling that his very considerable business success had been purchased at the expense of an atrophied inner life, so that now he experienced himself as hollow and exhausted and had, for the past year, been strenuously attempting to remedy this condition. Neither a flirtation with Eastern mysticism nor a period of psychoanalysis had proved effective and he was left with serious doubts concerning his "spiritual worth."

S spent the first few hours of his session enjoying a variety of sensory phenomena and especially his experience of the range and intensity of light and color perception. He spoke frequently and with great enthusiasm about the "luminous quality" of objects and repeatedly marveled at the "aura" which he saw as emanating from his hands. About three hours into the drug experience (start of recollective-analytic materials), he began to speak compulsively of the "wasteland" of his life, enumerating the many lost opportunities for personal development he felt had marked the last twenty years of his life and bitterly condemning himself for his one-sided dedication to materialistic pursuits.

S described himself as having been a spiritually precocious child and adolescent, much given to prayer and meditation as well as to theological reflection. The death of his father when S was twenty-one years old left him the sole support of his mother and six brothers and sisters all much younger than himself. Thus, instead of being able to pursue the career in literature and philosophy that he had planned, S was forced to take over his father's business interests and at this he showed himself surprisingly adept. The praise and material rewards that came to him worked to increase the industry with which he applied himself to the business and by the time he had reached the age of forty he found himself wealthy and respected. But he also found himself with enormous material responsibilities and the feeling that the rich inner life he once had prized so highly was shrunken and virtually extinguished. This description of his present inner state profoundly distressed the subject, who repeatedly declared that: "I'm all dried up inside . . . dried up like a desert . . . dried up . . . dried up . . ."

S now obviously stood at a forking of the psychedelic road, with breakthrough one possibility, the other a circular self-reinforcing depression that would be both unrewarding and painful. To avoid this latter possibility, S was urged to lie back and close his eyes and was told (note close surface relation of images): "Perhaps instead of thinking of a desert, you will find it possible to think of a void. Think now of a void, a black, silent void. A void beyond life, beyond existence, beyond you, beyond me, beyond everything. Now there is a light coming faintly into this void. A light that is beginning to dimly illuminate the landscape. Tell me what you see there." What follows is the record of the subject's utterances as they were recorded by the guide. The story is told in terse sentences comprising a polyglot mythology of the child-hero with whom the subject identified. The actual (symbolic level) "incarnational" sequence took about forty minutes to unfold:

"Yes, the light is coming up. I see a woman lying on top of a mountain. . . . She is struck by a thunderbolt . . . and out of this union . . . I am born. A race of ugly dwarfs seek to destroy my mother and me . . . so she hurries down the mountain . . . hides me in a swamp . . . A serpent with great jaws flicks out his tongue . . . draws me into his mouth. . . . I am swallowed. . . . I am passing down inside the snake. This is horrible. Incredible demons line the shores of the snake's insides. Each tries to destroy me as I float by. . . . I reach the end of the tail and kick my way out . . . raining very hard in the swamp . . . I am drowning. . . . No. . . . I am caught in a net . . . being pulled out of the water. . . . An old fisherman has caught me in his net. . . . The serpent rises out of the water . . . grown into a huge sea monster . . . opens its jaws and snaps them shut on half of the fisherman's boat. With the next bite it will swallow both of us. A thunderbolt comes out of the sky and smashes the boat in two, leaving half of it stuck in the monster's gullet. The fisherman takes me in his arms and swims with me towards shore. . . . The sea monster pursues us. . . . Just as we reach the shore it snaps off the fisherman's leg. The fisherman continues to hold me and crawls with me in his arms to a nearby hut. His wife is there. She nurses her husband and puts me into a cradle. I am raised by this couple as their own son. They are very kind to me . . . tell me I must be very special seeing as how I was drawn from the water. . . . They call me Aquarion. The years pass. I am now four years old but already I am tremendously strong and powerful. . . . Also, I know the language of birds and flowers . . . talk to the animals and plants and learn many strange things. They tell me I must avenge myself on the sea monster who tried to destroy me and bit off my fisher-father's leg. I dive into the water to go and find the sea monster. . . . For many hours I swim around and finally I find it. It is swimming towards me at tremendous speed. It has grown gargantuan and horrible ugly . . . opens its jaws to consume me but I evade them and get a strangle hold on its throat. For many days we battle together. . . . The sea is crimson with our blood. . . . Great waves are created by our combat. . . . I am the conqueror . . . tear open its belly . . . I slay the internal demons. . . . In its stomach I find the leg of my fisher-father. I take the leg back to land and fit it onto his stump. It instantly joins and he is whole again. My parents take me to the temple to give thanks for my victory. . . . We approach the high priestess with a thanks offering . . . tell her my story. When she hears of it she swoons. . . . She comes to and says to me, 'My womb was quickened by the thunderbolt. You are the son of promise whom I hid so long ago.' She raises her hands to the heavens and . . . she says . . . 'Speak, O Lord, to this your son. Speak to his strength and his glory. He hath prevailed over the Evil One. He hath delivered the deep of its Enemy. Set your purpose upon him Lord.' A great thunderbolt shatters the air. . . . A thunderous voice speaks: 'Aquarion, my son, you are now your own man. Go forth into the Wasteland and bring forth fruit. Know that I shall be with you always and where once there had been drought . . . wherever you pass . . . there shall spring up a Green Land.' "

S recounted this classic and fully developed scenario of the child-hero in a hushed monotone, as if he were reciting the forbidden liturgy of a mystery rite. He seemed to be speaking from far away, or from so deep inside of himself that one had the general impression that his was a disembodied voice. His body and face remained impassive, almost death-like during the recital, giving one the eerie feeling that the subject was living in another time and place while his body and its vocal cords served as the feeble link from one world to another. It took him almost an hour to "rejoin the living," during which time he lay with his eyes open, speaking not a word and apparently reacting to nothing. He said almost nothing else for the rest of the session, except at the very end when he bowed slightly to the guide, smiled, and said "Thank you." Several days later he felt more like talking and said that the session had been the most important, most profound and most intense experience of his life. His "inner state," he reported, was burgeoning "like a spring garden" and he felt that his life had been "transfigured" by the "new being" which had emerged out of the depths of his psyche. He felt that his experience had been so transparent an allegory that interpretation would be ridiculous.

This frequently occurring phenomenon of the "transparent allegory" is one of the most important and most curious met with in the psychedelic drug sessions. Psychodynamic materials which in the context of the dream would emerge as ambiguous or inscrutable events and (presumed) opaque symbols, represent themselves on the *symbolic* level of the drug-state as unveiled mysteries in which the drama of the self is played out within a lucid series of sequential stages bearing the subject along to a moment of powerful resolution. So continually explanatory is the symbolic process on this level that it sometimes happens that the subject, should he "miss the point," is immediately "provided" with an eidetically imaged diagram or illustrative cartoon. He may even receive a series of such clarifying images and keep on receiving them until he fully understands, when the main sequence will resume just where it left off.

The fact that S's symbolic drama was rooted in the thematics of a great number of child-hero legends served to enhance the emotional power and meaningfulness of the experience. The student of comparative mythology will recognize in this subject's experience patterns common to the legends of Sargon, Gilgamesh, Marduk, Moses, Heracles, Perseus, Dionysus, Cyrus, Jesus, Krishna, Parsifal, and a host of Year-Daimons, as well as important themes in the poetry of T.S. Eliot (whose poems, especially "The Wasteland," S greatly admired).[8] Each of these legends as well as the subject's own symbolic creation reflects the allegory of the self in its search for wholeness. As Jung has observed, the various child-heroes "may be regarded as illustrating the kind of psychic events that occur in the entelechy or genesis of the 'self.' The 'miraculous birth' tries to depict the way in which this genesis is experienced. Since it is a psychic genesis, everything must happen non-empirically—e.g., by means of a virgin birth, or by miraculous conception, or by birth from unnatural organs. The motifs of 'insignificance,' exposure, abandonment, danger, try to show how precarious is the psychic possibility of wholeness, that is, the enormous difficulties to be met with in attaining this 'highest good.' They also signify the power-lessness and helplessness of the life-urge which subjects every growing thing to the law of maximum self-fulfillment, while at the same time the environmental influences place all sorts of insuperable obstacles in the way of individuation. More especially the threat to one's inmost self from dragons and serpents points to the danger of the newly acquired consciousness being swallowed up again by the instinctive psyche, the unconscious." [9]

Several years now have passed since this subject's session and the divine child, he says, "continues within" him. He feels that the need no longer exists to maintain a dichotomy between his inner spiritual and his outer professional life—since the "Green Land" is continuous and compatible with both. The child-hero remains effective as his "activating symbolic agent," helping him to preserve the "whole man" he has become. Thus again, in this case, we encounter the impressive but little understood phenomenon of timeless, universal symbols and themes emerging into consciousness in a particular dramatic form adapted to the requirements of the psychedelic drug subject who becomes the drama's protagonist and thereby is transformed.

The Forest in the Psychedelic Allegory. One of the more frequently occurring settings for the symbolic drug-state dramas is that of the forest. This, of course, is not surprising since, as Zimmer has put it, "All that is dark and tempting in the world is to be found again in the enchanted forest, where it springs from our deepest wishes and the soul's most ancient dreams." [10] In the context of the psychedelic state, the meanings of the forest are various and complex; but for many subjects it would seem to indicate the realm of the soul itself wherein the self may find its deepest meaning.

Those mythic dramas occurring in the forest setting are mostly

European in type and largely Celtic—abounding in princes, maidens, castles, executioners, dragons, dungeons, secret words, talking horses and birds, enchanted frogs and the like.[11] The subject confronts these familiar figures from the Celtic mythology with a shock of recognition —seeing in the figures now revealed as inhabitants of his own deep psyche enigmatic bearers of ancient answers to the riddle of existence.

In the following case we have an example of a subject whose symbolic drama takes the form of the Celtic-type myth or fairy tale. In the course of its elaboration the subject develops elements relevant to her own life situation and finally arrives at insights providing a basis for important changes in her outlook and behavior. The subject, S-5, was a newspaperwoman in her late twenties (peyote).

After a period of several hours during which she did little more than remark that her images and perceptual changes were aesthetically not at all up to what she had expected, S closed her eyes, grimaced, and began to describe at length a sequence of images in which she became increasingly involved. She now found herself, she said, in the courtyard of an old and evil-looking castle which lay just at the edge of what seemed a vast forest. The atmosphere was medieval and the castle was complete with moats and turrets and towers from which blue and red pennants were flying. The courtyard in which she stood was crowded with a holiday throng of extremely ugly people who she likened to figures in paintings intended to portray the character- and physiognomy-destroying effects of gluttony, drunkenness, etc. Like herself, these figures were dressed in costumes which she described as belonging to the Middle Ages.

The crowd's attention was focused upon a young woman who stood on a platform just behind a large block of wood, and at whose side was standing a masked executioner holding a huge ax. Next to S was standing an immensely fat woman with brightly rouged cheeks, or cheeks reddened by the wind, and S asked her what was going on, receiving the half-chortled response: "Why, it's heads-off day!"

No sooner had S received this answer than the young woman fell to her knees, placed her head on the block, and the executioner lifted up his ax, then severed the head with a single blow. The head fell to the ground and lay face upward, and S recognized the face as her own. However, she had no time to think about this since the young woman's body began running around the courtyard like that of a decapitated chicken, splattering the onlookers with blood. The crowd cheered and jeered and the body finally fell at S's feet, one of its hands grasping S's ankle in a painful death grip. S tried frantically to free herself from this clutch, but to no avail. Then the brawny executioner strode towards her and pulled the hand free of her ankle. S felt that her ankle had been severely bruised by the headless body's steely grip and then discovered that she was unable to walk. The executioner then said he would take her to a place where she could rest. He picked her up and, holding her under one powerfully muscled arm, he carried her up a flight of crumbling stone steps to a room at the top of a tower where he placed her on a couch.

S now observed the executioner closely and saw that he was a huge, brutish, cruel-looking man. He wore the traditional executioner's black sack over his head, with slits cut in it for eye holes, and another slit for the mouth through which she could see that his lips were fat, red, and sensual. There seemed to her to be something strangely familiar about this man, and suddenly it came to her that in a curious, distorted way he resembled her own husband.

The executioner smiled at her, revealing broad, thick teeth and asked if she was hungry. When she said that she was—for suddenly S had discovered that her appetite was ravenous—he walked to a kind of heavy oaken sideboard on whose panels many "menacing" symbols had been carved and returned with a large bowl filled with grapes. S took two of these and was about to swallow them when she noticed that what she held in her hand were two intense black eyes that fixed her with an unwavering malevolent glance. She screamed, leaped to her feet, ran down the steps, through the now-empty courtyard, and into the forest. (S now was totally involved in the drama. Her images were vivid, she was breathing heavily, her face was reflecting powerful emotion, and her body, although she remained in her chair, went through motions appropriate to the unfolding events.)

S ran for "a long time" through the darkness of the forest, her terror at first increased by glowing eyes and dim but sinsister and threatening forms that appeared at the edges of the path along which she was running. Then, gradually, as she felt herself safe from the executioner, the forest lightened, the dim forms seemed "neutral" and then "maybe even friendly," the trees lost their grotesquely gnarled appearance, and at last she reached a pleasant glade where the sun shone down upon the grass and decided to rest for a while under a shade tree. She seemed to fall into a kind of half-sleep, during which she "dreamed" that she wandered in a forest that was "a place of great security." Only, eyes hung in clusters like grapes from certain trees having almost-human forms and she felt a strong impulse to eat two of these but could not bring herself to reach out and pluck them from the clusters. She "awakened" from this "dream" and discovered that a man was standing over her.

This man was inquiring if something was wrong, and at once she told him she had injured her ankle while running through the forest. He said that he would like to help her and she noticed that he was younger, better formed, and more handsome than the headsman. He was also a kindlier figure and yet he, too, wore a mask and had a curiously distorted appearance. She then thought that he resembled in some way the headsman, and that he also resembled her husband, and began to grow afraid.

The man picked her up under one arm, carried her to the bank of a beautiful river or stream, and gave her some clear, cold water to drink. He asked if she was hungry, she discovered that her appetite was ravenous, and she said she would like to have something to eat. He brought her a bowl of grapes, she took two, and was ready to put them into her mouth when she noticed that they were not grapes but rather two melancholy-looking brown eyes. She became very frightened, cried out, leaped up, plunged into the stream and then was borne along on its waters for a long time. Finally, the waters washed her up on a shore at the edge of the forest where another castle stood. This castle seemed newly built and had about it nothing of the evil aspect of the first castle. She discovered that in jumping into the stream she had injured her ankle, and now hobbled painfully towards the castle, where she hoped to find help and sanctuary.

She entered the open door of the castle, walked down a long, narrow, high-ceilinged hall, and entered a room where she sat down on a long wooden chest which had panels on which many strange but somehow "good" symbols had been carved. A man entered the room and she noticed that he was younger, better-looking and gave the impression of being "much warmer and more human" than the headsman and the man in the forest. However, he was wearing "a kind of purple Halloween mask" that covered his eyes, except for the eye slits, and had at its bottom a piece of cloth that hung down to just above his lips. His face was not distorted, but veiled by the mask, and she had the feeling that she would recognize his face if he only would take off the mask.

The man asked her in a gentle way what she was doing in the castle and she explained that she had injured her ankle, had had many terrible adventures, and now had no place to go so that she hoped she would

be permitted to stay in the castle for a while. The man smiled and
nodded and then instructed her to follow him. She started to get to her
feet but her ankle collapsed beneath her and she fell to the floor. He
then picked her up, holding her in both his arms, and carried her into a
dining room containing a long table. He placed her on a chair and asked
her if she would like something to eat, whereupon she discovered that
her appetite was even more ravenous than it had been before. When she
admitted this, he brought her a bowl of grapes. She picked up two of
them and started to put them into her mouth when she noticed that
what she held were two clear, penetrating blue eyes. Her impulse was to
throw them down and run away, but now it seemed to her that she
could not run anymore and she placed the eyes on the table in front of
her and said she no longer was hungry.

She asked the man to remove his mask. He then told her that he was
not wearing a mask and that she was unable to see his face for just the
same reason she had been unable to see the faces of the other two men.
She needed new eyes to see with, he said, and she again was being
offered those eyes. Now it was up to her to accept what was being
offered. Upon hearing this, she suddenly picked up the eyes, popped
them into her mouth, and swallowed them down at a gulp. At once, she
saw before her the unveiled face of a very handsome and "wholly
trustworthy" young man who bore a striking resemblance to her husband. At the same time, she knew that he was also the man at the first
castle and the man in the forest. But the man at the first castle had not
really been an executioner. There had been no execution and the be-
heading of the girl whose face was her own face had represented a
projection of her own fears with regard to the man and his intentions
toward her.

S now sat up and with great intensity began to interpret the eidetically imaged sequence. This sequence, she said, with its dreamlike,
nightmarish flavor corresponded to aspects of her own life wherein she
had been seeing "everything as if from in a nightmare." Her distortion
of the three men reflected the distorted view of her husband she had
been taking in her daily life. She had misinterpreted his every attempt to
help her to see things in their proper light and to his every act of
kindness towards her she had attributed a fiendish motivation. Whenever he had denied such motivation, and insisted that "This is not at all
why I am doing these things," S had stubbornly refused to believe him.
Now, she thought that he had been trying to give her "eyes to see
with."

S then began to vividly recall an "almost forgotten" incident that had occurred a few years earlier and did much, she thought, to explain some particulars of her drug-state drama. She recalled that she and her husband were on vacation and had gone for a horseback ride in a large wooded area. He was riding his horse at a fast pace and was some distance ahead of her when she, trying hard to catch up with him, had been knocked from her horse by a tree limb and had fallen to the ground, badly spraining her ankle. Her husband had not noticed her fall and had kept on riding. For several hours she had remained on the ground in great pain, all the while building up a fantasy concerning her husband's motive in thus "abandoning" her. She thought that her husband had seized on the opportunity presented by her fall to ride back to the hotel and initiate an affair with an attractive woman guest who had shown interest in him. Then she decided that her husband probably thought she was badly injured and was leaving her alone in the woods with the hope that she would die. Finally her husband returned and told her that he had ridden some distance before noticing that she was not behind him. Then, in looking for her, he had become lost and had had much difficulty in relocating the trail. This story, which S now viewed as "wholly plausible," had been rejected by her at the time in favor of the version constructed while she lay weeping on the ground. Afterwards, she became increasingly suspicious and "downright paranoid" about her husband's behavior and motives. By the time of her session, she felt, this had even resulted in her seeing him in a distorted way. She had begun to visually perceive him as looking "almost like the brutal executioner," instead of seeing him as "rationally" she knew him to be—i.e., his appearance was close to that of the good-looking young man in the second castle. But now, the distortions had "dropped away" and in her "mind's eye" she "saw" a picture of her husband that she felt was the true—and attractive—one. S felt that "my unconscious has been playing me tricks," but now she was "over all of that." In fact, in the ensuing months it became evident that the subject's relationship with her husband was enormously improved. Ten years after her peyote experience S continues in a marriage she describes as "very happy" and believes would certainly have ended in divorce "had I not been shocked back into my senses."

This case is especially interesting in that it well may shed light on the mythopoeic process, particularly as it is involved in the genesis and elaboration of the fairy tale. Its details clearly disclose how ugly and threatening figures and settings serve to represent in a fictionalized but life-analogous sequence the problem persons, conflicts, and anxieties of the individual. It further shows many points of both similarity and difference between the drug-state symbolic drama and the dream—the former utilizing readily decipherable symbols as the plainly analogous sequences unfold; the latter, with its usually opaque or heavily veiled symbols withholding from us in most cases its detailed meaning and relevance.

In this case of S-5, the classic symbolism of the subject's experience progresses steadily from the dark to the light, from the ugly and threatening to the beautiful and comforting, as S moves in the direction of enlightenment. The first pair of grape eyes offered her are black and malevolent, in keeping with the other components of her situation. The second pair are brown, in keeping with the other components. Finally, the eyes become an acceptable blue and their clear and penetrating quality suggests to her the kind of vision she needs and wants. She then has only to eat the eyes to incorporate their capacity for clear and penetrating vision into herself. Similarly, the men grow progressively handsomer and more reassuring; the second castle is much pleasanter than the first; and so on.

As the subject later explained in some detail, the forest was for her a place of catharsis. The first castle lay on the edge of this forest—was "a kind of hell at the outer edges of the possibility of redemption." The ugly, vicious-looking people in the courtyard, who had gathered there to applaud the execution, were personifications, she felt, of her own self-destructive tendencies and also of the "evil and ugly suspicions" she had entertained with regard to her husband. She felt that the execution itself was a warning that she was threatened by a psychosis if she continued to create delusional patterns concerning her husband's motives. By such behavior, she was putting her head on the block and asking to lose her head—i.e., become psychotic—"at the hands" of the distorted version of her husband she had fabricated.

When S ran into the forest she passed successfully through its dark, menacing areas and moved towards a place of light, experiencing what she later saw as her "first catharsis—a liberation from most of the morbid, destructive ideas." She "needed to get into nature and there fall asleep to the old self." After she awakened, everything looked better than before. Her "second catharsis" occurred when she leaped into the stream and was borne along by its waters, finally to be washed up on a shore near "the other edge of the forest," where stood the castle representing the terminus of the redemptive process. She experienced the waters of the stream as a cleansing of her spirit and later remarked that she had emerged from the waters with a feeling of having been reborn. She now was sufficiently wise (having seen the evils of her former condition) and strong (having been cleansed and reborn) to be able to take the offered gift of clear vision. However, she remained crippled (the injured ankle, which also referred to the horseback riding accident) so that she could only approach the gift of vision with the help of her husband who carried her towards it, holding her in both of his arms (not under one arm, as had happened in the previous episodes). The experience of the forest, she felt, "meant principally in my case a restoration to my own nature, through the contact with Nature. The forest was terrifying in the beginning because of my alienation from nature—both my own nature and Nature. All of its terrors are products of such alienation. It then follows that the closer one gets to one's nature, and to one's basic roots in Nature, the more the forest becomes home and its plants and creatures take on a friendly and lovely appearance. But man is something more than Nature, and must finally rise to some extent out of it, leaving behind him, although not without regret, some of its more primitive aspects—the things of the forest, for example. We have to keep our rapport with Nature, even while our own nature has to rise above it. The castle was, on another level, what man has built in rising above nature. It preserved its contact with Nature by remaining on the edge of the forest—but this second castle was 'above and beyond' Nature, while the first castle, also on the forest's edges, was almost 'below' it, and showed me that man's nature is such that he may not only alienate himself from Nature, but also descend to an unnatural level where he goes beyond Nature by sinking to depths that leave him at the very bottom of everything, looking back up at what he has lost with mixed feelings of fear and regret. Then he has to 'climb back up' through the forest, which will be a terrible ordeal in the beginning. He has to re-experience all of Nature, good and evil alike, but then he at last becomes one with it, is at home there again, and is able to stand with one foot at least out of, and beyond, the forest."

In fact, the experiences of various drug subjects suggest that the forest often has such a meaning, and that the forest is peopled with ogres and other fearsome monsters about to the extent that the person (and perhaps the culture) has become estranged both from his own nature and from Nature. This sense of being estranged from one's own nature is also a fairly common one with the drug subjects. What they mean by this, it would seem, is a sense of having been deflected away from proper goals, of having become bogged down in "unnatural" pursuits—i.e., artificial and meaningless entertainments, striving for status through acquisition of "symbolic" things, etc.—and of having relinquished candor for hypocrisy, individual freedom for the security of the collective irresponsibility of the mass. The forest, then, is a place where individuation is restored, while at the same time the individual regains his sense of *being one* with that Nature of which he is a part and which is also the very ground upon which he stands. Individuality re-stored, and the sense of oneness with nature regained, the forest is depopulated of its monsters; then, if the experience is sufficiently pro-found, the person returns to a world that also has been depopulated of monsters, no longer experiencing himself as anxious or hostile where no real threat or enmity exists.

The forest in drug-state allegory also can be a place of childlike enchantment—a place where infantile wishes meet with immediate mag-ical gratification, where pleasures have about them the soft, moist qual-ity of dreamy suckling and no intensity intrudes to awaken even by the sharpness of rapture the voluptuous passivity. The security is of the womb or of a maturity-rejecting absorption in childish symbols having about them all the seriousness and substance of caramel-coated red apples and pink cotton candy. Here, the forest is dotted with Hansel and Gretel cottages and licorice trees, while Bambi-like fawns frolic in the pale green glades and an occasional resident dwarf or goblin peeps innocuously out from between bushes frosted with multi-colored icings. Sometimes the eidetic images of the forest resemble those Disney car-toon films in which real persons move against the artificial backgrounds or, conversely, comic-strip persons and animals move against a "real" background. This last, of course, is an extreme form—indicating an extreme regression on the part of the subject.

In less extreme versions of the fairy-tale enchanted forest the setting may function principally as a means of demonstrating quickly to the subject his immersion in immature attitudes which he must now go beyond. Then, the subject seeks to find his way out of the forest and his decision to do this is also a decision to "grow up" and assume the attitudes and responsibilities demanded by maturity.

In the following case we have an example of regression and "recog-nition" in the "enchanted forest" by a subject who saw her main prob-lem as an incapacity to love on a mature level—an incapacity she felt she had "extended" until she felt cut off in other areas of her life as well. This, in turn, had resulted in a "drinking problem," since only when slightly intoxicated did she feel capable of giving to others the large amounts of love, understanding, and concern that she wanted to give. She felt "blocked by something inside" of herself from giving this love of which she knew she was capable. And the "blocking" she attributed to the negative influence of her mother, a rigid perfectionist, who had demanded that the subject adopt a stoic philosophy and ascetic way of life, along with goals so impossibly high that the subject could only fail repeatedly to achieve them and, then, finally rebel. But the mother's constant criticism had made the daughter extremely self-conscious, and the mother's belittling of emotional states as compared to "analytical reason," had taken its toll of the subject's capacity for emotional response. Although her mother had been dead for many years, the subject continued to have a strong sense of her mother's presence as a traumatizing influence, referring to her as "my Super Ego-Mind-Mother."

This subject, S-6, age thirty-nine, was the wife of an extremely successful lawyer (LSD: 200 micrograms). She had had three previous LSD sessions with another investigator. During one of these there had occurred a profound "rebirth" experience. This, she said, helped her considerably but did not give her in full measure the capacity for involvement or ability to love that she so much wanted. Subsequent unguided experiences with peyote did not give her her "breakthrough" either. Psychotherapy indicated that S had no severe psychiatric problems but perhaps, in accordance with her early training, was trying to exceed her natural limitations and was drinking too much because of her frustration at her inability to do so. Her "drinking problem" was a problem only within her own family. Otherwise, she was functioning in a superior way in her day to day life and gave the impression of a warm, vivacious and—ironically—much "involved" person. She understood that the session was not intended to be therapeutic but rather would require her co-operation in furthering the research of the guides. She expressed a particular hope that she would have a "religious experience."

About thirty minutes after having taken the LSD S experienced a variety of sensations. The roof of her mouth seemed to be dissolving and, at the same time, there was a heightening of sensitivity in the pelvic area. She then felt herself to be hollowed out "like an egg that has been punctured so that its insides are pouring out." This meant, she said, that "I am emptying out. I want to fill the emptiness with Oneness, with the Thinker-feeling synthesis. But do I want feeling even if it brings anxiety with it? A part of me would settle for peace." S was silent for about fifteen minutes and then said that she was "waiting for the curtain to go up." Shortly afterwards she found herself on a moor, where "a lovely, lambent, luminous mist swirled" around her and was "implicit with the promise of sunrise." It was a pearly gray mist and had "a quality of tenderness, of softness." S was happy there because she knew she had only to wait and the pale silver sun would rise when it was time. She fell silent again and, when asked how she felt, said: "I feel good. The sharp edges of me are gone . . . the edges that are always bumping into me. But this place where I am now is not where I'm going to be, it's just a place along the way."

About ten minutes later (and a little less than two hours into the session), S announced that she was in "an enchanted forest." In this forest were all of the elements of the child's fantasy, although the fact escaped her at the time: Hansel and Gretel houses, candy trees, pastel landscapes. She had many innocuous adventures, proclaiming that she felt "like the protagonist of every myth that ever has been." One of these themes occurred repeatedly, as S began to sense that this soft, dreamy world might trap her and prevent her from reaching her goals. She spoke of Odysseus, enchanted by Circe, and unable to devise a way to escape the enchantment. The forest now became "a dangerous enchantment . . . This isn't life. This is like being in a beautiful quicksand. I want to wake up! I have to wake up!"

For many hours, almost the whole day, S wandered in the forest, repeatedly seduced by its beauty only to rediscover her danger and cry out her need to "awaken from this dream-like enchantment." After several hours, asked what it was she wanted to awake to, she responded that: "The mist is always here, but occasionally it lifts. Then I am able to see the Citadel, the Kingdom, and the Power and the Glory, high on a pinnacle in crystal-clear air. I long to reach it. I know that if I reach it I will experience awakening. The air will smell fresh and cool and the blossoms will be scented. I will feel as if I have taken a cold shower in magic water. There will be a coolness, a cleanness, a purity that I have never felt totally." Throughout the remainder of her session, S was largely caught up in a struggle to reach the Citadel. The forest-Citadel image was finally, at the very end of the session, replaced by another, similar image; but the session ended with S having failed to reach her ultimate goal.

In several follow-up reports S offered additional and instructive materials concerning her experience of the forest. She writes:

"First of all, the landscape the whole time was largely pink and white. The air was white, not translucent, and yet I could see perfectly. Perhaps I could better describe it by saying that there was a core of clarity in which I moved and which extended around me for some distance, but then the wall of white fog started, so that I was enclosed in a little world of my own clarity. This circle of clarity moved with me when I moved, rather like a spotlight following a player on a stage, so that I never actually went into the mist where I would have been blinded by it.

"The landscape (and all this was partly visual, partly 'mental' images) was Disney-like. . . . There were gingerbread houses, and spotted young deer like Bambi dancing through the forest. The trees had sort of Disney shapes and the people whose presence I felt, although I did not meet any, were Cinderellas, Sleeping Beautys, and Marys with their little lambs. All of this was quite charming. There was no feeling of lurking wolves to bother Little Red Riding Hood, or any kind of fairy-tale monsters. Hansel and Gretel were there someplace, but there wasn't a sign of the witch! There was, because of this, and because of the pink-and-whiteness, a real enchantment.

"There came a time when I left the tiny world of clarity and went deeper into the white mist. At first, there was a peace, a cessation of striving, of struggle, a blissful nothingness; just swirling mist, shutting me off from discord, and strife, and noise, and confusion. I felt that I could rest there forever content, safely blanketed by the enveloping fog, provided for and protected from life.

"Meanwhile, back at the womb . . .

"Gradually this peace was disturbed. I began to resent the pervasive mist. I wanted to be free of its clinging tendrils, its staleness. I began to wander through it. . . . I began to come out of the mist and then I saw the Citadel, the impregnable place of *real* security, the home of Love and Purity and Awakening, high on a rocky peak, brilliant and glowing with jewel-deep colors in the unbelievably brilliant clarity of the air. I moved toward it, up the steep hill, until my body was in the clarity from the knees up. I couldn't see me below the knees; I was still enveloped in the white enshrouding mist.

"And that's as far as I got! In my LSD sessions to date I have gone from being surrounded by a constricting black girdle to a gray barrel and now to a white fluid mist. Next time total clarity maybe?"

As indicated by her "Meanwhile, back at the womb . . ." remark, S subsequently recognized the regressive character of her experience of the forest. In communications written several weeks after her session, and which we here combine, she comments on this regression:

"That (Bambi, Cinderella, *et al*) part of the enchanted forest was childhood, immaturity. It was a world of superficial prettiness, of unreal values, of fairy tale rewards—a world, in short, that I suspect most of us inhabit. . . . I am amused in thinking of the prevalence of pink and white, the colors I tuned in on, although other colors were there. What else is a little girl's bedroom?

"I have since had a strange and lengthy dream and what I gleaned from it was this: The Disneyland core of the forest, which was surrounded by the dense mist was, in its own way, a land of enchantment. But it was the land of childhood or immaturity in which the inhabitants still believe in fairy-tale endings—'they married and lived happily ever after,' etc. As long as these illusions last the forest is a lovely place to live, and the air is good, and there are clear streams, and mushrooms and berries, and easy laws which everyone knows and obeys because those are the laws they want—the 'rules' of the 'game.' But there comes a time for some of us when this changes, when the air becomes noxious, the mushrooms turn into toadstools, the berries are poisonous, and the streams polluted. Then one must move on.

"Move on, if you like, on pure faith alone, leaving the core of enchantment and walking alone into the mist, seeking the Citadel. It is a hard thing to do. The forest's inhabitants are full of dire prophesies. 'You must not go,' they say. 'No one who left has ever come back. There are monsters who live in the mist, and roots to trip you up, and quicksand to swallow you. If you go away from here, from us, you will die a horrible lonely death.'

"But what we know, we searchers, is that if we stay to eat the toadstools, to breathe the poisoned air, to drink the stale water, we will *surely* die. The risks hidden in the mist are better than certain death, and clarity and love and purity lie at the end of the mist.

"So we start our trip, armored only in the hope that if we dash our foot against a stone, Someone will support us.

"I think that those for whom the forest has become unlivable, but who, for lack of courage, or faith, or hope, stay behind, become our alcoholics, our drug addicts, our neurotics, and our psychotics—and, obviously, our suicides.

"Well, that's it, for what it may be worth to you. It is worth a great deal to me, and I am finding my way out of the mist."

Such are some of the meanings of the forest in this seventh decade of the twentieth century.

A Note on Consciousness and the Symbolic Drama. Participation by the subject in the symbolic drama requires the effective, harmonious **coexistence** and functioning of not less than seven distinct states **or** types of consciousness. These seven, to which others doubtless could be added, we will enumerate briefly as follows:

A residual environmental and "guardian" consciousness: monitors the symbolic drama but does not otherwise participate in its unfolding. This faint consciousness in effect stands sentinel in the "real world" in order that the person otherwise may become fully engaged in the symbolic sequence. It constitutes the subject's link with the "real world" and, in a way not disruptive of his engagement in the symbolic sequence, is the means of his continuing awareness of himself as physically existing in an objective environment distinct from the environment of the drama. It reminds him, too, that these psychical events in which he now more or less fully participates are *only* psychical, or imaginary, and have as their precondition the psychedelic drug he has taken. This residual environmental consciousness is able, should the need arise, to intrude itself vigorously to disrupt and even terminate the drama in case events in the external world require that the subject function in that world.

Imagistic consciousness: the consciousness that visually perceives the eidetic images (actually, the consciousness that *is* the eidetic images) and so seems to serve the person as his "organs of sight" in the world of the drama.

Dramatic consciousness: the consciousness that "thinks about" and "keeps track of" what is going on in the "world" of the symbolic sequence. It is more or less comparable to its counterpart in the everyday world with the exception that additional important functions are likely to be required of it. First, since the subject does not *hear* what is said by the persons who speak to one another in the drama, this consciousness is responsible for communication and serves, in effect, as the hearing apparatus and voice of the subject. To further clarify, it might be explained that there is in the drama no sense of telepathic or other extraordinary communication. Only in recollection is the subject likely to become aware that no words were spoken aloud or other sounds heard as they are in the course of life in the "real world." Rather, at the time of the drama, this aspect of the imaginary world seems perfectly natural and one has no sense of not speaking and hearing in the ordinary way. Moreover, when the eidetic images are lacking but the drama nonetheless unfolds, this consciousness has to serve also as the eyes of the subject, so that he *knows* the "visual" content of the experience in the same way that he knows the "auditory" content. In the absence of eidetic images, then, there will have to be "mental images" which seem to fall within the functional province of the dramatic consciousness. This consciousness also may affirm the there-ness of unseen presences and the occurrence of events not actually experienced in the drama. For example, S-6 "felt" that Cinderella, Sleeping Beauty and the others were in the forest, but S did not "meet" them.

Somatic consciousness: consciousness of sensations experienced in terms of the drama—pleasure and pain sensations, odors, etc., experienced in response to the imaginary dramatic stimuli. There also may be a residual normal somatic consciousness, providing the subject, for example, with a faint awareness of his body as touching the couch upon which he is lying.

Somatic-kinesthetic consciousness: consciousness of one's body as moving in response to the dramatic stimuli or in terms of the action of the drama. These movements are mostly token approximations, their range limited by the body's situation in the real world. Here, too, there may be a residual consciousness that these movements are being performed in the real world—upon this couch, and thus are visible to whatever other persons may be in the room. In some cases, this particular residual consciousness then operates to inhibit movement, "advising" the subject that his movements are such as later may be a cause of embarrassment, or perhaps that he is in danger of falling off the couch.

Affective consciousness: consciousness of responding emotionally to the dramatic stimuli. In addition to consciousness of making emotional responses appropriate to the events of the drama, there may be consciousness of another kind of affective state which has few parallels outside the psychedelic drug experience and, even there, is only met with under certain conditions. This is the affective consciousness experienced in those instances where the drama reaches a resolution of the sort that may be transformative of the person. It is that affect experienced at the time when "everything falls into place," when the crucial relevance of the drama to the life stands revealed, or when this is about to occur. Here, the subject becomes acutely aware of a powerful emotional "atmosphere" or "climate" that seems to press heavily, but not at all unpleasantly, in upon him. It is as if, by sheer weight, this affect were exerting a pressure to impress upon his psyche the important insights being "given." This emotion, unlike some experienced in terms of specific dramatic events, is "quiet," but it is not for that reason any the less profound or forceful. Since it is almost always a very different affective consciousness from any experienced apart from certain symbolic- and integral-level drug-state stages, it is difficult, if not impossible, to describe to the person who has not experienced it. But the intense affect somehow manages to convey to the subject a sense of controlled prevoluntary purposiveness and complete beneficence.

"Spiritual" consciousness: this state of consciousness, the experiencing of which we feel well may have contributed to the idea of an indwelling human "spirit," is a strange and almost always hitherto unexperienced awareness carrying with it a curious nonspatial and a-temporal "flavor of eternity." The consciousness discloses itself in the subject's gradually intensifying sense of participation in the drama through a psychical component of the self of which no previous awareness existed and which is sensed as having as a precondition of its emergence the falling away of the spatial, temporal and other existential categories serving to delimit the existent in the "real world." The consciousness then is finally of universals, of essences and noumena somehow constituting the ground of the subject's, and of the world's, particular existence. Again, we have here an awareness which emerges with few exceptions only under certain conditions of the symbolic and more uniformly throughout the experiencing of the integral level. Almost always unprecedented in the experience of the subject, it will rarely have any precedent in the experience of the reader either, so that we may be trying against insurmountable odds to communicate what is incommunicable and requires to be experienced.

This orchestration of states of consciousness should be kept in mind when, in the next chapter, we consider the authentic varieties of the religious and mystical experience.

In the psychedelic experience the progressive deepening and ultimate transformation of conscious life are less the result of self-transcendence "towards the world" than of the gathering enrichment consequent upon increasing knowledge with improved understanding of more of what the self contains within itself. In the case of the symbolic drama the expansion basically involves a movement beyond the limits of the particular-personalistic and towards the personal-universal—a movement towards broadening contexts and more universal formulations that has, however, as its precondition the achieving of adequate knowledge with sufficient understanding of that which then may be surpassed.

As we have shown, if the subject has been able to confront and then go beyond the significant literal and empirically grounded data of his life, he then may move to a level of possible symbolic encounter with broader and more profound aspects of his nature. Here, the self reveals itself to consciousness more completely than has been possible hitherto, with consciousness "living" the ensuing symbolic drama in terms of patterns that have become simultaneously personal and universal. Beyond the surface and the literal, then, seems to lie *in potentia* for consciousness the self's larger vision and comprehension of itself; and, also *in potentia*, a dynamism possible of drug-state (and possibly non-drug-state) activation and which, to the analytical consciousness, increasingly represents itself as an entelechy now "liberated," activated, and functioning. Further, this entelechy appears to achieve its effects by means of symbolic systems most often formally structured along archaic lines as myths, rituals and other motile and plastic forms appropriate to the end of realizing the transformation of the particular in the universal.

When one inquires as to why this entelechy emerges clothed in the archaic symbolism of the mythic form it further may be suggested that in the symbolic mythic drama (as in the drug-state religious experience) consciousness is confronted with a context one of the essential characteristics of which is a primordial state wherein space and time remain undifferentiated; that this primordial state is characteristic of the deepest levels of the psyche; and that the mythic drama is just that temporally and spatially undifferentiated form into which consciousness most easily and effectively may be drawn with the result that a new consciousness is born. Moreover, consciousness, no sooner entering as participant into the drama, finds itself also in this primordial "eternal" state which by disallowing the preconditions of individuation (i.e., particularity in real space and time), allows for involvement in the universal myth as distinguished from the strictly individual factual or fictional sequence and in the essential as distinguished from the exclusively particular existential reality.

That the symbolic dramas occur on a depth level of the psyche "deeper" than that on which occur such phenomena as revivification of past experiences, recovery of lost memories, and other factual historical materials seems evident both on the basis that the latter recollective-analytic level materials and experiences characteristically precede the symbolic level phenomena and are a prerequisite in most cases of meaningful symbolic level experience, and also on the basis that the transformative effects of the recollective-analytic experiences and materials, like their counterparts in psychoanalytic psychotherapy, provide insights essential to growth, remission of symptoms, and even elimination of neuroses, but cannot abruptly and in a fundamental and positive way transform the individual as may the symbolic level experiences and, still more, the experiences on the yet deeper integral level.[12]

Thus, in providing a means of access to these deeper symbolic and integral levels of the psyche the psychedelic drugs open up the possibility of working in areas little or not at all touched by psychoanalysis and other therapies unable to penetrate beyond those psychical levels where the encounter is with the literal life-history materials and related affect; they also open up the possibility of work on these levels that aims not at restoring the sick to health, but at enabling the comparatively healthy to realize growth potentials thwarted by processes science has not yet even begun to describe, much less to understand.

Nine:
Religious and
Mystical Experience

One of the most important questions raised by the psychedelic drugs is whether authentic religious and mystical experiences occur among the drug subjects. To this question the answer must be Yes—but we feel an extended discussion is warranted and that many qualifications are in order.

In our experience, the most profound and transforming psychedelic experiences have been those regarded by the subjects as religious. And in depth of feeling, sense of revelation, semantically, and in terms of reorientation of the person the psychedelic religious and religious-type experiences certainly seem to show significant parallels with the more orthodox religious experiences. These parallels alone would be sufficient to demand extensive and careful study.

Undoubtedly it would be the supreme irony of the history of religion should it be proved that the ordinary person could by the swallowing of a pill attain to those states of exhalted consciousness a lifetime of spiritual exercises rarely brings to the most ardent and adept seeker of mystical enlightenment. Considering the present rapid assimilation on a mass cultural level of new discoveries, therapies, and ideologies, it then might not be long before the vested religious interests would finally have to close up shop. And no less renowned a prophet than the late Aldous Huxley has suggested that humanity at large may in fact come to avail itself of psychedelic drugs as a surrogate for religion.

Since his statement appeared in 1954, the controversy has raged between those like Huxley, Gerald Heard, and Alan Watts who believe that in these chemicals the evolutionary acceleration of man's spiritual nature is now at hand, and other writers such as R.C. Zaehner who contend that these drugs at the most produce a very minor sort of nature mysticism and moreover tend to vitiate higher forms of religious and mystic expectations.[1]

Before considering this debate in the light of our own findings, it should be of value to examine briefly something of the history of artificially induced states of mystical and religious consciousness. We do this in order to demonstrate to the reader the unbroken line of continuity in the history of "provoked mysticism."

Since the time when man first discovered that he was a thinking organism in a manifold world, he has sought to marshal his analytic capacity to control the manifold and discover its natural laws. As a parallel movement to this analytic process there developed as an undercurrent another way of knowing—one that sought to discover man's essential nature and his true relationship to the creative forces behind the universe, and to discern where his fulfillment lay. For the sake of achieving this integral knowledge men have willingly submitted themselves to elaborate ascetic procedures and have trained for years to laboriously master Yoga and meditation techniques. They have practiced fasting, flagellation, and sensory deprivation, and, in so doing, may have attained to states of heightened mystical consciousness, but also have succeeded in altering their body chemistry. Recent physiological investigations of these practices in a laboratory setting tend to confirm the notion that provoked alterations in body chemistry and body rhythm are in no small way responsible for the dramatic changes in consciousness attendant upon these practices. The askesis or ascetic discipline of fasting,[2] for example, makes for vitamin and sugar deficiencies which acts to lower the efficiency of what Huxley calls the cerebral reducing valve.[3]

Similarly, the practice of flagellation will tend to release quantities of histamine, adrenalin, and the toxic decomposition products of protein—all of which work to induce shock and hallucination. With regard to sensory deprivation, the work of D.O. Hebb at McGill University in Canada and that of John Lilly at the National Institutes of

Health in Washington demonstrates on the laboratory level how the elimination of external sensory stimuli can result in the subjective production of fantastic visionary experiences similar to those reported by St. Anthony during his vigil in the desert or the cave-dwelling Tibetan and Indian hermits who live out great segments of their lives in complete isolation. Other techniques of "provoked mysticism" include breathing exercises rhythmically performed to alter the composition of the blood and provide a point of concentration, extended chanting (which increases the carbon dioxide content of the blood), hypnosis, prayer dancing (employing body oscillations which induce trance and presumed physical changes), the spinning frenzy of the whirling dervishes, and so on.

The most comprehensive and consciously controlled system of disciplines is, of course, the Hatha Yoga which incorporates the practices of posture regulation, breathing exercises, and meditation. Its immediate aim is to bring under conscious control all physiological processes, so that the body can function with maximum efficiency. Its ultimate aim is to arouse what is called *kundalini*, a universal vital energy which is supposed to gain its access to the body at the base of the spine. When aroused and controlled, it is said to activate the psychic centers and thus make available to the yogi unusual powers. It is claimed that if this energy can be directed to the head center (the thousand-petalled lotus), a mystical state is attained and the yogi becomes aware of a mystical unitive consciousness. To this end the early Sanskrit psychophysical researchers developed a remarkable knowledge of physiological processes and their relation to body control.

Thirty years ago, in a volume entitled *Poisons Sacrés, Ivresses Divines*, Philippe de Felice provided considerable documentation to support the ages-old connection between the occurrence of religious-type experiences and the eating of certain vegetable substances. He wrote that the employment of these substances for religious purposes is so extraordinarily widespread as to be "observed in every region of the earth among primitives no less than among those who have reached a high pitch of civilization. We are therefore dealing not with exceptional facts, which might justifiably be overlooked, but with a general and, in the widest sense of the word, a human phenomenon, the kind of phenomenon which cannot be disregarded by anyone who is trying to discover what religion is and what are the deep needs which it must satisfy.[4]

De Felice advanced the thesis that one of the earliest known of the substances, the *soma* of the Vedic hymns, may have been indirectly responsible for the development of Hatha Yoga. The *soma* appears to have been some kind of creeping plant which the Aryan invaders brought down with them from Central Asia about 1500 B.C. The plant occupied an integral position in the myth and ritual structure of Vedic religion, was regarded as divinity, and was itself ritually consumed to bring the worshiper to a state of divine exhilaration and incarnation. "We have drunk soma and become immortal," hymns the early Vedic author. "We have attained the light, the gods discovered." According to de Felice, as the Aryans moved deeper into India the gods proved more difficult to find as the *soma* plant, like fine wine, would not travel. The exercises of the Hatha Yoga school, he suggests, may have been created as an attempt to fill the "somatic" gap and achieve that physiological state of being conducive to religious states of consciousness similar to those brought on by the ingestion of the sacred food. The larger implication of this thesis is that vegetable-provoked mysticism exists as a state prior to askesis-provoked mysticism—that early man may have come upon his first instances of consciousness change through his random eating of herbs and vegetables. Certainly this thesis can never move beyond the realm of conjecture, although the fact remains that naturally occurring mind-changing substances are found the world over and are much more likely to have been experimented with before the creation of any system of mind-changing exercises.[5]

For millennia man has been involved in the ritual ingestion of substances reputed to produce an awareness of a sacramental reality and has come to incorporate these substances into the myth and ritual pattern of the culture in which they occur. The words *haoma, soma, peyote,* and *teonanacatl,* all of which refer to God's flesh, are significant semantic referrents to the religious experiences believed to be inherent in the sacred foods.

One of the major archaeological discoveries of recent years has been the digging up on the Guatemalan highlands of a great many stone figures representing mushrooms out of whose stem emerges the head of a god. Thus the mushroom appears to have been hypostatized as deity as early as 1500 B.C. These figures occur as Aztec artifacts as late as the ninth century A.D. However, the earlier figures are technically and stylistically of finer craftsmanship, indicating a flourishing cult in the early pre-classical period. By the sixteenth and seventeenth centuries of our era reports of such a mushroom cult occur in the writings of Spanish explorers and priests. They naturally regarded these rites as demonically derived celebrations and soon made certain that they were driven underground. The rites, as noted, continue to survive today among the Mazatec Indians of southern Mexico where the ancient liturgy and ritual ingestion is still performed in remote huts before tiny congregations.

In recent years the cult has been subject to a great deal of publicity owing chiefly to the efforts of that well-known mycophile R. Gordon Wasson. In thirty years of search for the secret of the mushroom throughout the world, he and his wife believed that they uncovered the mystery among the Mazatec communicants. They persuaded a *curandera* or cult shaman to allow them to participate in the ceremony and swallow the sacred food. Recalling his experience, Wasson wrote that "as your body lies in the darkness, heavy as lead, your spirit seems to soar and leave the hut, and with the speed of thought to travel where it listeth, in time and space, accompanied by the shaman's singing and by the ejaculations of her percussive chant. What you are seeing and what you are hearing takes on the modalities of music, the music of the spheres . . . as your body lies there . . . your soul is free, loses all sense of time, alert as it never was before, living eternity in a night, seeing infinity in a grain of sand. What you have seen and heard is cut as with a burin in your memory, never to be effaced. At last you know what the ineffable is, and what ecstacy means."[6]

In a monumental study of the mushroom, *Mushrooms, Russia, and History*, the Wassons claimed to discover its sacramental usages in cultures widely distributed from the Levant to China; and they state that it even was known to the Norsemen of the Icelandic culture.[7] In addition to the Mexican cult, the rite continues today among certain shamanistic tribes in Siberia, the ritual object of the cult being the hallucinogenic mushroom *Amanita muscaria*. Because this variety of mushroom occurs widely throughout Europe, Wasson has advanced the hypothesis that it might provide an answer to the secret of the Elusinian mysteries. From certain Greek writings and from a Pompeian fresco there are indications that the initiate drank a potion and then, in the depths of the night, beheld a great vision. Aristides, in the second century A.D., speaks of the ineffable visions and the awesome and luminous experience of the initiates.[8] Wasson finds significance in the fact that the Greeks frequently referred to mushrooms as the "food of the gods," *broma theon*, and that Porphyrius is quoted as having called them "nurslings of the gods," *theotrophos*.[9]

However interesting is the notion of a mushroom-inspired Hellenic mystery, we suspect that Wasson's mycophiliac zeal exceeds his academic rigor when he suggests that Plato came upon his theory of an ideal world of archetypes after having spent a night at the temple of Eleusis drinking a mushroom potion.

The history of transcendental experience bears testimony to the thin line that often separates the sublime from the demonic, and to the frequency with which the one may cross over into the other. In demonic terms the visionary foods were extensively used, for example, by witches, especially during the period 1450 to 1750. As remarked, the witches drank and rubbed on their bodies concoctions the principal ingredients of which were the *Solanaceae* drugs contained in such plants as the thorn apple, mandragora, deadly nightshade, the henbanes, and others. The drug concoctions were employed at the Sabbats to produce hallucinations and disorientation, and also were taken at home for the purpose of inducing dreams and imagery of flying, orgiastic revels, and intercourse with incubi. So vivid were the nightmares and hallucinations produced by these drugs that witches frequently confessed to crimes they had only dreamed about but thought they had committed in the flesh.

The peyote ceremonies of the Native American Church have received sufficient treatment elsewhere in this book.

The historic sacrality of the visionary vegetables has since given way to the modern notoriety of the synthetic derivatives—especially, LSD, psilocybin, and mescaline. With regard to religious experiences as otherwise, one confronts these contemporary compounds with a host of puzzling questions. How, for example, may one reconcile the extremes of enthusiasm on the part of those who claim to find in these drugs a near-panacea for all ills and the key to mystical illumination with the vehement antagonism of those who are convinced that at best the drug-state mimics schizophrenia while at worst the drugs may wreak irreparable havoc with the psyche and possibly also irreparably damage the brain? Again the whole question arises as to whether these substances are consciousness-expanders or merely mind-distorters? In Savage's well-known phrase, do they provide "Instant Grace, Instant Insanity, or Instant Analysis?"[10] Finally, there is the tragic-comic denouement that these altercations have won for the drugs a pariah mystique. The problem with such a mystique is, of course, that it dictates that the pariah must go underground and there fester in cultic movements.

The contemporary quest for the artificial induction of religious experiences through the use of psycho-chemicals became a controversial issue with the publication of Huxley's *Doors of Perception* in 1954. In that book Huxley with his usual genius for the quixotic offered the suggestion that visionary vegetables in their modern synthetic forms could provide a new spiritual stimulation for the masses: one that was surer than church-going and safer than alcohol.[11] The actual experimental testing of the claims for the psycho-chemical-as-religious-surrogate occurred in 1962 on an occasion now known as "The Miracle of Marsh Chapel." As a part of his work on a Harvard University doctoral dissertation in the Philosophy of Religion, Dr. Walter Pahnke, an M.D., set out to test a typology of mysticism based on the categories of mystical experience summarized by W.T. Stace in his classic study of the subject.[12] Pahnke designed his experiment to test this typology on subjects who were given psilocybin in a religious setting. The subjects in question were twenty theology students who had never had the drug before and ten guides with considerable psychedelic experience. The theology students were divided into five groups of four persons, with two guides assigned to each group. After a preparatory gathering the groups moved upstairs to the chapel and the three-hour Good Friday service that awaited them. It was on this occasion that two of the subjects in each group and one of the two guides were given 30 micrograms of psilocybin, a fairly strong dose of that drug. The effects of psilocybin are very similar to those of LSD. The second guide and the two remaining subjects received a placebo containing nicotinic ingredients which provided the subject with a tingling sensation but produced no psychedelic effects. The drug was given in a triple-blind framework, meaning that neither subjects, guides, nor the experimenter knew which ten were getting the psilocybin and which ten were members of the control group and received placebos. The Good Friday sermon was preached and the subjects were left in the chapel to listen to organ music and to await whatever experiences they were to have.

What subsequently occurred has been described as "bizarre," "outrageous," and "deeply inspiring." As Pahnke's dissertation has not yet been published, we will not to be able to describe at this time the events that transpired in the chapel. However, it is permissible to say that nine subjects from the psilocybin group reported having religious experiences which they considered to be genuine while one of the subjects who had been given a placebo also claimed to have experienced phenomena of a religious nature. Typical of the responses was this excerpt from a report written shortly after the experiment by one of the subjects: "I felt a deep union with God. . . . I carried my Bible to the altar and tried to preach. The only words I mumbled were peace, peace, peace. I felt I was communicating beyond words."

In order to provide some material for a meaningful critique of this experiment the subjects' reports were read by three college-graduate housewives who were not informed as to the nature and background of the reports, but were asked to assign to each a rating of *strong, moderate, slight,* or *none,* according to which of these terms best applied to a subject's statement in the light of each of the nine elements of mystical experience listed in the mystical typology provided by Pahnke. According to Pahnke, the statistical results of these ratings indicated that "those subjects who received psilocybin experienced phenomena which were indistinguishable from if not identical with . . . the categories defined by our typology of mysticism.[13]

Various other studies would seem to attest to the mystico-religious efficacy of the psychedelic drugs. For example, in an attempt to explore the "revelatory potentialities of the human nervous system," Dr. Timothy Leary and his associates arranged for 69 full-time religious professionals to take psilocybin in a supportive setting. Leary has subsequently reported that over seventy-five percent of these subjects stated after their sessions that they had experienced "intense mystico-religious reactions, and considerably more than half claim that they have had the deepest spiritual experience of their life."[14]

In another study by two Californians, a psychiatrist and a psychologist respectively, Oscar Janiger and William McGlothlin reported on a study involving 194 LSD subjects (121 volunteers and 73 as part of a program in psychotherapy). The drug was given in a nonreligious setting so that presumably religious expectations did not influence the subjects as was the case with the Leary experiment. Below is a statistical abstract of their findings, based on a questionnaire answered by the subjects ten months after their sessions:

	JANIGER-MC GLOTHLIN (NONRELIGIOUS SETTING) N= 194 Percent
Increased interest in morals, ethics . . .:	35
Increased interest in other universal concepts (meaning of life):	48
Change in sense of values:	48
LSD should be used for	

becoming aware of oneself:	75
gaining new meaning to life:	58
getting people to understand each other:	42
An experience of lasting benefit:	58

It also should be added that ten months after having taken the drug twenty-four percent of the 194 subjects still spoke of their experiences as having been "religious."[15]

Two other similar studies should be mentioned because of the remarkable percentages reported with regard to the subjects' feeling that they had had a religious-type experience. Both experiments were conducted by psychiatrists but whereas one provided a supportive environment for the session, the other not only was supportive but also was structured in part to provide the subject with religious stimuli. This second procedure resulted in significantly higher percentages of subjects reporting religious experiences.[16]

	DITMAN AND HAYMAN (SUPPORTIVE ENVIRONMENT)	SAVAGE (SUPPORTIVE ENVIRONMENT AND SOME RELIGIOUS STIMULI)
	N= 74 *Percent*	N= 96 *Percent*
Feel it (LSD) was the greatest thing that ever happened to me:	49	85
A religious experience:	32	83
A greater awareness of God or a Higher Power, or an Ultimate Reality:	40	90

Taken altogether these findings must be regarded as remarkable. In the five studies just cited between thirty-two and seventy-five percent of psychedelic subjects will report religious-type experiences if the setting is supportive; and in a setting providing religious stimuli, from seventy-five to ninety percent report experiences of a religious or even mystical nature.

The reader is surely by this time wondering what to make of the claims of these researchers. Are they psychedelic Svengalis employing suggestion to play upon the sensitized psyches of their hypersuggestible subjects, imposing whatever delusions they might need or wish to impose? Or may it be that they themselves are deluded and fail to understand that in present-day America a man or woman will put a check next to "had a religious experience" if a drug has helped him or her to feel in some impressive way "different" than usual? There can be no doubt that the psychedelic drugs give the subject experiences very "different" from any the average person is likely to have had. For the most part the drug-state resembles neither the effects to be gotten from alcohol nor those resulting from amphetamines and tranquilizers. Does the present-day subject, then, having little or no familiarity with what is meant by the terms "religious" and "mystical" (other than something undefinedly exciting), adopt these words by default to describe the novel phenomena he has encountered during his session (and finds conveniently present on the questionnaire)? The Eastern scholar R.C. Zaehner offers a sophisticated version of this argument in his book attacking Huxley's position, *Mysticism, Sacred and Profane*. In this work Zaehner presents a closely reasoned and scholarly look at the classical records of religious and mystical experience and concludes that drug-induced mysticism falls so far short of the experiences of saints and holy men that a subject is badly misleading himself if he feels that he has undergone an authentic religious experience. "Preternatural" experience, the experience of transcendence and union with that which is apprehended as lying beyond the multiplicity of the world, is very common experience indeed, Zaehner argues. Not only is it common to nature mystics, but it recurs regularly with poets, monists, manic-depressives, and schizophrenics. Whether one is dealing with the "cosmic emotion" of the nature mystic, the "almost hysterical expression of superhuman ecstasy" found in a poet like Rimbaud, the bliss of subject-object dissolution, or the rapture of psychologically dissociated states, one is dealing exclusively with "preternatural" phenomena and not with authentic religious or mystical experience. Zaehner deems all psychedelic drug experience, be it madness, monism, or nature mysticism, to lie entirely within the province of such preternatural experience.

The further implication of Zaehner's thesis is that these drugs can never induce theistic states of religious and mystical experience which he regards as the supreme and authentic religious experience. The other two forms of mystical experience which Zaehner recognizes, nature mysticism in which the soul is united with the natural world and monistic mysticism in which the soul dissolves into an impersonal Absolute, are infinitely inferior states of religious awareness as compared to theistic mysticism in which the soul confronts the living, personal God.

Here Zaehner's position is clearly open to criticism. Apart from questioning the value hierarchy which Zaehner ascribes to the three kinds of mysticism, one might take him to task for suppressing the evidence for drug-induced theistic mysticism. As is well known, the peyote rituals of the Native American Church are frequently productive of theistic religious experiences. James Slotkin, an anthropologist, has noted that the Indians during these ceremonials "see visions, which may be of Christ Himself. Sometimes they hear the voice of the Great Spirit. Sometimes they become aware of the presence of God and of those personal shortcomings which must be corrected if they are to do His will."[17] (Slotkin, it should be added, had observed the Indians' rites and been a participant in them.) And, in any case, the phenomenon of specifically theistic versions of psychedelic mysticism is an ancient and widespread tradition.

Needless to say, Zaehner's arguments have provided ammunition for many theologians and churchmen who refer to religious experiences induced with the help of psychedelic drugs as "chemical religion," "cheap and lazy religion," "instant mysticism," etc., and who charge that the use of the drugs for such a purpose amounts to "irreverently storming the gates of heaven." However, there is no avoiding the fact that Zaehner's critique has the ring of an eleventh hour *tour de force*. One philosopher sympathetic to the use of the drugs for religious purposes says that "Zaehner's refusal to admit that drugs can induce experiences descriptively indistinguishable from those which are spontaneously religious is the current counterpart of the seventeenth-century theologians' refusal to look through Galileo's telescope or, when they did, their persistence in dismissing what they saw as machinations of the devil. . . . When the fact that drugs can trigger religious experiences becomes incontrovertible, discussion will move to the more difficult question of how this new fact is to be interpreted."[18]

In our own experience, the evidence would seem to support the contentions of those who assert that an authentic religious experience may occur within the context of the psychedelic drug-state. However, we are certainly less exuberant than some other researchers when it comes to the question of the frequency of such experiences. It is not here a question of our having had fewer subjects who claim to have had a religious experience—over forty-five percent have made this claim; rather, because of the criteria employed, a large number of these claims have been rejected by us. The difference therefore is one of criteria rather than of testimonial opulence.

In our attempt to develop unbiased criteria for the authentic religious experience we have employed the usual measuring devices; however, we have also found it important to place some emphasis on what we have termed the "depth level" of the experience. The literature of nondrug religious and mystical experience appears to lend considerable support to this criterion. It is significant to note, for example, that in this traditional literature the writers repeatedly deal with and emphasize the stages on the way to mystical enlightenment and describe these with metaphors suggesting striking analogies to the psychodynamic levels hypothesized in our psychedelic research. Again and again, the literature reveals comparable gradations or levels of experience as the mystic moves from acute bodily sensations and sensory enhancement to a heightened understanding of his own psychodynamic processes, through a stage inhabited by visionary and symbolic structures, until at last he achieves the very depths of his being and the luminous vision of the One. This level is described as the source and the ground of the self's unfolding and represents the level of confrontation with Ultimate Reality. The most important of the experiences reported by William James in *The Varieties of Religious Experience* are of this type in which the person seems to be encountered on the most profound level of his being by the Ground of Being. Religious experience can be defined, then, as that experience which occurs when the "depths of one's being" are touched or confronted by the "Depth of Being." Mystical experience differs from this in degree, not in kind. This latter occurs when one's personal depths dissolve into the "transpersonal" depths—when one is unified at one's deepest level with the source level of reality.

Mystics and religious personalities have repeatedly warned against accepting states of sensory and psychological alteration or visionary phenomena as identical with the depths of the spiritual consciousness. These warnings go unheeded today by many investigators of the psychedelic experience who seem to accept the subject's experiences of heightened empathy and increased sensory awareness as proofs of religious enlightenment. Doubtless some of these experiences are analogous in some way to religious and mystical experiences. But religious analogues are still not religious experiences. At best they are but stages on the way to religious experiences. And a major problem in this research to date is that it has been conducted by persons unfamiliar with the nature and content of the religious experience. Thus claims are made that can be misleading.

For example, a subject may have a euphoria-inducing experience of empathy with a chair, a painting, a person, or a shoe. This may result in protestations of transcendental delight as chair, painting, person, and shoe are raised to platonic forms and the subject assumes himself to be mystically enlightened. Too often in these and similar situations the guide will offer reassurance to the subject and so reinforce his belief that he is having a religious experience. But by doing this, the guide may prevent the subject from descending to a deeper level of his being where a genuinely religious and transformative experience then might be had.

Given this type of misunderstanding, it is no wonder that the psychedelic drugs have resulted in a proliferation of "fun" mystics and armchair pilgrims who loudly claim mystical mandates for experiences that are basically nothing more than routine instances of consciousness alteration. The mandate being falsely and shallowly derived, the subsequent spiritual hubris can be horrendous, the subject announcing to whoever will listen that all mystic themes, all religious concepts, all meanings, and all mysteries now are accessible and explainable by virtue of his "cosmic revelation." It is frequent and funny, if also unfortunate, to encounter young members of the Drug Movement who claim to have achieved a personal apotheosis when, in fact, their experience appears to have consisted mainly of depersonalization, dissociation, and similar phenomena. Such individuals seek their beatitude in regular drug-taking, continuing to avoid the fact that their psychedelic "illumination" is not the sign of divine or cosmic approval they suppose it to be, but rather a flight from reality. Euphoria then may ensue as a result of the loss of all sense of responsibility; and this can and often does lead to orgies of spiritual pride and self-indulgence by those who now see themselves as the inheritors of It! In fact, they come to spend several days a week with It! And all mundane concerns, all earthly "games" seem superfluous and are abandoned insofar as circumstances will allow.

The situation is complicated by the fact that many such persons are caught up in a quasi-Eastern mystique through which they express their disenchantment with the declining Western values and with the proliferating technology, the fear of becoming a machine-man, and the yearning for some vision of wholeness to turn the tide of rampant fragmentation. This vision they pursue by means of a wholesale leap to the East without, however, having gained the stability, maturity, and elasticity needed to assimilate the Eastern values. Few have the spiritual sophistication of a Huxley or have spent as many years of study and training in quest of methods of achieving the spontaneity and integration elaborated in the teachings of some schools of Vedanta and Mahayana Buddhism. Thus the leap out of the "games" and everyday "roles" of Western reality is usually into a nebulous chaos seen as Eastern "truth." It is an added misfortune that the psychedelic drugs may genuinely give some inkling of the complexity of Eastern consciousness, although the vista usually uncovered is no revelation but merely a glimpse—one that would require years of dedicated study before it could be implemented and made effective in day-to-day existence.

To at least some extent the responsibility for this seduction of the innocent must lie with such authors as Huxley, Alan Watts, and others who in their various writings imposed upon the psychedelic experience essentially Eastern ideas and terminology which a great many persons then assumed to be the sole and accurate way of approaching and interpreting such experience. Armed with such terminology and ideation, depersonalization is mistranslated into the Body of Bliss, empathy or pseudo-empathy becomes a Mystic Union, and spectacular visual effects are hailed as the Clear Light of the Void.[19]

It should by now be evident why the authors discount as belonging to the class of authentic religious and mystical experience a good many cases in which the data of altered sensory perception and other ordinary drug-state phenomena are hypostatised by the subject as having sacramental or religious significance. Among our own cases, that of the young woman in the opening chapter who perceived the objects around her in terms of "holy pots" and a "numinous peach" is clearly not an example of religious experience as the rest of her account goes on to make clear. This subject is indulging in a commonplace practice of psychedelic subjects—the describing of various uncommon experiences in terms of sacramental metaphors.

This is not to suggest that religious insight and religious-type experience never occur in combination with an experience of sensory enhancement. The interpretation accompanying the perception may result in revelatory insights. A famous case in point is the divinity school professor contemplating a rose: "As I looked at the rose it began to glow," he said, "and suddenly I felt I understood the rose. A few days later when I read the Biblical account of Moses and the burning bush it suddenly made sense to me." Thus within the framework of the psychedelic experience one man's glowing rose can be another man's epiphany.

Analogues of the Religious Experience. The sensory, ideational and symbolic analogues of religious experience are not religious experience; but, at the same time, these may be productive of insights enabling the subject to live more easily and fruitfully than he was able to do before. In order to illustrate this point, we will reproduce here a description by a subject of an experience of extended sensory awareness bordering on nature mysticism and verbalized by the subject mainly in religious terms. Although the subject was at the time indifferent to religion, she found it necessary to make use of metaphors drawn from the religious vocabulary in order to formulate and communicate her responses.

The subject, S-1 (LSD), a housewife in her early thirties, was taken by the guide for a walk in the little forest that lay just beyond her house. The following is her account of this occasion:

"I felt I was there with God on the day of the Creation. Everything was so fresh and new. Every plant and tree and fern and bush had its own particular holiness. As I walked along the ground the smells of nature rose to greet me—sweeter and more sacred than any incense. Around me bees hummed and birds sang and crickets chirped a ravishing hymn to Creation. Between the trees I could see the sun sending down rays of warming benediction upon this Eden, this forest paradise. I continued to wander through this wood in a state of puzzled rapture, wondering how it could have been that I lived only a few steps from this place, walked in it several times a week, and yet had never really seen it before. I remembered having read in college Frazer's *Golden Bough* in which one read of the sacred forests of the ancients. Here, just outside my door was such a forest and I swore I would never be blind to its enchantment again."

The subject remained true to her vow and as of two years after the session continued to experience not only heightened sensory appreciation but also a kind of awe and reverence whenever she walked through her "Holy Wood." Thus, although the subject cannot be said to have had a religious experience in the forest, she unquestionably had an experience of the sensory transfiguration of a part of her everyday world so profound that she found it necessary to use the vocabulary of the religious life to describe her experience. Further, although S considered herself to be basically agnostic, her experience in the forest caused her to feel in herself an awakening to dimensions of reality to which she previously had been indifferent. Subsequent to the session she continued to remark in herself a growing interest in "spiritual matters," as she describes:

"Since that day I have had brewing in me a sense of the relevance of that forest for the other areas of my life and the life of my family. For I have come to realize that my way of seeing and hearing and smelling the forest in a way that was greater than any way I had ever seen and heard and smelled before was not because the forest was in any special way 'different' or even more 'sacred' than the rest of the world but because the rest of the world (and this includes myself and my children) was perceived by me with the eye of ordinary expectation. With this expectation life becomes just something that somehow you muddle through with no thought or hope of it ever being anything else. But that forest proved me wrong. I saw there and I knew then that there were dimensions to life and harmonies and deeps which had been for me unseen, unheard, and untapped. Now that I know that they are there, now that I have awakened to the glorious complexity of it all I shall seek, and perhaps some day, I shall find."

It is interesting to compare this subject's account of discovering unsuspected dimensions of life with the classic account of William James in which the great psychologist similarly evaluates his nitrous oxide experience in terms of a revelation of the levels of existence:

"One conclusion was forced upon my mind at that time, and my impression of its truth has ever since remained unshaken. It is that our normal waking consciousness, rational consciousness as we call it, is but one special type of consciousness, whilst all about it, parted from it by the filmiest of screens, there lie potential forms of consciousness entirely different. We may go through life without suspecting their existence; but apply the requisite stimulus, and at a touch they are there in all their completeness, definite types of mentality which probably somewhere have their field of application and adaptation. No account of the universe in its totality can be final which leaves these other forms of consciousness quite disregarded. How to regard them is the question —for they are discontinuous with ordinary consciousness. Yet they may determine attitudes though they cannot furnish formulas, and open a region though they fail to give a map. At any rate, they forbid a premature closing of our accounts with reality. Looking back on my own experiences, they all converge toward a kind of insight to which I cannot help ascribing some metaphysical significance."[20]

As noted, there are various odd and pathologicomimetic states of mind which seem to be especially productive of unfounded claims of religious and mystical experience. Depersonalization and empathy, for instance, can cause an ordinarily secular-minded subject to sound like a garrulous Hindu sage who has been transplanted into Southern California. It is not infrequent to hear these psychedelic Swamis intoning such "wisdom" as:

"The not-self of me yields to the Void of Becoming."
"You and I are One. One and God is All."
"We are Mind-ed by God and Self-ed by each other."
"My Isness is of God. My Supposed-to-be-ness is of Man."

Of course not all experience which falls short of being authentic religious experience is on so sophomoric a level. And some actually superficial experiences may sound quite authentic when taken out of their context in the session. Such is the following example which involves the not-too-rare psychedelic experience of feeling that one has been raised to a transcendental plateau from which it is possible to look down upon one's own mental processes in Olympian fashion and as if with the "eye of God." This Olympian perspective then leads not infrequently to religious or pseudo-religious phenomena.

S-2, a thirty-four-year-old sociologist (LSD), writes (with initial reference to his eidetic imagery):

"The surface of my mind, upon which I—evolved to a superconsciousness—looked downward, was revealed as a vast illuminated screen of dimensions impossible to calculate. I observed the myriad multiform ideas and images passing across it; and sensations and emotions, flowing inward and outward—whatever occurred within the psyche; perhaps, within the still larger, more complex totality of the self.

"From above, with absolute concentration, observing and sustaining all of this, I was—directing everything, controlling the internal events as one might control the carefully preconceived flights of innumerable aircraft, keeping each on course, preventing all miscalculations and wanderings that might lead to missed objectives and collisions and needless expenditures of energy.

"The light that illumined these images grew brighter and brighter until I was almost frightened by the intensity of the brilliance. I saw that perfect genius would require the perpetuation of the capacity so, from above, to visualize and direct and regulate. Perfect genius would be an unwavering perfect control of the positions and velocities of ideas and images, instantaneous pre-arranged channeling of impressions—all the internal events, from conception, held in view and directed.

"But then, in a flash of illumination, I understood that this perfect genius of which I conceived was nothing more than a minute and miserable microcosm, containing but the barest hint of the infinitely more complex and enormously vast macrocosmic Mind of God. I knew that for all its wondrous precision this man-mind even in ultimate fulfillment of all its potentials could never be more than the feeblest reflection of the God-Mind in the image of which the man-mind had been so miraculously created.

"I was filled with awe of God as my Creator, and then with love for God as the One Who sustained me even, as in my images, I seemed to sustain the contents of my own mind. It seemed to me that I stood in relation to the whole of the universe in somewhat the same relation as the universe, itself no more than a greater microcosm, stood to the Macrocosm that is God.

"Thus recognizing my own total insignificance, I marveled all the more at the feeling I now had that somehow the attention of God was focused upon me and that I was now receiving enlightenment from Him. Tears came into my eyes and I opened them upon a room in which it seemed to me that each object had somehow been touched by God's sublime Presence."

Read as here presented in the foregoing quotation this description might appear to be the report of a major revelation—an authentic religious experience. However, in the context of S's entire session, it loses most of its impact and importance and must be seen as no more significant than some other and not at all religious experiences of this subject. S was not changed in any important way by the "enlightenment" he said he had received, and a few days after the session S himself had relegated it to his personal stockpile of "interesting episodes."

Symbolic Analogues.   Since religious and other phenomena of the symbolic level have been discussed in the preceding chapter, we will consider here only a single aspect of symbolic analogues to religious experience—the eidetic images of an apparently religious nature experienced by almost all subjects. If taken uncritically, these images would seem to provide *prima facie* evidence of religious experiential content. However, the larger part of this imagery occurs without accompanying religious emotion, and we must conclude that it is a phenomenal curiosity of the drug-state and does not establish or portend any activation of religious or mystical states of consciousness. The following is a statistical breakdown of the kind and frequency of "religious" images as they have occurred among our drug subjects:

RELIGIOUS IMAGERY

	$N = 206$ subjects
	Percent
Religious imagery of some kind:	96*
Religious architecture, temples and churches:	91
Religious sculpture, painting, stained glass windows:	43
Religious symbols: cross, yin yang, Star of David, etc.:	34
Mandalas:	26
Religious figures: Christ, Buddha, Saints, godly figures, William Blake-type figures:	58
Devils, demons:	49
Angels:	7
Miraculous and numinous visions, pillars of light, burning bushes, God in the whirlwind:	60
Cosmological imagery: galaxies, heavenly bodies, creation of the universe, of the solar system, of the earth (experienced as religious):	14
Religious Rituals	
Scenes of contemporary Christian, Jewish or Muslim Rites:	8
Contemporary Oriental rites:	10
Ancient Greek, Roman, Egyptian, Mesopotamian and similar rites:	67
Primitive rites:	31

Certain comments should be made with regard to these statistics. Of the four percent of the subjects who did not report any religious imagery at all, these persons were, with two exceptions, completely imageless or imaged only geometric forms. This would seem to indicate that if a subject is able to image at all, then some kind of "religious" imagery is almost certain to occur as a part of the total eidetic image content.

The preponderance of imagery relating to religious architecture re-

* To the nearest percentage.

flects not so much a religious interest as an aesthetic appreciation of this generally most imposing and interesting of all architecture.

We will also note that some aspects of these statistics are more than slightly enigmatic. Why, for example, do ancient and primitive rites occur in the images so much more often than do the contemporary ones? Is it because the old rites reflect and minister to deep-rooted human needs that the modern rites do not, or is there some other explanation? Why do angels run such a poor second to devils? Here, it would seem that the devils and demons may be personifications of negative components within the psyche. Sigmund Freud, for one, undoubtedly would have remarked with great interest this apparent preponderance of negative over positive personifications of unconscious elements.

Another phenomenon of considerable interest is the fact that mandala (symbolic geometric diagram) imagery scores only eight percentage points less than imagery pertaining to traditional religious symbols. In this statistic one may be encountering evidence of the radical individuating tendency of the psychedelic process. The mandala is, after all, a highly personal symbolic form; in fact, the symbolic condensation of the thematics and dynamics of the person's own nature. It is the coded formula of the subject's personal mythos. The significant percentage of mandala imagery then may be testimony to one of the key phenomena of the psychedelic experience: the discovery and creative utilization of personal patterns of being against the backdrop of universal structures and sanctions.

The Integral Level. When we examine those psychedelic experiences which seem to be authentically religious, we find that during the session the subject has been able to reach the deep integral level wherein lies the possibility of confrontation with a Presence variously described as God, Spirit, Ground of Being, Mysterium, Noumenon, Essence, and Ultimate or Fundamental Reality. In this confrontation there no longer is any question of surrogate sacrality. The experience is one of direct and unmediated encounter with the source level of reality, felt as Holy, Awful, Ultimate, and Ineffable. Whether this Presence resides forever immanent in the integral realm of man's being or whether this realm provides the Place of Encounter between man and Presence remains a meta-question requiring no answer. The important thing is that the encounter does take place—in an atmosphere charged with the most intense affect. This affect rises to a kind of emotional crescendo climaxed by the death and purgation of some part of the subject's being and his rebirth into a new and higher order of existence. Specifically, the subject tends to feel that his encounter with Being has in some way led to the erasure of behavioral patterns blocking his development, and at the same time provides him with a new orientation complete with insight and energy sufficient to effect a dramatic and positive self-transformation.

Our major criteria for establishing the validity of these most profound religious and mystical experiences are three: Encounter with the Other on the integral level; transformation of the self; and, in most cases, a process of phenomenological progression through the sensory, recollective-analytic and symbolic levels before passing into the integral. In the case of these authentic experiences this progression has been at the same time a rich and varied exploration of the contents of these levels providing a cumulative expansion of insight and association until, at the threshold of the integral, the subject has experienced a comprehensive familiarity with the complex network of his being such as he had never known before. This process is greatly intensified and approaches culmination during the subject's passage through the symbolic level.

Comparative studies in the history of religion demonstrate the tendency in the life of a given religion or culture for the myth and ritual complex to exist as a stage prior to the development of the individuated religious or mystical quest. Indeed, it is a matter of cultural and psychological necessity that the myth and ritual pattern should dominate and precede the emergence of the mystic way for the one serves a more comprehensive role in the organic ordering and revitalizing of society and psyche, while the other involves a movement away from the social complex to a region of radical individuation.

It is significant then that in the levels of phenomenological progression revealed in the psychedelic experience, the symbolic realm with its abundance of myth and ritual material is, in most cases, experienced as preceding the level of integral and mystical reality. This relation of the symbolic to the integral will be illustrated in the following case.

The Authentic Religious Experience. In the highly unusual case to follow we present a detailed account of what we consider to be an authentic religious experience. It is also a transforming experience, one that profoundly and beneficially changes the person. The movement is continuous, beginning in the first of three psychedelic sessions, and reaching culmination in the third as the subject attains to the integral level. This case should be read as exemplifying better than any other we present the guided progression through the various hypothesized levels toward the climactic, transforming confrontation—here, a confrontation with God.

The (LSD) subject, S-3, in his late thirties, is a successful psychologist who has achieved much recognition in his field. Before offering any account of the sessions it will be necessary to discuss the background of the subject at some length. We should add that we have received from thoroughly reliable sources confirmation of many of the strange autobiographical materials first supplied us by the subject.

As we have found to be very often true, in its broad outlines the life of this subject may be seen as the re-enactment of a myth—in this case, the myth of the rebellious angel Lucifer who challenged the power and authority of God Himself and was cast down into Hell as a punishment for his pride. One of the most extraordinary elements in this case is the very early "choice" of the particular myth and the thoroughness with which the myth has been acted out in the subject's life.

In considering this case it may prove helpful to keep in mind several key points. S, since earliest childhood, has displayed a high degree of intelligence accompanied by a rich imagination continuously expressed in both his overt behavior and his abundant fantasy life. He has shown a constant tendency to represent his life to himself in terms of symbolic analogues. And he has long regarded the progression and details of his life as "a kind of 'art work,' initiated by a fertile childish imagination and subsequently 'improved upon' by an older imagination armed with immense amounts of esoteric data."

S is the only child of well-to-do Protestant Anglo-Saxon parents with whom his relations are good. As it has been described to him, he came into the world with long silky black hair growing over much of his body. His face at the time of his birth was wizened, he had teeth and resembled a tiny, ancient man. Shortly after his birth he developed pneumonia and "was born with or soon got a bad case of jaundice." His skin was wrinkled and yellow and his relatives thought him an extremely odd-looking baby, "a little old Chinaman," although his mother insisted she thought he was "quite beautiful." S was not expected to survive, but "surprised" his family and the physician "by somehow pulling through."

As a child, S was precociously intelligent, imaginative, and self-reliant. By the time he was four he could read and, at the age five, was reading pulp fantasy and science-fiction magazines as well as the usual children's books. Myths and legends of many lands, along with the works of Poe were read to him or by him. As far back as he is able to remember, S always felt himself to be "alien, not really a member of the human race at all, but someone who belonged someplace else and got into this world by accident or under strange circumstances." However, he soon found it expedient to keep "the secret" of his "difference" to himself and to "make believe" he was "like other children." Or, when unable to deceive himself, he would "consciously pretend" to be "a human child." Whether this began as a game he played with himself, S cannot be certain; but this seems to him a likely explanation.

Also as far back as he can recall, S felt an irresistible attraction toward "what others regarded as evil," although S himself "at no time accepted this value judgment." All through his childhood his "sympathies were always with the bad guys" in films, on the radio, etc. In playing with other children he selected games in which he could take the role of the robber or some other villain. His precocity was such that he was easily able to "manipulate most other children" and also, much of the time, the adults around him. Until rather recently he has continued to see his relations with others in terms of their manipulation by him—a manipulation that was usually not a means to some end, but rather was an end-in-itself.

At around age six, S greatly distressed his mother by declaring his disbelief in God. He attended Sunday School under duress and excelled at memorizing passages of Scripture; but, in reading the *Bible*, he "was always turning to the erotic incidents and to anything that concerned the Devil." His fascination with the Devil was constant throughout his childhood and much of his adult life. At the age of twelve, he made the first of his many "unsuccessful attempts" to sell his soul to the Devil. He found books on demonology and sorcery, studied them, and identified with the demon Ashtaroth. He practiced black magic, "sometimes with apparent success."

At age thirteen, S had his first sexual experience. Thereafter, he was "constantly out after sex." He became exceedingly promiscuous and had remained so up until about one year before his session. He also "read omnivorously about sex," especially prohibited sex practices and aberrations. All of this he did "because society, and especially the church, regarded sex outside of wedlock as evil." Whatever was thought to be "evil," S would do—although he stopped short of activities likely to result in serious trouble with the police. At the same time, S "never did believe that sex was evil." He never experienced any feelings of guilt in connection with his "evil" practices and "probably" never has known what it is to feel consciously guilty. Yet, no one has ever suggested that S is a psychopath. For all his "manipulation" of others, he has frequently been of great help to his friends and associates and is regarded by many as a kind, compassionate person.

As he grew older, S became "a real scholar of evil." He searched assiduously for "all the banned books" and read them. In school, his intelligence (I.Q. about 165) permitted him to earn good grades without effort and left him time to "stir up lots of mischief." At the university, he was considered to be an outstanding student. He was drawn to the study of psychology, and especially to psychoanalysis, because his own mental processes seemed to him "mysterious and unlike those of other persons."

Although an atheist with scientific interests, S continued his studies in satanism, witchcraft, "black" occultism, etc. His atheism was militant and for a time he also was a nihilist. His militancy "attracted disciples" and others often remarked that he had "some strange kind of power." He had much sexual success with coeds and "preached a doctrine of total debauchery." However, he preferred his contacts with socially low-level girls and spent much time in "almost skid-row surroundings" that seemed to have a very great fascination for him.

"As a nihilist," S "believed in nothing at all," and "the effect of this" was to cause him to lose the "power" that others always had recognized in him. The "next effect" was a "crippling anxiety neurosis" that came on when S still was in graduate school. He was "just barely able to control" his anxiety to the extent required to let him finish school. Whenever confronted by "a person in any position of authority" over him, S would "inwardly tremble" and felt that at any moment the trembling "would be exteriorized and then degenerate into total panic." Yet, when confronted by such situations, he "somehow always got through." And even when the neurosis was at its worst S remained a forceful personality who "always managed to have a few disciples on the string."

In his practice as a psychotherapist, S was unusually effective. Here, he felt, the "upper hand" was his and consequently the "anxiety problem did not come up." Outside the therapeutic situation, however, S's "neurotic symptoms intensified" until, for a few brief periods of his life, he found himself almost unable to enter a store to make a purchase. If he found himself in a position where he "had to *ask* anybody for anything," he became extremely agitated and feared he would be unable to speak. This condition, which was intermittent, was at its worst during a period of three to four years. The neurosis "seriously handicapped" S and caused him a great deal of misery for almost a decade.

At age twenty-eight, S embarked upon a lengthy self-analysis that continued for some seven years. His method was eclectic, but mostly psychoanalytic and Freudian. He worked with auto-hypnosis and relaxation techniques in an effort to suppress his physical symptoms (trembling, tachycardia, etc.) while he "attacked the neurosis itself" with his self-analytic method. During the whole duration of the neurosis S continued to be promiscuous, but could only overcome his anxiety with the woman he approached as "suppliant" by drinking very heavily. He felt that this necessity presented the added threat that he would become alcoholic.

About four years previous to his LSD sessions, S "achieved important breakthroughs" in his self-analysis. He did not "cure" the neurosis but developed techniques "for detecting a symptom at its inception and immediately suppressing it." He felt that the cause of the neurosis no longer was operative, so that the task was really one of breaking down habits and conditioned response patterns. His anxiety, he felt he had learned, was in fact a "rage unable to express itself because known to be an irrational, inappropriate response." This rage occurred whenever S was "in any sense in a subordinate position." Then the rage, which he could not express, "would come to the surface as symptoms" which S initially had "mistaken" for anxiety. Later, what he feared was the symptomatic behavior itself, and "then the anxiety became real." After his "breakthroughs" he continued to work at the self-analysis for another year, then abandoned it as no longer needed. He continued to be "very promiscuous," but "more out of habit than need."

About one year before his sessions, S had several experiences he felt to be of great importance. He long had recognized religious tendencies in himself but had always suppressed "this need" or "deflected the need towards the Devil." Now, however, he felt that his lifelong preoccupation with the Devil was "juvenile" and made some strenuous efforts to tap "that genuine source of strength and inner peace men call God." S felt that on several occasions he had "broken through to this Source." Each time, after such a breakthrough, he noted "definite gains towards improved adjustment and self-mastery." But he never could manage to subdue his "inner devils, who whispered that all of this was merely hypocrisy and self-delusion."

S then had a curious kind of "mystical experience." His "totem animal" for many years had been the wolf. This wolf, with which S identified, represented "a wild, untameable freedom." The wolf was, like himself, "a solitary beast, self-reliant (and as S wanted to be), strong and snarling his defiance at the world." This personal totem was abandoned when S, reflecting upon his "wolf-identification," suddenly knew beyond all possibility of doubt that the wolf in himself now was dead. In almost the same instant, closing his eyes, he saw before him a vivid eidetic image of a huge, beautiful tiger and knew with equal conviction that the tiger now was his totem. Following this incident the tiger appeared to S in a succession of dreams. During the dreams S was "somehow made to understand" that the transition from wolf to tiger represented a distinct advance for him and that the neurosis was coming to an end.[21] From the moment of this change of totems onward, S continued to make "steady gains" in the form of "a healthier outlook than ever before and better relations with other persons." He continued to "seek God" and the feeling that this was "something to be ashamed of" troubled him much less than before. He felt that for the first time in his life his mental health was "very good, though not perfect," and that the more severe of his problems had been left behind him "once and for all."

Such, very briefly, are the general outlines and some relevant details of this subject's strange background. The information was not available to us previous to his session and, in this subject's case, no amount of interviewing could elicit what he did not want to tell. He was far too practiced and knowledgeable a veteran of dissimulation to reveal either in conversation or testing any information he preferred to withhold. Nor was there, at the time of his first session, any longer any serious disturbance to be diagnosed.

The First and Second Sessions.   Because S's last two sessions are more important and require rather lengthy summation, we will pass very briefly over the first.

During that first session, S spent several hours experiencing the various phenomena of the sensory level. He adjusted to the drug-state[22] quickly and kept up a witty and intelligent running commentary on his images, visual distortions, ideas about "psychodynamic mechanisms" involved in the sensory phenomena, etc. He expressed some desire to examine his own psychology, but produced nothing of much importance. We agreed with S that, at this point, his psyche already was so well explored that he might as well go on to something else.

Some three and one-half hours into the session, S abruptly ceased his brief venture into the recollective-analytic realm and experienced many phenomena characteristic of the symbolic level. He felt the evolutionary process in his body and also imaged rudimentary life forms, then observed with much interest the development over the aeons of new and more complicated varieties of plant and animal life. He observed dinosaurs in ferocious combat and a series of "abortive humanoid forms, failing to develop so as to enable them to survive." He repeatedly observed "very decadent half-human beings" and great twisting masses of serpents, writhing in a brilliantly colored mass, "inextricably intertwined." He remarked that this latter image often had been seen (eidetically imaged) by him outside of the drug-state, but never so vividly.

The most dramatic moments of this session occurred after some five hours, when S imaged a great ball of fire that exploded in outer space and molten-looking but "immaterial" sheets of flame rained down upon the earth—"a kind of fiery deluge." These sheets of flame became a blazing, glowing cylinder that surrounded "the edges of the earth." The cylinder "cooled," became a silvery mist, and then appeared to evaporate. "After this," S declared, "the Presence of God was upon the earth" and the attempts of evolution to bring forth man were crowned with success. Henceforth, the "pull of Nature upon man was downward." It was as if whatever force had itself failed at creating man, now set itself the task of undoing God's successful creation. Concerning this conflict, S described himself as being "very ambivalent . . . wanting to side with God, but somehow allied with the other force that incessantly strives to turn order into chaos." S felt that this conflict he now described was basically his own, but "infinitely more complex" than his statement of it would suggest. With great emotion he announced that "this is of vital importance to me" and that he "absolutely must get to the bottom" of what he felt was being disclosed to him about his own nature.

From this point on, the drug effects rapidly diminished and no material of any importance was produced. After the session, S continued to insist very strongly that "something has been started, some process that it is very important I see through." He felt that this could only be accomplished if he had another LSD session.

While only rarely in our work have we found it desirable to give a subject more than one session, in this case we shared the subject's conviction that "something big is in the wind." Since all were agreed that another session was in order, we scheduled the second for the following Saturday, just seven days from the date of the first session. On the occasion of this second session, S declared he would "waste no time with the exotica"—the sensory level phenomena—and almost at once resumed his first-session preoccupation with symbolic level materials. His session from that point on was largely on this symbolic level with, however, frequent and important movements "back up" to the recollective-analytic.

Early in the session, S reported feeling his body to be that of a huge, happy dragon lying upon the surface of Mother Earth. He also reported the recurrence of a surface numbness or anesthesia which he now related to the tough hide of the dragon. This anesthesia, as before, could be penetrated by music, which provided intense pleasure sensations "as if each nerve end were being simultaneously stimulated"; but whatever he touched was felt "as by one whose whole body is encased in a thin rubber glove." Bach's *Brandenburg Concerto No. 4* was played and S was urged to permit his body to "dissolve." At first he was "overwhelmed by a bombardment of physical sensations, by tangible sound waves both felt and seen." The sensations were "erotic" and his intellect too now seemed to be "almost wholly genital." He closed his eyes and described great sinuous, jeweled shapes undulating through space. "Everything" was "coming in waves and from all sides." "Great waves of stimuli" were "crashing against the permeable rock" S now felt himself to be. He reported that "everything is happening now on a great universal scale. I can dissolve. Now I understand what is meant by being a part of everything, what is meant by sensing the body as dissolving. I have a knowledge of all my particles dissolving and becoming incorporated into a sea of particles where nothing has form or even substance. In this sea there is no individuality."

It was not clear at this point whether S was moving toward an authentic or a pseudo-mystical experience. He was urged to continue the dissolution process and almost at once announced that he was resisting the process. "At the same time as I dissolve," he said, "I feel myself to be some kind of huge monument, some great stone edifice." Again, he was urged to "let go," to dissolve not only the body but also the self. To this he responded that "There are two ways of doing it. I can take everything into myself, or I can let myself go totally into what is not myself. This decision is the most difficult problem of all. I must see what I can do."

S then was momentarily diverted by images of "a huge beautiful ballet in which all of my physical and mental states are personified.

There are thousands of dance figures, each one of whom is myself. I am able to feel myself into each one of them, but am also able to combine them all and feel them as a totality." He then quickly returned to the "dissolution theme" and described an image of "horizons that go out and out and out. These expanding horizons are what I see and feel and am. This became possible when something was pulled away from over my head. A kind of net was lifted from the top of my head, and caught in the net and pulled away with it were many ugly things. Once the net and all that garbage had been pulled away the horizon could begin to go out. I now have no horizon at all. I have a feeling and knowledge of being physically boundless. There is an oceanic quality, yet sometimes I get washed up by some irritating passage in the music. I get washed up into dirty little bistros on tropical islands in the ocean."

Again S was urged to stop resisting, to allow himself the experience of boundless being. But now he found himself surrounded by "darting, oriental, snake-like things, moving in circles around me so that I cannot go beyond them." He began to breathe heavily and gave the impression of being involved in some great internal struggle. His face reddened, he started to perspire, and the facial expression resembled that of some mythological hero locked in mortal combat. After some minutes he reported experiencing a "titanic struggle." His senses were unwilling to relinquish their "hold upon the earth." He complained of being "in bondage to serpentine, oriental forms that press down upon consciousness strangling its horizon." S struggles against these forces and, in so doing, experiences sensations more intense than any he has known. His effort, he now says, is directed towards "containing God." But the "Idea of God is too big to contain. One tries to know God by extending oneself outward in all directions as a circle radiates outward from its center along an infinite number of lines." S is told that he should not struggle any longer but simply "Be the circle extending outward, let yourself extend outward to meet God if that is what you want." S then wondered about the advisibility of this, saying that "If God is real, one would not dare to meet Him unless properly prepared." He laughed loudly and said that "My ego is still in pretty good shape. I find myself sitting down before the Majesty of God, but as a member of the House of Lords. The meeting place is long and narrow and contains a few minds who have elected God to His high office. We acknowledge our submission to His power, but only reluctantly."[23] He adds that "Should I allow God to enter me, then I would expand as if filled with a wind, and finally I would burst."

After a silence of some minutes, S remarked: "I am locked in a titanic struggle. The creatures are enormous and symbolic. Whether I am losing or winning I don't know, because I don't understand the symbolism or what the outcome should be. Great colossi are fighting. Tigers and other beasts, hundreds of feet high, tear at one another's throats. These are the forces of myself, forces threatened with dissolution should I abandon myself to God. The forces also have cosmic meaning—meaning beyond the meaning they have in my own psychology."

At this point, S reviewed a good deal of the material summarized at the beginning of this case. He tried to put his conflicts into conventional psychological terms, but declared himself unable to make a convincing formulation. Only religious terms were "relevant and valid" and "The big, essential conflicts are with God. Any others I am able to take care of by myself." Concerning his "conflict with God," S said that he found himself "impelled by a basic instinct of survival to fight against God. Should I be overthrown in this, then my I would be gone. To preserve itself my I must wage war against God. Once I give in, I am subject to God. My I is only able to preserve its singularity by blowing itself up very large and fighting against everything. . . . Either I meet God on equal terms, or I cannot meet him at all. I feel like a terribly battered boxer who gets knocked down again and again but keeps on getting up and coming in for more punishment. I am a battleground of the most titanic forces. All this time colossal tigers and enormous dragons are snarling at one another's throats. These forces I know to be symbolic and involved in my conflict with God, yet I still cannot say exactly what they are."

S reported that he was continuing to experience very intense sexual sensations and said that he feared abandoning himself to God because God might "take away" his "sexuality." The subject was now at the start of what proved to be a three-hours-long "battle with God." The psychical climate of this "battle'" was intensely emotional as at times S would "rage against God" and against his own "impotence in this terrible struggle." During much of this time he continued to describe what he was experiencing and we must condense the monologue:

"What Infinity takes away has to be infinite also. I would be sucked at both ends by God should I give myself up to Him. I am both giving all that I can and all that I have is being taken away. I have done all I can. God must sustain me if this effort is to continue . . . Yes, yes I need God. I need Him out of the need that everyone has who knows he cannot stand alone against all of the forces of the universe. God has raised all these forces up and God alone can sustain them. But I don't see why I should have to fight all these terrible battles. Rather I'd pass unnoticed like some grain of sand on the beach. I see the promise of giving in to God, and also the threat if I do not. But I have started out with nothing but my bare hands and through the years have piled up plenty of weapons. If God tries to fight me in my own world, He will find me plenty tough to handle. And God, to fight me, has to be willing to assume certain human proportions. He has to dwindle down and make Himself almost human, come into the human sphere, to contend with those who can't fight Him on more potent levels.

"It is unfair! Unfair! I have no chance at all in this fight! [Here, S became extremely angry.] How do I keep my self-respect if I give in to God? God stands with His foot on one's neck and will only take it away if one makes an abject surrender to Him. This I cannot do! All around me these damned tigers and dragons and herculean figures are fighting, trying to tear each other to bits . . . If we can neither give in to God nor successfully resist Him, then we have to settle for some smaller, less satisfying place in the scheme of things. But one doesn't accept it placidly. One always resents the fact that God is so much greater—and, even more, that God should make us aware of His greatness. One is ultimately defeated by God because one is defeated by an Idea that is greater than oneself.

"My mind goes out as far as it can go, and beyond that is God. I am beaten down again and again by it. My mind reaches out to encompass all and when it fails I get mad and start complaining that someone is greater than I. If I can't encompass all, at least I can defend myself. I can put on a suit of armor. When some small nation is threatened by a bigger neighbor and can't develop good enough offensive weapons, then it puts up good defenses. Still, there should be the possibility of some kind of agreement. To accept God seems to me to mean only surrender and this I haven't been forced to do. Every minute I fight very hard and am very, very tough. I am like an old general who has been through many wars, knows all the tactics and has developed his arsenal. . . . The more one acquires, the more one has to protect. What ultimately threatens can only be God, for ultimately God is whatever is other than oneself."

At this point the subject launched into a lengthy and scathing attack upon Christ. Christ was seen as "the archetypal demagogue, the personification of the socialist concept in religious terms. . . Given all that man has learned in the last two thousand years, I consider that my mind is greater than God's mind personified in Jesus. God had to reduce Himself too much in order to make Himself comprehensible to the human masses. In Christ, God reduced himself to such miserable proportions no man of intelligence can accept Him."

Asked if God might incarnate in man again, S responded: "Only if man evolves to a scope sufficiently great that God needn't degrade Himself too much by personifying. What the hell is the matter with me? Why do I keep fighting this thing? For as long as I can remember if a fight was clearly futile, then I wouldn't get into it. I would only fight if there seemed to be some real chance of winning. But now I fight and I know I can't win. I've fought battles today like no man ever fought before. I have this possibility of seeing God as Chairman of the Board. At best, then, one can be no more than a member of the Board. It is important to know that one would then be inferior only to God, not to other people. I have fought God all my life. Other members of the Board are satisfied with money, power, that kind of thing. I have always wanted much more. I want the whole *Idea of God*. If one has that, the rest will follow. But the Idea of God is always just what one can't have. I can only know what is in my mind and the Idea of God is much too big to be contained by my mind." S again, at this point, launched into a furious attack on Christ and Christianity, returning from this to discuss his futile struggle against God. Time and time again, he notes, he has hurled himself "against the God-Idea in an effort to assimilate or encompass it." Time and again he is "battered to the ground," then gets up and fights some more. It is a "futile fight" he "cannot win," but his "pride" compels him to "get up and keep trying." Also, now, he recognizes a certain value in this struggle. Even as he continuously flings himself against the Idea and is "knocked down" by It, his "consciousness is enlarged" and his "head is flattened out and gets bigger just from ramming it against the stone wall of the effort to comprehend God." Should he abandon this effort, then he would have "no more motivation to keep enlarging [his] horizons. One can vegetate in self-renunciation and assimilation into God, but by so doing one admits that one has no absolute value. If a man stands alone, apart from God, he exists as something separate and so has a certain value, however petty in relation to God's value."

Having continued in this vein for several hours, and still only four hours into the session, S suddenly appeared to have very largely shaken off the drug effects. He announced: "I seem to be coming out of it," and said that he was feeling very tired but wanted to move around a bit. He sat up on the edge of the couch where he had been lying and then got up and walked around the room. He felt that his brain had been "greatly stretched" and likened the top of his head to a flowerpot with a plant growing in it. This plant ("ideas") had grown too large for the present dimensions of the pot ("mind"), was top-heavy, and felt as if "it might be pulled out by its roots." The pot now would have to grow still more in order to be able to support the plant; also, the plant now needed "better roots to support this new superstructure."

After pacing the room for several minutes, S said that the drug effects again were being felt but not so intensely as before. He sat down and began to try to analyze what had happened. As a part of this effort, he dredged up a wealth of memories from his childhood, including some left untouched even by his long self-analysis. He wondered if the "battle with God" could have been "a smokescreen thrown up to prevent any coming to terms with the real problem?" But he doubted that this was so and felt that he had been dealing with what for him was the "fundamental issue."

S felt that the answer to the "riddle" of himself must lie in finding the reason for his "early and almost instinctive tendency" to align himself with whatever forces society regarded as evil. This tendency, he felt, "*should* point to deep-rooted feelings of guilt acquired at a very early age." But he had never experienced conscious guilt and had never tried to "provoke punishment." On the contrary, he had "always exhibited extraordinary talent at not getting caught in any wrong-doing." And, when caught, he had been "extremely skillful and effective at evading punishment."

S now saw for the first time his "whole life as a recapitulation of Lucifer's struggle with God." S, like Lucifer, has wanted to be God and has been punished for his pride. Pride has been his main fault and no matter how much he has suffered for it, he has been unwilling or unable to give it up. His hunger for God, which has "been conscious only from time to time," has been a hunger "to devour God"—"to become God." His "main and driving passion" has been "the full richness of the Idea of God." This goal has at times been variously defined, but in one form or another it has been what has driven him to constantly try to expand his consciousness, to try to acquire all knowledge, to try to "bring everything" into himself.

Since childhood, S said, he had "created phantasies, worn masks, dealt in illusions." He was "like Genet, but where Genet's hangup is sexual," S's problem has been his "preoccupation with evil." He was, as a child, "a little philosopher of evil, a little Marquis de Sade, a kind of born criminal." To be this was to be unacceptable to others and so he was forced to wear masks, deal in more and more illusions. His anxiety, he thought, might derive in part from this: his fear that his mask was not good enough, his hiding place not hidden enough, so that others might find him out, see through him, and then reject him. Yet, he wanted to be accepted by others as he "really" was, and so would reveal to others just as much of himself as he could, while always stopping short of "that degree of revelation" that would cause the others to reject him. He always had the sense of not being human, of "coming from someplace else and not belonging in this world at all." He manipulated others and, for a long time, wished to make others evil just as he was evil—"so that then they could accept me?" To do this, he was obliged to try to "make evil appear very attractive to others, to show others that if they would do something evil they would get pleasure from it, so that it was good after all—so that *I* was good after all?" Yet, when others succumbed to his persuasion, his sense of having manipulated them tended to make him scornful of them. They were weak and he was strong, and "what is it worth to be accepted by weaklings?" He apparently wanted others to remain "good" in spite of all his tempting of them, but he also wanted these "good" others to accept him in all of his "evilness." Again and again, S noted, he reviewed the facts of his life to find himself in the position of Lucifer—trying to be God, tempting man and then despising (punishing?) man for succumbing to this temptation. His own great sin was pride and his evil-doing may have been a revolt against his realization that he could not be God. If he could not be God, then he would be the very antithesis of God, the master of all that God "has rejected." He would carve out his own domain, even if that domain were a wasteland, and be God there. And he must try to enlarge his kingdom by taking away a part of God's kingdom—i.e., by "seducing others away from God's Good and persuading them to accept (his) evil, come into (his) domain, which can exist apart from God's because consisting of what has been rejected by God." He would "lead the whole world away from God, into evil, and thus win a kind of victory over God," demonstrating his "own power as against God's power." (S, in addition to his other proselytizing, has attempted to do this by writing novels and philosophical works which, however, he has not published.)

Yet, S remarks, at various times in his life "things have happened" to change the course of his life. He has come to see that the struggle with God is one he cannot possibly win. He has recognized the painfulness and the self-destructive results of the struggle. He has had a painful anxiety neurosis "inflicted upon" him. This he conquered by acquiring "enormous amounts of knowledge" in the fields of psychology and psychiatry, among others. This knowledge he then used as "a weapon against God," just as his extensive studies in sorcery could be seen as an effort on his part to provide himself with weapons by means of which he might "prevail against God by magical means." But even when he rejected God altogether—when he considered himself an atheist—he sometimes "felt a conscious need for God." Increasingly, in his later years, he has come to feel that he "cannot stand alone against God." He has "lost the dynamism" of his evil, but this "has only opened up an inner void since having let go of much of the will-to-devildom" he has not "filled the void by accepting God." This void, he recognized before his session and has "tried in many ingenious ways to come to terms with God, to be accepted by God while still not surrendering to God," and while preserving himself as "a separate entity not entirely controlled by God."

S feels that his life has been changing for the better precisely as he has become more willing to "accept the God-values and give up the Devil-values." For example, the residue of his anxiety has continued to diminish. His activities have prospered. Yet "problems remain," and he wonders whether freedom from problems at the expense of giving himself over to the "other side" could be worth the price? This would perhaps be a self-denial and a self-humiliation. God has "no right to force such a choice upon man." One is either crushed by God or one surrenders to God. S has considered it better to be crushed, no matter how painful the crushing. However, he now repeatedly emphasizes his awareness that it is stupid to fight battles one cannot win. His "stubbornness and pride" are "surely the main source" of his difficulties. But "is giving up the stubbornness and pride and behaving not stupidly" better than the "abject surrender that seems to be the only other alternative?" He is "unable to conceive of the problem in other terms," although he recognizes that this may be his "own deficiency and perhaps there are other alternatives" he is "not able to see."

Considering the tiger and dragon that clashed repeatedly in his images, S "would hazard a guess" that the dragon represents, on one level, his masculinity; the tiger, the feminine aspect of his character. The dragon also stands for S's sexuality, "a very complicated and knowledgeable sexuality," and the tiger for a "rather corrupt heroic-ascetic aspect of the self." The tiger also represents "occult weapons." Yet, "it is still more complicated than this, much of the symbolism is beyond my present understanding."

His unusual amount of sexual activity S now "very clearly" sees as being "something that I did to be doing something that in the world's terms was wrong although it wasn't wrong on my own terms. It was also an effort to break through a kind of barrier against really *touching*. This I always have had and the anesthesia I have felt during the sessions reflects this. The anesthesia is ineffective against music, because the music is not something I reach out and try to touch. Also, I have had so many sexual relationships for the ordinary reasons: physical pleasure, warmth of human contact, and so on. But to go to such an enormous amount of trouble as I have always gone to! To read so many hundreds of volumes, to sleep with all of those hundreds of girls! And all of it was only secondary, having no profound meaning for me. It was mainly a superimposition on Some Other Thing, an outgrowth of my need to do evil. I didn't want to do really bad things, for example I didn't want to kill anybody, but I wanted to do things as bad as I could within the limits of those laws likely to be enforced. That was why I became an atheist, a nihilist, slept all around the time and became a student of sexual perversions and all sorts of crime. I felt this constant compulsion to build up a great store of knowledge of everything that man, and especially the Christian religion, said was evil. I was as driven to do this as if it were the most basic and powerful impulsion within me."

During this period of problem-formulation on the recollective-analytic level, S frequently emphasized how important it seemed to him to be able to see his life in terms of the Lucifer myth. "On these terms," he is "able to make sense" of much of his life. However, his "initial choice" of the myth still remains "an inscrutable mystery." Why, even as a tiny child, had he always cast his lot with "the forces of evil?" Why the tremendous fascination with the Devil, demons, black magic? As the session was coming to a close S remarked that he felt that he now for the first time really understood the futility of struggling any longer against God. He could not hope to "be God" but this "need not undermine" his "position as something other than God." Between him and God, during the session, had been "the wall of the Idea of God." This Idea of God was "by definition" beyond his comprehension. However, should he "stop trying to comprehend the God-Idea," then he might be able "to confront God directly."

S felt that his session had been extremely productive, but had "raised more questions than were answered." He felt, as did we, that he was "getting very close" to understanding himself in terms that would be more helpful and more transformative than any he had achieved by approaching "the problem" through "more conventional"—mainly psychoanalytic—means. A third session was scheduled for the following week.

The Third Session. While waiting for the LSD to take effect, S read an account of his previous session. He asked that a recording of "innocuous" eighteenth-century lute music be played for him and said he wanted "nothing profound or emotional." He closed his eyes and saw himself and the guides in an ornately furnished drawing room, all suitably attired for the occasion. At this point the telephone (not cut off as it should have been) jangled and S leaped to his feet. He felt that the call had "ruined everything," and that now he was "going to come out of it." He thought at this time that the session had been going on for about two hours, although he had reported his "first feeling of the drug effects" about ten minutes previously.

For almost an hour S reacted to the phone call, claiming that it had irrevocably wrecked his experience. We doubted this, and suggested to the subject that he "descend" to the point he had reached in the last session. S then, in a bored and rather patronizing manner, described an image of a circular staircase with jeweled walls. But this feeble symbolization of his psychic descent could not hold his attention. He announced he was resisting and again repeated that "I think I am in some danger of altogether throwing off the drug effects." S then was urged to try to discover why he was resisting the experience. It was proposed that he try to find some image for this resistance. He was silent for a moment, then said "Sinking ship . . . I see a sinking ship and I am afraid of sinking the ship." He interpreted this image as being "partially related" to his previous session when he had fought against God in an effort to preserve his own identity. Shortly thereafter he admitted fearing at the start of the session that the confrontation with God was "imminent." He was now "so well prepared" for this confrontation that it would "have to happen right at the beginning or not at all." His resistance was "partly an attempt to block" his "greatest expectation just when the confrontation" seemed "most imminent." But he also was "very fearful about meeting God." "Little did I know," he said later, "that God was biding His time."

S now reported "a strange alteration of the emotional tone of the experience." The lute music now seemed "much too innocuous" and the *Brandenburg No. 4* was played—this being the same concerto to which S had responded so powerfully the previous week. Now, however, S reported that the concerto "sounds very simple this time. Almost a simple little 'pop' tune. Yet always before Bach's music has seemed to me almost as complicated as the God-Idea. This is amazing!"

Asked what images he was seeing, S responded: "I envision wave after wave of comic-strip monsters bearing down upon me. I am not at all impressed." This was striking when compared to the intricately detailed and formidable monsters seen by S in the earlier sessions. The monsters had dwindled to "comic book status," somewhat as the Bach concerto had become "simple, almost 'pop' music." One wondered if the subject now might be apprehending the things of this world and of his image-world as from the perspective of deity? S now remarked that:

"Instead of myself going out and away from myself as in the last session, everything is coming in upon me." It was suggested that he try to reverse this process, but S responded by saying that he was "caught up in very sensual feelings." Returning to his discussion of the Bach, he said that "This is the first time that I've ever felt that this music is brought down to proportions that I can contain. I see how the music loses by this. I see that to try to contain the Idea of God would be to infinitely shrink and cheapen its proportions, or else one would have to stretch one's own comprehension to the bursting point. A greater richness is to be had when there is something beyond comprehension, something that continues to challenge." S then listened to a concerto of Beethoven. He was more impressed and found Beethoven "for the present more complicated than Bach, or perhaps it is only that the scope is greater." He described an image of "someone outdoing both Bach and Beethoven by sitting and pushing buttons on an electronic graph computer." Asked why he was insisting on reducing everything to simple or conquerable proportions, S replied that he was aware of "a great sense of a personal will-to-power" that was "blocking" him off from both the experience of God and his own deeper levels. "In terms of the music I seem to have to reduce everything in this world to manageable proportions before I can hope to go beyond the things of this world and meet God."

At this point a change of environment seemed advisable and S was led into the adjoining room—the scene of most of his "titanic struggles" of the last session. The enormously complex Bach *Toccata in C* was played and the subject was given a little figurine of a sweet-faced child mermaid who is holding a fish. S contemplated both music and figurine for a while and then remarked: "My mind is getting another lesson. I can see with regard to this music how easy it would be for God to contain it and also, given my present physical feelings, how easy it would be for God to dominate the world by just stimulating certain sensations. One man might control the whole world by giving people sensations they've never had before and can't get elsewhere. God has declined to do this and has left man free to go beyond his sensations and control them by means of his thinking and creating."

S then became intensely interested in the little porcelain mermaid and stared at her for several minutes. He looked up and remarked that "Maybe I can open myself up to God by understanding who I am and perhaps I can do that through this very ancient and wicked little child." (As noted, this figure is a kind of personification of childish innocence; and it quickly was evident that S was projecting himself as a child into the mermaid figure.) He continued:

"I see that her wickedness is the result of inheritance. Hair is growing over her whole body and this hair is like a wolf's hair. (In fact, the merchild's hair is mostly obscured by the fish and her body has no hair on it at all. S is here referring to what he has heard about himself as an infant, as noted in our earlier summation of the background to this case.) It should not be that a mermaid has such hair. I see under the face of this child the face of Pan, the faces of corrupt priests. Her face turns into a death's head, into a succession of grimacing devils."

S then was told: "Look past all that to what is still farther underneath. Look past your distortions to see what really is there in her face."

S responded: "I see still greater, more complex, more beautiful but less describable evils. I perceive them in terms of the child's face which reflects a whole series of works of art, and I see the mermaid also in terms of the material the artist has used to impose upon it her form. I see the infinite number of forms that might have been imposed upon this material. I see how the basically beautiful material can be beautiful or ugly in its form, good or evil, vulgar or shaped with great refinement."

One of the guides (G) asked him: "How do you relate this understanding of form and matter to yourself?"

S: "I made the terrible mistake of thinking that the fault lay in the matter rather than in the forms imposed upon matter. I thought (S now speaks with very great emotion) that matter was evil. Now matter stands revealed to me as basically beautiful, but subject to whatever one chooses to do with it."

G: "Keep going deeper, and back in time, and see if you can find out when and how it was you first got this idea that matter is evil. Where did this idea begin with you? Go back to the source."

S: "I am in a silent subterranean place. I have the sense of some kind of machine and of operating the machine. But yet this machine is inside of me. I think that only from within this protective bathysphere-like thing do I feel safe to look around. Down here all of the things that have been so much a part of my drug images on the more conscious level are present. Dragons and snakes, especially, are at home here and are not fighting. This is where I come from. It is as if always inside of my head I somehow knew that this is my own world—the place I came out of and up from when I was born. A world so different from the face of the earth."

G: "Go ahead and describe this world."

S: "I feel that I am speaking from a deep, quiet place. There are, in this world, no straight lines ever. Everything is sinuous and serpentine, often undulating, very graceful and rhythmic. Things appear to be very hard and brilliant on the surface, yet I know they are soft and that I could crush them if I squeezed them in my hand. Everything looks hard but could be crushed if it were felt. I've always seen this world before, in my images when I am lying in bed, in my dreams, and again with this drug. I find this world to be beautiful and if I can retain the insights I am getting, there will be some fundamental change in my whole being."

G: "Why will this change occur?"

S: "Because it is a perception of everything as not only potentially beautiful, but as basically beautiful in its own right and as formless matter. The forms one imposes on matter are one's own fault and not the fault of the Creator of matter. One is given this beautiful substratum of reality and what one does to it after that is one's own decision. This world which I now perceive as 'down there' is a particular world imposed upon the plastic reality."

G: "Keep trying to find out more about this world. Find out just where it is and what it means."

S: "One seems to rise up out of it into birth in this world in which my body now is."

G: "Try again to find the source of your original idea that matter is evil."

S: "I was told that matter was evil. This teaching I have associated with Christianity. Perhaps I learned it when I was very young. It seems to me that when I was born I already was very old. I was cold and shivering—not from lack of human warmth, but because of what I already had seen in other places. It seems to me that when I was born I already was old and that I remembered things. Almost at once I forgot a great deal, but not the forms that have kept coming back to me in my images."

G: "Try to recapture those memories you think you lost just after you were born."

S: "Down here the colors, the forms, the emotional tone, everything is familiar. It is a very sensual and corrupt beauty. If only I can hang on to my awareness that matter basically is beautiful! . . . that beauty is inherent in the material that is plastic, malleable, so that the material can be shaped into any kind of form at all."

G: "But your feeling that matter was evil, where did it begin?"

S: "I think it may have been my initial reaction to the world. It wasn't just the environment where I found myself. It was something I knew . . . I already knew it . . . I felt . . ."

Here, the subject stopped talking and put his thumb into his mouth. For all of the rest of the period during which he discussed his infancy, he kept his thumb in his mouth and occasionally sucked on it. Asked to continue, he went on speaking with much emotion.

S: "I had the sense then (at birth) of cheating somebody by living . . . as if somebody wanted me to die, but I was aware of this and made up my mind that I would live in spite of it. I feel also that my father, I'm not quite sure if I mean my human father, flung me snarling and gnashing my teeth like some kind of dragon or mad dog against the whole material world . . . so that I would subdue it all and doubtless so that I could give it to him. I felt that this was what was expected of me. I had to batter down everything, bring back everything. It seems to me that I was born shivering, snarling, and gnashing my teeth at the world like some kind of mythical animal . . . like some kind of oriental dragon . . . a yellow, miserable infant covered with long hair . . . some kind of little Mongol tyrant sitting on a throne of diapers. Yet, as this baby, I was stuck with all of the adhesions of the past, all of this corruption and anger that I had dragged up with me from below. As soon as I saw the world I snarled at it like a wild beast.

"Later I forgot some of the sense of identification I had with this world down below. I had roots that ran through all of my body, roots reaching down toward this world underneath. I have felt that one could dive into a swamp and go down and down and finally get to a place that would be home. Whenever, during my life, my mind would lose its direction downwards, then all kinds of impulses would come up from below to pull me back and remind me who I was. Thus I wasn't like any of the others. I didn't belong to the human race. I think I must have come up from down there because the images are so deeply rooted in my mind."

G: "Itemize these recurrent, deep-rooted images. Describe for us again this world you keep mentioning."

S: "There are snakes, alligators, dragons, beautiful reptiles. They are lying on the bottom of a kind of sea, but I don't think it is water. At the edges of this place where they are there are tigers walking along the shore. Up on the beach all kinds of wild orgies are going on. Lots of sex, people getting drunk, and tigers eating the people. Tigers getting drunk on blood and then slaughtering one another."

S is now urged to try to descend to a level even more basic than this one. He says he "can do that" and reports: "I don't know how far down I am, but it is very, very far. I see myself down at the bottom of a pit and each one of its four walls slants inward towards the bottom and each wall is a single great stone slab. There are gray boulders on the floor. I have been hurled down to the bottom of this place, where I also feel myself to be. Everything I would ever want to have is looking down at me. God is up at the top and I am at the very bottom. God is the light at the top, the light over one's head. I have a feeling of having been punished and shoved down into this hole for having done something. It was something that happened before I was born as the person I now am.

"Even when I was successful and seemed to be a good child, really I was being bad because my actions were never motivated as others thought that they were. Whatever decision was made about me was made very early. I know that I am the product of hereditary factors, not environmental ones. I was born already in many ways determined. All of my life I have felt stretched apart by something trying to go up and something pulling down. I would make a little progress up, then snap back down like a pair of suspenders somebody has let go of. Always I sensed something pulling me down. I seem to see this pull downward in terms of the dragons and other beings of the 'down there world,' and in human terms of derelicts and skid row bums. I associated with the dregs of humanity so much because of what they satisfied in me—that is, this need to associate myself with something resembling or representing what I had come up from, the dragons and snakes. But always there was something in me too that wanted to get beyond this—to go in the direction of gobbling up the whole world."

G: "How would you describe this direction?"

S: "The movement was up, but it was my father who decided that the movement was 'up.' My father . . . again I'm not quite sure who I mean by my father, whether my human father or someone else . . . saw this up-movement as one towards power and possession and knowledge and a kind of expansion of consciousness generally, but to satisfy selfish-wants. I was pushed by my father in this direction. But I became aware that I saw some goals as worth pursuing in their own right, not necessarily because of the benefits I was going to get. At one time I saw these goals very clearly, but then I mostly lost sight of them. I was constantly being torn in three directions: Heaven, Hell and my own self all pulling me in opposite directions."

G: "What was your position in this world you feel that you came from?"

S: "I see myself down there and I may have some special kind of status. Nobody interferes with me down there." (S's image here changed and again he was down at the bottom of the pit, which he described in more detail.) "I am down at the bottom of this great stone dungeon with big goatskins hanging from walls that reach hundreds of miles up into the sky. I came into the world with a rage against it. The self I have been in this world had to pay for what someone did in some other time and place. I see myself as acting out all kinds of universal dramas and can't separate my ordinary self from these legendary selves."

G: "What are these legends you participate in?"

S: "Faust, and the Grail, and Lucifer being cast down out of Heaven." Asked about any connection between the Devil and the Grail, S declared that "The Grail is one of the things that the Devil always wants."

G: "Why don't you now go down still deeper, down to a level where you might meet God if you still want to do that."

S: "I don't know if I should. I'm afraid. If one goes down far enough one is likely to run into all the fires of Hell. If I am unable to contain God, no more am I able to contain the Devil."

G: "Why don't you try? Maybe you will find that the Devil has no more power over you?"

S: "I have the feeling of going down to see someone I always have known and whom I know very well. I see him with all his historical faces. His power was over me from the very beginning. From the day I first came in to the world I was full of the sense of his power. I could always feel his power running through me, going down like licking flames or the roots of trees, going down into the ground. There were all these impulses running down my body to there, and other impulses coming up into me from down there. I seem to have known the Devil from a very long time ago. The Devil is a literal Devil. I feel that the Devil created the earth and this seems at odds with my understanding that the substratum of reality is beautiful."

S then got up to go to the bathroom and came back reporting: "Whenever I looked at myself in the mirror during the other sessions I was always surrounded by darkness. But now I am surrounded by light. I saw myself in the mirror before as looking like the Devil. My image in the mirror was each time that of the Devil. And I have seen it often before in my life, without any drugs. As of several years ago I started seeing this Devil image in the mirror less often. But now I see my own face surrounded by light and somehow the face is changed in other ways I can't yet describe. This seems to me to be some kind of defeat for the Devil and at the same time I feel a hope with regard to myself that I never felt before. The hope seems to be a kind of awareness of the possibility of my being delivered from all the punishments I feel I've had to bear for what I never did . . . as if I were the one who had to bear the burden of the Devil into the world as a little child and then had to live with it."

All of this time S had given the impression of speaking from within some deep recess of himself. He began now to analyze some of the material but continued to speak as if from this deep level. He speculated as to whether "all this is a strange kind of fairy tale or has a deeper reality?" Even though he has "always borne the burden of the Devil," he has had a sense of "being bound by what seemed to be and yet not to be ethical restrictions." S "could only go so far and no more. I see I am not referring to morals, but to something more tangible. Something always prevented me from doing anything too bad. This was never a fear of getting caught, since I felt I was clever enough to get away with most anything. But there were literal boundaries of my own being that I couldn't reach beyond. I could only move within my own natural limits that seemed to have been given."

G: "Do you understand now anything more about the anxiety neurosis?"

S: "Why should I always have felt it with people I had to come to and ask them for something? I thought that it was probably my rage that I had to control and this rage then was turned to anxiety. Because there was never anything for me to fear. These would be people to whom I would feel infinitely superior. And I had good, objective reasons to feel superior to them. But finally what I began to be anxious about was the anxiety itself. I thought this helpless rage of mine, that should never have been and could not be expressed, was going to push me into a psychosis. If there was any other ground for anxiety, I haven't been able to find it. Maybe it partly was an unconscious fear I had that others would manage to find out who I was, discover these connections I had with something down below. Situations would come up where I was certain I was going to panic. But some strength would come into me or something would happen to spare me and then I felt as if God had reached down and given me a reprieve. Many times I have felt protected by God when I did the most incredible things. I have been in places where I certainly should have had my throat cut. But some little miracle always would happen. I felt I was being saved for some purpose. I felt I must be a special case or else I wouldn't be tormented to the limits of my endurance, but always just to the limits of my endurance."

S then remarked that he had a sense of being out in the middle of a lake by himself. The guides were on the shore and could not swim in these particular waters. The drug subject, he observed, is always out in the middle of the water and the guides can at most be on the shore. It seemed apparent that S now was preparing to "descend" to the integral level where the subject has a strong sense of experiencing what can never really be shared with others, so that although the subject may speak about what is being experienced, he still feels himself to be fundamentally alone. As he approached the threshold of this integral level, S remarked upon a gathering emotional intensity, expressing his surprise that such an emotionally charged psychical environment also could be experienced as "a state where all that is happening is good and supremely in one's best interest."

At this point, as is likely to happen when the subject reaches the threshold of the integral level, S made a kind of final summation of the data collected on the several levels and formulated mainly in symbolic-analogic terms. Speaking in a clear and almost matter-of-fact voice, he remarked that "The whole broad outline of my life, and also many of my life's particulars, now are seen by me much more clearly than ever before. I am able to see it all as being essentially an acting out of these dramas I was caught up in. I know that there are other ways of looking at my life, but I have a very strong feeling that this is the way I can deal with the facts most effectively.

"Once certain premises are accepted as in some way true, then everything makes perfect sense. I thought that I was some kind of devil and now, whatever the cause of that belief, I have managed to emancipate myself from the belief and from most of its effects. All of my life I have been trying to cut loose from something at the bottom of myself that prevented me from going where I wanted to go and also from knowing what I wanted to know. What I wanted to know was, essentially, God. But before I could get to know God I had to cut loose from most of what bound me to the Devil. I am sorry that what I have learned cannot be put into terms that would seem to me more scientific. I continue to have some resistance to understanding myself in these terms of God and Devil, Heaven and Hell, although I believe that these terms are the only ones really acceptable to me and effective as instruments of change. I would prefer not to have these naked truths stated so bluntly, but rather frosted over with lots of high-sounding medical terminology. But some part of my mind is especially well equipped to communicate with God and Devil. As the cords that have connected me to the Devil are being cut away, so does my anxiety diminish. I have experienced some of this during the last several years. I felt sometimes during this period that God was tossing me bones to lead me along as if I were a dog. I was afraid it might be a seduction, but allowed the possibility that it might be something else. Whenever I have seemed to be successful in dealing with God in personal terms, I have noticed I experience effects in my favor. As I cut through the cords or roots my anxiety diminishes. As my anxiety diminishes, I have the strength to cut through more of the cords. What was once a vicious circle thus has become a process working for me. I see that what I want most at this stage of my life is strength. Not strength to be used to subdue other persons, but strength enough to let me be master of myself. With the knowledge I have I can then use my strength to help others."

The time now seemed to have come for this subject to experience whatever was to be the culmination of a process that had developed continuously and with minimal meandering throughout the three sessions. S was told that there was now no more reason to resist and no justification for resisting—that he must now have his confrontation with God if he was going to have it. S agreed with this at once and lay back with his eyes closed, somehow conveying the impression of one in a state of extraordinary calm who, at the same time, was being infused with a vitality and a spiritual force not possessed by him before.

As might be expected, the psychedelic subject is not, at such a time, very communicative. In this case, S spoke very calmly but also in terse and rather cryptic phrases, a high degree of emotion becoming apparent only toward the end of his experience. The guide must not interrupt at such a time to ask for amplifications, and so it is necessary to reconstruct later what has occurred. Much is undoubtedly lost in so doing, but much more would be lost were one to keep interrupting and asking for details.

As since reconstructed, S now imaged and physically felt himself to be standing in an immense and brilliantly illumined hall where shone a preternatural light predominantly an "indescribable blending of white and gold." The Presence of God was tangible and overpowering within this hall and S understood that he was about to be initiated into some kind of order as yet not defined. Before him he saw a very large "occult" circle, etched into the highly polished substance of the floor. Many complicated symbols encrusted with precious stones were seen around the inner edges of the circle. And beyond the circle, through which he must pass, S perceived two tall, rectangular and gleaming white boxlike thrones. In one of these was standing, facing towards him, an enormous and exceedingly beautiful tiger; and, in the other, stood a lion of equally awesome stature and beauty. Emblazoned on the front of the boxes or on their pedestals were metallic jewel-studded *bas reliefs* of the tiger and lion, respectively. The initiation, S now understood, was for the purpose of investing him with "The Order of The Lion."

As his attention was drawn to the lion, S perceived from the corner of his eye that the tiger, now dead and apparently having been sacrificed, was being hauled up out of its box by braided ropes slipped under its forelegs; and, once clear of the throne, the tiger was lowered until it disappeared from his view.

S's attention continued to focus upon the great-maned archetypal lion standing majestically in its throne-box and facing towards him. Then, it seemed to S, he was transported to the rear of the box, stepped into it, and found himself to be identical with the lion although preserving the sense of his own identity as human. His body was the body of the lion and yet it remained his own body. His face was the face of the lion and yet it remained his own face. And during this "brief" identification, which seemed to him to last no more than a second, S suddenly knew that he had stopped being what was represented by the tiger and had become, instead, what was represented by the lion. He had left behind him the "blood-lust, anger, and unrestrained sensuality" of the tiger. The lion was "a more mature form, along the same lines of development as the tiger, but older, wiser and stronger—a creature destined to become wiser still, and who would not be controlled by his passions as the tiger had been."

S now once again assumed his own form, the lion was gone, and S stood in the place where previously the lion had been standing. He felt that now he was permitted to speak, and he suddenly found himself "asking all sorts of stupid questions of God"—i.e., was all of this "real" or was it "only a fantasy?" When he did this the lights in the hall were dimmed, and S felt that God had withdrawn in disgust at these questions. However, he was somehow reassured that what had been given to him would not now be taken away.

S at this point began to speak to us and seemed to be both awed and very upset. He said that the initiation images had been "much different from all of the other images" he had seen. He said of these images that "everything had a strange, dreamlike quality and I know that the content will pass away like a dream and be forgotten if I fail to tell you enough so that you can remind me of the major details afterward." He then related to us in much-condensed form the events just described.

We now urged S, since he felt that he had behaved so badly, to "Go back and tell God you are sorry. Remedy right now any mistakes you feel that you made." S then experienced the Presence of God for a second time, and on this occasion with much greater emotion than before.

The image was of "a great hand (God's hand) that the lion (S) rubs against with his cheek and nuzzles." S began to weep and later said that this image meant to him that the relationship between God and man was revealed to him in terms he was able to accept by means of this image. "The lion," he now *knew*, "can take full pride in being a lion and has no reason to be disturbed that he is not a man. The man is totally other than the lion and the lion is only able to exist as what he is. Any comparisons the lion may make can only be comparisons between himself and other beings like himself. There can be no degradation or humiliation in not being something that is entirely different from oneself. I see in this image that I can love God without being diminished as a man any more than a lion need be diminished as a lion by loving a human person. To weep is something I have never permitted myself to do. But now I am weeping and it is good. These tears are tears of joy—the very first tears of gladness I have ever wept in my whole life."

While S remained in this affect-charged state, it seemed advisable in what time remained in the wake of his God confrontation to deal with some of the "symbolic symptoms" described by him. The most outwardly dramatic moments of the session then occurred when S was asked to deal with his "roots."

G: "You have mentioned many times your 'evil roots,' those roots going down to the place you feel that you came from. Do you still feel those roots now?"

S: "My roots extended down to that other place. I have had to cut myself away from my roots one by one. I have a sense now of having cut through so many of these roots that there may not be too many of them left."

G: "Good, then maybe now you can pull free. Try pulling free. *Pull free now!*"

S: (Waves his feet in the air, makes jerking motions with his feet and legs, etc.) "I feel like I really am free! But it was so easy! I broke them off where they came into the soles of my feet. They were dry as dust and just crumbled when I started to pull away from them. Like dried old umbilicals, attached to the bottoms of my feet, and I've broken them all off. Why didn't I know before that they were ready to crumble? How long could they have been like that? Why, now I am free!" S was smiling, very excited, and looked extremely pleased and happy.

G: "And this hold that you say the Devil has had on you? What about that?"

S: "Satan has no more power to control me! I still have habit to fear, but the organic link is gone! What I just kicked loose was the whole serpent identification and the dead crumbling umbilical cord that still was tying me down to Hell. I seem to have shattered every physical connection with the place below. Look! (S gets up and stamps his feet against the ground.) I am crumbling the last remnants of the connection under my feet. I shake off the last of the dust and I step free of it all. My perception with regard to matter was what triggered everything off—seeing in the face of the little mermaid that it could be shaped in so many ways according to the way I looked at it. Intellectually, of course, I was aware of this before. But now I really knew it to be so and it seemed that from there I could go on to other real knowledge."

S now walked around the room, picking up his feet, shaking them, and declaring he was freeing himself from the last remnants of the "dust" that linked him to the "down below" aspects of his past. He looked at us, smiled very happily, and said: "It is over." The session had lasted less than five hours and the drug effects were cut off about as abruptly as lights go off when someone flips the switch.

The After-Effects. However awe-inspiring the strictly religious elements of the transforming experience, the subject's most immediate interest is almost always in himself and the ways he feels that he has been changed. Later, when some of his euphoria has passed, he returns to a more sober consideration of those moments of the session that were truly profound and climactic. For the present, however, the subject is intensely happy, even blissful as he continues to discover and itemize the various signs by which he knows he has been transformed.

S, for instance, discovered that with the "sloughing off" of his "roots" he experienced a sensation of lightness and also felt that the bottoms of his feet were "all new, like the feet of a new-born babe." He went to the bathroom again and found that his mirror image was substantially changed. His face appeared to be simultaneously younger and more mature. He had lost his "characteristically tormented look" and his upper body appeared to him to be more trim, more muscular, and better shaped. "Above all," he felt that his "whole general outlook" had been "changed for the better." He felt "an extreme contentment" and the sense that he had been "reborn and moved far beyond the limits imposed on the old self by restrictions that now have been dissolved."

Changes noted by S the next day included the following:

The previously noted mirror image changes were retained and the face seemed also "stronger" than before. The body seemed to have been energized and to be more compact, better co-ordinated, and also lighter than in the past. The bottoms of the feet continued to feel "like those of a child, tender and sensitive, a very, very good feeling."

All of the senses seemed to be more acute, and objects were apprehended as "presenting themselves more forcefully" and as "being less opaque, more easily yielding up meanings."

Looking down from a terrace high over the city, S found that a street scene he had always thought drab now was seen by him as "colorful and happy." A "mild anxiety" about "falling or jumping from high places" no longer was experienced except for his noting that it did not occur.

Sitting in a chair, S felt that he was sitting "less on the chair than *with* the chair." In all of his "relations to externals" he experienced a heightened sense of "unity and harmony."

His emotional state was one of "tranquility, a quiet kind of happiness and a security coming from the knowledge of having accomplished something enormously worthwhile, of having made some very great advances." "The mind" was "active, stimulated, but without any sense of the 'manic' involved in the stimulation."

S felt that he had "gone beyond" the Lucifer myth and so had gained a much greater measure of freedom to be himself.

He noted that "There is some occasional skepticism as regards the permanency of these benefits, but it is easily shrugged off. One feels that there is no need to analyze what has happened—It is what it is, and should simply be accepted. One should wait and see what develops, expect the best, and not pick at and try to tear apart the whole experience—as perhaps can be done with any experience, no matter how valid, thus reducing or entirely forfeiting the gains. However, there is much less a fear of losing the gains than there is a feeling of 'rightness' about letting the experience progress on its own terms. These terms were never primarily analytical, and possibly just the opposite of analyzing, breaking down. By opposite I mean that everything was directed toward fitting the pieces together into a harmonious whole, toward integrating and synthesizing."

Only two "negative side-effects" were reported by the subject. On the evening following his session, S was walking by the river and became aware of "a strange feeling of rootlessness, of having no real sense of direction." This was "only very mildly disturbing" and was understood by S as being the result of "cutting away the old roots." This feeling of rootlessness was accompanied by "a very positive feeling of greatly expanded freedom." He "rejoiced in the feeling of being free to go anywhere, of not being controlled," and felt "secure enough in the knowledge that the rootlessness was temporary and awaited my developing new and positive directions."

The second "side-effect" occurred four days later and was "intensely distressing, but also very brief." S had awakened during the night and "felt exceedingly uneasy." He walked into the next room and "for about thirty seconds experienced what can only be described as a sort of 'metaphysical panic.' During these few seconds it seemed to me that nothing any longer held me to the earth and that because of this I might simply blow away into what I thought of as a 'void.' This feeling passed when I told myself that it was the natural result of not being tied down any longer by the old roots, while I had not yet had time to attach myself to the world in a positive way." The "metaphysical panic" had not, a year later, recurred and S felt at that time that any danger of recurrence had passed. He was now "too strong, too happy, too much at home in the world to feel cast adrift and susceptible to being blown away."

Separated from his last session by the temporal distance of one year, S felt that he could offer "more objective" evidence in support of his conviction that important changes in himself had occurred.

He noted, for example, that his work capacity was greater than before and that this could be measured both by the volume of patients he was able to handle and by an increased literary output. "Subjectively," he felt that the quality of the literary output was higher and that he was being more effective in his therapeutic work.

S felt no wish to be promiscuous and had "fallen in love." He was planning to be married to a woman he felt to be his equal in every respect and no longer sought out the society of persons he regarded as inferior to him. He felt more "gregarious" and had translated this into action by participating in social activities for which he previously had "never had any time."

Where before he had felt it necessary to "stay on the wagon," S now was able to drink moderately and even "get a little high on occasion" without feeling the need to drink more and without engaging in any behavior offensive to others or damaging to himself.

"Subjectively" again, S felt that he had retained almost all of the gains reported just subsequent to his session. The mirror image and the felt body image remained improved. He seemed to have more energy and this had led to greater physical activity which, in turn, had improved his level of fitness and the general state of his health. He felt "fully human, a *bona fide* member of the species." "Devils" no longer whispered in his ear—i.e., each positive thought or perception no longer was swiftly followed by a kind of "negative reflex" with the positive idea such as "How good everything seems!" at once "provoking" such a thought as "You are kidding yourself. The world is an ugly and wicked place!"

In general, he felt, "a destructive response to the world has been replaced by a response that is essentially creative."

Comments. No more than the subject will we attempt to analyze this case in any orthodox way. Conventional psyche-analysis is not a part of the psychedelic experience as we have worked with it. There is no purpose that requires such analysis and neither would conventional analysis very often be successful in one or even several psychedelic sessions.

S, at one year after his session, continued to regard himself as "transformed" and to behave as he feels he could only behave as a consequence of an authentic transformation. These two criteria: *subjective certainty* that a transformation has occurred, and *behavioral changes* of a positive character supporting the certainty of transformation, seem to us to be sufficient evidence that the person *has in fact been transformed*. This does not mean that all questions are thereby answered.

We have said that this is an authentic religious experience. By that we can only mean that it is authentic in terms of such criteria as we are able to devise for measuring whether such an experience is or is not authentic. Someone else may say that "God can't be found in a bottle" and go on from there to say that one cannot have a religious experience without God. *Ergo*, whatever else may be involved in this case, it is not a religious experience. Definition then excludes the possibility that we are correct and the discussion ends there. However, anyone arguing in this way must also, we think, rule out most of the "religious experiences" of many famous mystics and saints, since these persons, too, induced in themselves physiological changes instrumental in bringing about confrontation with God and mystical union. Drugs are quicker and perhaps more effective than fasting and other ascetic practices, but the principle would seem to be the same.

Unfortunately, the high emotional content, sense of awe and reverence, and other elements of a psychedelic subject's religious experience cannot really be conveyed in such a way as to validate the content of the experience so far as a reader is concerned. Thus, we can only provide certain facts we consider to be relevant and then offer our evaluation of those facts and the evaluative criteria employed. Some of these criteria are also subjective and not susceptible to objective measurement. For example, we cannot hope to convince anyone by speaking of the "emotional feel" of a subject's authentic religious experience as compared to those experiences we, as observers, dismiss as inauthentic. The "contagion" of the authentic experience moves from the subject to those physically present and cannot be further communicated by means of the written word. The skeptic who easily dismisses the first-person accounts to be found in, say, Bucke and James, will not be impressed with regard to religious content by our data either.

It will be clear from this case as from others that our schema of psychical drug-state levels does not describe a phenomenological pattern of progression invariably followed by the subject. In the case just given, S certainly does not move in orderly fashion from one level to the next. Rather, he "plunges" into various "depths," "comes up" to "surface" at a "higher level," then "descends" again, and so on. The value of our schema is *methodological*, permitting us to recognize within limits "where" the subject "is" so that we are able to have some idea of what is possible at that "place"; and permitting us, too, to direct the subject toward "deeper levels" where we know from experience that certain phenomena and effects are likely to be possible. Whatever the present defects of this method, whether in lack of precision or otherwise, it nonetheless is effective to a degree we have not found any other method to be.

In the foregoing case the subject's active, intelligent, and highly developed imagination has enabled him to erect upon a rather commonplace foundation an exceedingly complex and certainly fascinating superstructure. But if we do not miss the forest on account of the lushness of the foliage, we are able to see clearly enough those typical elements with which the guide may work to lead the subject toward self-understanding and, hopefully, profound and beneficial self-reorientation.

In moving toward these goals it assuredly is helpful if the subject has gained by more conventional means some real understanding of his mental processes and problems. Individuals (including psychoanalysts) who have been analyzed often do particularly well as psychedelic subjects. However, as subject, the person must be prepared to go far beyond the search for traumas, dissection of motives, and so forth, and operate in ways enabling him to profit to the full from all of the tools he now has at his disposal.

Particularly the subject now must work with symbolic representations, not with the stark and unadorned facts of his existence. He must be enabled to formulate his problem in symbolic terms in order that the problem may be resolved on a symbolic level where it no longer is necessary to deal with the literal factual materials so often productive of resistances not met with when the materials are symbolically represented.

Once the person is able to perceive his life in these symbolic terms—in terms of a myth, as S saw his life, or perhaps in terms of the need to participate in some rite of passage—then the ground has been laid for participation in the symbolic actions. One may "go down," as S did, to the "place" where one has one's "roots" and there, in symbolic form, encounter materials which set in quickening motion a mobilization and orchestration of powerful, beneficent forces. The symbolization of the life, that is, initiates a process wherein image, ideation, sensation, and finally, affect, work *for* the person and, when final orchestration is achieved, bring about some degree of positive transformation. Observing the development of this process, it becomes difficult to avoid the speculation that there exists within the person some entelechical impetus tending towards positive integration.

That the "entelechical" process so often moves toward confrontation with the most potent and beneficent of all man's symbols—God—scarcely should surprise us. Neither should we be surprised when we know how often the movement is just toward this "Symbol," that the God *is* potent and that the confrontation with God, the authentic religious experience, *does have* the power to transform.

Psychedelic Drugs and Mystical Experience. Of mysticism it often has been said that it begins in mist and ends in schism; and to this statement, the psychedelic variety is no exception. A part of the blame for the historical abundance of misty schisms may lie with the ambiguities inherent in the mystical experience itself. As writers and mystics alike have noted, there are two distinct and differing types of mystical experience available—the inward and the outward way. Variously termed introvertive and extrovertive, introspective and extrospective, both involve the apprehension of an Ultimate Unity with which the seeker unites or identifies. The outward way differs from the inward in that whereas the one attempts to discover the Ultimate Unity in the external world, the other introspects into the depths of the self therein to meet and yield to the Ground of Being. Mystics and writers are unanimous in declaring the inward way the superior mysticism. The outward variety is considered at most a preparation for the true mystic pilgrimage inward.

In his classic study of mysticism, the noted philosopher W. T. Stace distinguishes between the two types of mysticism and terms them extrovertive and introvertive. He suggests seven common characteristics of introvertive mystical states of mind as evidenced from a wide sampling of the literature of mystical experience. According to Stace, these seven characteristics are:

1. The Unitary Consciousness, from which all the multiplicity of sensuous or conceptual or other empirical content has been excluded, so that there remains only a void and empty unity. This is the one basic, essential, nuclear characteristic, from which most of the others inevitably follow.

2. Being nonspatial and nontemporal. This of course follows from the nuclear characteristic listed above.

3. Sense of objectivity or reality.

4. Feelings of blessedness, joy, peace, happiness, etc.

5. Feeling that what is apprehended is holy, sacred, or divine.

6. Paradoxicality.

7. Alleged by mystics to be ineffable.[24]

Extrovertive mysticism differs from the introvertive variety in only the first two characteristics. In extrovertive mysticism, according to Stace's typology, there is no Unitary Consciousness but only a unifying vision "expressed abstractly by the formula 'All is One.' The One is, in extrovertive mysticism, perceived through the physical senses, in or through the multiplicity of objects." The nonspatial and nontemporal character of introvertive mysticism has no place in the extrovertive variety in which there is a "concrete apprehension of the One as being an inner subjectivity in all things, described variously as life, or consciousness, or a living Presence. The discovery that nothing is really dead,"[25] is also a crucial revelation for the extrovertive mystic.

In the psychedelic drug-state there also may occur major and minor forms of mysticism, these being roughly equivalent to Stace's descriptions of the extrovertive and introvertive varieties. The drug subject is also prone, however, to another experiential possibility of mystical awareness, one which is nothing more than an analogue of mystical experience differing from the religious analogues already described mainly in the degree of identification and the intensity with which the subject responds to persons, objects, and various drug-state phenomena. These mystical analogues we do not regard as authentic mystical or religious experiences. At best they are experiences of intense empathic communion often rendered more impressive still by such accompanying drug-state phenomena as ego loss and body dissolution. That these are profoundly moving and impressive experiences explains in part why it is that they are so often confused with authentic states of mystical awareness.

In our investigations we have discovered that religious professionals are especially given to this kind of confusion, perhaps because of their strong desire to have first-hand experience of a phenomenon with which they may have had only theoretical familiarity. As often has been true in the past, at the opportunity of moving from theory into practice the scholar and theologian will all too often mistake the sow's ear for the silk purse.

In discussing the extrovertive mystical experience as it occurs in the psychedelic state, we will limit ourselves to an examination of one of its most frequently recurring types—a type experienced by almost one half of all our LSD subjects and which we will term *cosmological mysticism*. Cosmological mysticism is essentially an ecstatic experience of Nature and Process which leaves the subject with a sense of having acquired important insight into, as well as identity with, the fundamental nature and structure of the universe. Rarely transformative of the person as integral level experience may be transformative, it is not a religious experience either, since it rarely involves an individual encounter with That which is perceived as God or Being. Pantheistic terms are frequently employed, but what the subject expresses is likely to be the pervasiveness of energy states rather than the plenitude of deity.

Cosmological Mysticism. In its best sense cosmological mysticism is an experience of Reality illumined from within; an experience in which, to quote Blake's words, "the doors of perception are cleansed" so that "everything appears to man as it is, infinite."[26] It is an experience that has inspired poets and nature mystics to revel in the Immanence in things and to speak of:

> . . . a sense sublime
> of something far more deeply interfused,
> Whose swelling is the light of setting suns,
> And the round ocean and the living air,
> And the blue sky, and in the mind of man:
> A motion and a spirit, that impels
> All thinking things, all objects of all thought,
> And rolls through all things.[27]

With the great mystics of the past this is familiar terrain and is regarded as a way station along the Mystic Path. The Protestant mystic, Jacob Boehme, was especially prone to the raptures of cosmological mysticism, for as Evelyn Underhill remarks:

"In Boehme's life . . . there were three distinct onsets of illumination; all of the pantheistic and external type . . . About the year 1600 occurred the second illumination, initiated by a trancelike state of consciousness, the result of gazing at a polished disk . . . This experience brought with it that particular and lucid vision of the inner reality of the phenomenal world in which, as he says, he looked into the deepest foundations of things . . . He believed that it was only a fancy, and in order to banish it from his mind he went out upon the green. But here he remarked that he gazed into the very heart of things . . . viewing the herbs and grass of the field in his inward light, he saw into their essences, use, and properties, which were discovered to him by their lineaments, figures, and signatures . . ."[28]

It is not uncommon for the psychedelic subject to feel that he, too, gazes into the very heart of things to discover therein the "essences, use, and properties," the "lineaments, figures, and signatures." He, too, may be certain that he perceives the "hidden unity in the Eternal Being" and knows directly the mysterious workings of Nature which science is only beginning to guess at. This sense of acquiring real knowledge of the processes of life while in the drug-state, is at first glance one of the more baffling phenomena of the state we have termed cosmological mysticism.

In a curious article entitled "The Religious Experience: Its Production and Interpretation," Timothy Leary asserts that "those aspects of the psychedelic experience which subjects report to be ineffable and ecstatically religious involve a direct awareness of the processes which physicists and biochemists and neurologists measure." Leary believes[29] that the data of the drug session provide psychedelic correlates remarkably similar to the most advanced scientific thinking with regard to 1) the ultimate power question, 2) the life question, 3) the human-destiny question, and 4) the ego question. Leary had defined religious experience as the "ecstatic, incontrovertibly certain, subjective discovery of answers to these four basic questions." He argues that since psychedelic correlates correspond so favorably to current scientific findings, the subject who achieves such information in the course of his session is undoubtedly undergoing an authentic religious or mystical experience according to the Leary definition.

Our own position is that while we have witnessed the same kind of phenomena Leary describes, we would be very hesitant to suggest as he does that in the ecstatic-psychedelic state genetic codes are unlocked, nuclear enigmas revealed, and the virtual infinity of intracellular communication lines perceived and in some sense understood. Further, we must argue that his criteria for what constitutes religious and mystical experience are not adequate as criteria for the authentic experience. As mystics through the ages have known and shown, much that is accepted as evidence by Leary is but a part of the exotica accompanying certain minor forms of mysticism.

To take a brief look at some of this exotica, we find drug subjects with little or no scientific training describing evolutionary processes in some detail, spelling out the scenery of microcosm and macrocosm in terms roughly equivalent to those used by the modern physicist, empathizing with primal states of matter and energy and then recounting this experience in terms more reminiscent of Heisenberg than of an hallucinatory state. Since this book already is replete with subjects' descriptions of just such experiences, there is no need to burden the reader with further "documentation" of this kind.

Still the question remains: Where is this information coming from? Is it a gift of God? of Grace? of hyper-neuronal ecstasy? Is it a result of our twelve billion brain cells astronomically interconnecting at the speed of light and now galvanized by a psychedelic drug to ever more prodigious computations—to tune in finally on the Process Itself? Or perhaps may it be, as some theorists propose, that the cell has its knowledge that Knowledge does not know? In regard to this last suggested explanation, it might be argued that it is a well-known fact of biophysics that there is a kind of purposiveness to all bodily processes, be they ever so microscopic. It might be, then, that in the sensitized psychedelic state the subject picks up some sense of this purposiveness from his physical processes which he then dramatizes in terms of the drama of birth, growth, decay, and death. Or could it even be that the subject becomes aware of the purposiveness and then transforms this insight into a scientific spectacular from information dimly remembered or subliminally recorded?

Whatever the explanation may be, we believe that it is fair to say that we are here facing the same problem that was met with in the preceding chapter. There, it will be recalled, we described several instances of remarkably accurate and sometimes esoteric historical descriptions provided by persons who seemed largely ignorant of that kind of information. Just as one might have recourse to a "collective unconscious" in explaining the historical evocations, so with regard to the present phenomena one can easily fall into a kind of Jungian physicalism, proposing *a priori* knowledge of energy and nuclear and cellular processes. Claiming unconscious *a priori* knowledge is a very seductive stance, but it does not exhaust the possibilities. A more probable speculation would propose the drug-induced activation of memory patterns dealing with scientific data. As we observed in the previous chapter, the average American is exposed through his reading of newspapers, magazines, TV-watching, to enormous amounts of exoteric and esoteric information concerning a vast range of subject matter. This information is haphazardly absorbed, consciously forgotten, but cumulatively stored in regions of the mind accessible under certain conditions. As the surprising emergence of historical data into a subject's consciousness may constitute subliminal triumphs of *Time, Life, Newsweek,* so the scientific arcana of cosmological mysticism may be similarly attributed.

Having offered some suggestions as to the "where" of this material, it still remains to inquire after the "why." Why should a religious or mystic-type experience have as an important part of its content the metaphors and meanings of science? The reason, we will speculate, is this: Since man has been man he has limned his understanding of life through mythological motifs, finding in the myth both dimensional perspective and the emotional force necessary to interpret his world. As the mythopoeics of one age become inadequate for a succeeding age, the myth assumes a broader and sometimes more factual base from which it either develops or decays. Today the mythic mantle has passed in many cases from gods and heroes and has fallen upon the extraordinary hypotheses of inner and outer space. The new scientific knowledge concerning molecule and galaxy, DNA and RNA, force field and wave length, creation and evolution, provides the *stuff* of myth-making and constitutes part of the present domain of "sacred knowledge." It is for this reason then that we believe that after the psychedelic subject has paid eidetic and ideational lip service to traditional (but demythologized) myths and deities, he often will center his emotion and conviction upon the re-mythologized vistas of sacramentalized science. As we have shown throughout this book, it is a commonplace for the subject to apprehend the world both mythically and empathically. Cosmological mysticism would appear to be the mythic and empathic apprehension of the world, often scientifically conceptualized by virtue of the subject's normal or subliminal familiarity with the terms and "sacred" hypotheses of the new science. Cosmological mysticism is also the mythopoeic eye ecstatically encountering these hypotheses (the dogmatics of the myth) in the data of the world and so experiencing these data as revelatory though coherent, mystical though precise.

Introvertive Mystical Experience. Among our psychedelic drug sub-jects the authentic and introvertive mystical state as described by Stace has appeared to occur at the deepest phenomenological stratum of the subject's experience. This deep stratum, of the integral level, may be reached rather quickly when the movement is towards introvertive mys-tical experience. Sensory level phenomena are especially rich and typi-cally include some variety of cosmological mysticism which may be an important first step towards the more profound mystical state yet to come. After that, the subject moves quickly through comparatively unimportant recollective-analytic materials to the symbolic experiences carrying him to the threshold of what for want of a better term we will call the *Mysterium* of the integral level. This Mysterium almost always is experienced as the source level of reality. Here, the semantics of theological discourse become the visceral realities of the subject; and such well-known concepts as the "primordial essence" and the "ulti-mate Ground of Being" take on an immediacy and clarity hitherto unknown.

Out of our total of 206 subjects we believe that six have had this (introvertive mystical) experience. It is of interest to observe that those few subjects who attain to this level of mystical apprehension have in the course of their lives either actively sought the mystical experience in meditation and other spiritual disciplines or have for many years dem-onstrated a considerable interest in integral levels of consciousness. It also should be noted that all of these subjects were over forty years of age, were of superior intelligence, and were well-adjusted and creative personalities. It would appear, therefore, that where there is an intellec-tual and other predisposition, a belief in the validity of religious and mystical experience, and the necessary maturity and capacity to un-dergo such experience, then we have the conditions favorable to the psychedelic-mystical state.

Reports from the subjects concerning the structure and development of their mystical experience show a remarkable similarity. Along with generally confirming the characteristics of the introvertive mystical ex-perience as Stace describes it, they also agree as to many particulars met with, too, in the classical literature of mysticism. In almost every case the experience is initiated with a sense of the ego dissolving into boundless being. This process is almost always attended by an experi-ence of the subject being caught up in a torrent of preternatural light. S-4, a forty-nine-year-old woman (LSD), gives a typical description of this light:

"My body became the body of bliss, diaphanous to the rhythms of the universe. All around and passing through me was the Light, a trillion atomized crystals shimmering in blinding incandescence. I was carried by this Light to an Ecstasy beyond ecstasy and suddenly I was no longer I but a part of the Divine Workings. There was no time, no space, no 'I,' no 'You,' only—the Becoming of Being."

Another common aspect of the experience is the subject's becoming aware of himself as continuous with the energy of the universe. This is frequently described with words to the effect that the person was part of a dynamic continuum. It is also experienced as a state in which the subject feels himself to be filled by divinity. We find this illustrated in the experience of another LSD subject, S-5, a fifty-two-year-old engineer, who writes:

"Although consciousness of self seemed extinguished, I knew that the boundaries of my being now had been dissolved and that all other boundaries also were dissolved. All, including what had been myself, was an ever more rapid molecular whirling that then became something else, a pure and seething energy that was the whole of Being. This energy, neither hot nor cold, was experienced as a white and radiant fire. There seemed no direction to this whirling, only an acceleration of speed, yet one knew that along this dynamic continuum the flux of Being streamed inexorably, unswervingly toward the One.

"At what I can only call the 'core' of this flux was God, and I cannot explain how it was that I, who seemed to have no identity at all, yet experienced myself as *filled with God*, and then as (whatever this may mean) *passing through God* and into a Oneness wherein it seemed God, Being, and a mysterious unnameable One constituted together what I can only designate the ALL. What 'I' experienced in this ALL so far transcends my powers of description that to speak, as I must, of an ineffably rapturous Sweetness is an approximation not less feeble than if I were to describe a candle and so hope to capture with my words all of the blazing glory of the sun."

It is characteristic of the subject during the mystical state to feel that the categories of time are strained by the tensions of eternity. "Everything was touched with eternity," said one subject. "Time was no longer. Eternity had burst in," said another. "Eternity had flooded the gates of time," said still another.

The subject experiences the world as transfigured and unified. He describes himself as having been caught up in an undifferentiated unity wherein the knower, the knowledge, and the known are experienced as a single reality. In the following case we have an account by a subject whose whole experience largely typifies the range of phenomena encountered in the psychedelic mystical experience. The subject, S-6, is a highly sensitive and intelligent woman in her late fifties. She wrote the following "Subjective Report" about twenty-nine hours after taking 75 micrograms of LSD:

"For those interested in the type of experience that was mine I should like to record, in the interest of 'preparation,' 'motivation,' that I have, for over twenty-five years, been drawn to the philosophy and literature of ancient China, India, and Tibet, and have practiced the science of meditation. After reading the published account of Aldous Huxley's experiences under mescaline, I hoped some day to have a similar opportunity to know the true meaning of an expanded consciousness. After waiting some years, this was given. Under guidance and in the company of beloved friends, I was given 75 gamma of LSD.

"Lying on a comfortable couch, in a room of great serenity, filled with roses, pansies, and hydrangea, I felt almost immediately a sense of profound relaxation and a great inner peace. I watched the sunlight on the ceiling as it played through the shadow of the windowpanes reflected there.

"Soon a shell-pink rose was given to me to observe. I sat up to do this and though quite prepared for the phenomenon given to most everyone under this influence, I was overwhelmed by the life that pulsated through this fragile, delicate flower. Its petals rhythmically expanding and contracting and hues of pink rushing into its heart and out again. It was spellbinding, and as I re-emerged into a three-dimensional world I looked with awe upon what I considered a live, fresh flower and realized that it was only a 'still life' in comparison to that which had been given. I asked whether my hand was trembling, so alive was this quivering rose. Later, I observed the rich, deep velvet tones of a large-faced pansy with the same 'inner seeing' only its heart became a fathomless tunnel of light.

"Now I no longer wanted the abstractions of this kind of glory, for deep within was the thirst for a greater knowing into the ancient Wisdom teaching I had long wrestled with. Closing my eyes, my position was suddenly shifted to some Oriental posture—legs folded across—palms facing up—wrists meeting under chin—it was pleasant—as if it were a prankish, almost impish moment into some former incarnation. Then followed this verbatim description (from notes made at the time) of what came out as 'The First Absorption'—The longing of my soul to experience the Reality of Oneness with the Absolute was my paramount hope and motivation in taking LSD—that some breakthrough might be given. Also, long had I contemplated whether Identity is sustained in the final Absorption. With these thoughts, I became a diffused light that broke into a brilliant glittering, quivering thing—then it burst—bringing a shower of dazzling rays—each ray filled with a myriad of colors— gold, purple, emerald, ruby—and each ray charged with a current— throwing off sparkling lights—there was the Ecstasy—all identification with self dissolved. There was no sense of time-space. Only an aware- ness of Being. At last I cried: 'I cannot endure this any longer. It is enough.' Someone whispered: 'You are given that which you can en- dure.' Then I wept. I recall there were 'instances' of a returning aware- ness. At no time was there a sense of the individualized self. I never knew when 'I' entered the stream. Only the emergence out of it.

"I joined the group who were having a late (?) lunch (there *is* no time) on the terrace. A friend asked whether I would like to have something and I said no and made a remark about those 'historic fig- ures' reputed to have lived a life without partaking of food and won- dered how this could be. Instantly, I became a vessel—a mighty force of energy, sparkling, crystal-like, and pure, came pouring into me. I remember thinking or saying—'This is the pure source of energy—right from the very mouth of Godhead.' The current entered into me— through the fingers first, then coursed through my entire body and all of me seemed electrified. I felt energized, knew to an overwhelming degree the meaning of regeneration and thought 'this is how it's done.' Why should this have to go into the earth, to be converted into food—to be digested and again converted into energy, when one may have it pure and glorified. I saw it dissipate itself into the earth and rise with incredi- ble speed into a spiral going up, up, up, and then I spoke of the Whirl- ing Dervishes and understood the Cosmic meaning of all nature dances and how man and nature merge into one.

"I was reminded that I had not yet known the joy of being outdoors, in the grass and under the trees. We went out beyond the house where I lay in the grass, felt its wondrous texture with my fingers and toes, then rose to stand under a cedar tree. Embracing its branches and burying my head, I was overcome by the crisp, pungent fragrance of the cedar. At that moment an icy wind began to blow over and through me and I was shifted to some solitary height, measureless, boundless, and inde- scribable. There I shivered and in that instant there came a repeat of the former, shatteringly ecstatic experience of an exploding shower of sparkling light, pouring into me illuminating rays of glittering jeweled tones—emeralds, amethyst, ruby, and gold.

"We returned indoors. I again stretched out on the couch, exhausted, spent. In conversation I mentioned everything that I had ever sought to experience in the realm of the 'other world' had been given—although the 'between worlds' had not. Instantly I became aware of a formless mass hovering above the gross body. At first it appeared with a cloud-like dimness—the texture gradually becoming more and more delicate and finally translucent. There was a sense of buoyancy—an inexpressible joy. I thought 'this may be suspended animation.' Unlike the two earlier experiences, this awareness had form. It was lovely and one knew why meditation at this level could be indefinitely sustained. I do not recall that 'it' had identity. I believe not.

"After the guides felt the peak had been reached, it was explained that I would descend quietly and cold cloths were applied to my head which now was throbbing. The ache became concentrated at the center of my forehead—between the eyes. This became so penetrating that I placed the third finger of my left hand on the spot and pressed down with all my strength. In so doing the finger became an iron shaft that kept pushing down, down, down. It was excruciatingly painful and remained so. All the while I felt something was 'being done.' The sense of several faceless, formless, and nameless presences were around the area making a concerted effort to keep the shaft going deeper and deeper. The pain increased and I cried out: 'No more today, please. Don't give it all in one day.' And suddenly the pain reached such intensity that it was no longer a pain. Questions were asked by voices in the room and someone mentioned the third eye episode and asked was it similar and what did it mean to me. I felt the shaft and said simply, 'an initiation.' It diffused itself by streaming to the base of the skull and dividing. The ache back of each ear was awful until it flowed into many little veins and entered some subterranean passage. The area between the eyes felt as if some surgery had been performed, the wound stitched and with the anesthetic waning, was left tender and sore."[30]

Although the experiences of introvertive drug-state mysticism are integral level experiences, they rarely yield any such radical transformation of the subject's inner and outer life as ordinarily results from the integral level religious experiences. The reason for this may be that those few subjects who are sufficiently prepared for and able to attain to introvertive mystical states are already persons of exceptional mental and emotional maturity and stability. The present potential of the person already has been in large measure realized. It is also possible, however, that the aforementioned tendency of these subjects to avoid or minimize work with psychodynamic materials may preclude the possibility of a transforming experience.

Apparently, introvertive mystical experience, at least in the case of the psychedelic subject, does not occur except in those instances where preparation has been considerable and a state or readiness for the mystical experience has been established. It may be significant that in each of our six cases of introvertive mysticism, the subject probably was, at the time of the session, near the peak of his or her preparation and readiness to undergo a profound mystical experience. Thus the function of the drug-state seems to have been that of giving the subject the final push off the mystical brink on which he or she already was standing.

We have said that the psychedelic mystical experience closely resembles the seven-point typology of mystical experience set forth by Stace. In fact, when Stace recently was asked if he thought the psychedelic mystical experience to be similar to traditional mystical experience, he responded that "It's not a matter of it being *similar* to mystical experience; it *is* mystical experience."[31] To this judgment we would like to introduce a qualification we feel to be significant to the future development and understanding of states of religious and mystical consciousness.

Our qualification has to do not with the *culmination* of the mystical experience—since we feel that the psychedelic and traditional varieties afford a virtually identical experience of non-sensuous, atemporal Unitary Consciousness—but with the developmental process of the experience, since here we have observed the psychedelic type to differ diametrically from the traditional. These differences of process are evidenced in the following important manner:

In nondrug introvertive mysticism, whether of the Eastern or Western variety, the seeker attempts a long, arduous process of gradually emptying his mind of all its empirical content; that is, of all events, associations, sensations, images, symbols—until the mind becomes a virtual vacuum which then can be "filled" with the Mystic Void. By thus systematically ridding the mind of its multiplicity the traditional adept attains to the pure essence of the Undifferentiated Unity, the One without a second. But in the psychedelic experience, it would appear that just the opposite happens. Consciousness expands and reaches outward to encompass a wealth of phenomena unprecedented in the subject's experience. The empirical content of the subject's mind is vitalized, the multiplicity compounded, and the fullness of awareness increases to an intensity that may seem almost too great to be borne. Then, with the crossing-over into the integral, consciousness abruptly and spontaneously contracts, narrowing to a focal point of awareness, which being so compacted then explodes into the mystic state of One Single Reality. The process is such that the phenomena condense into the Noumenon, the many into the One, the particulars into Essence.

While it is impossible at this time to make comparative qualitative judgments concerning psychedelic and traditional mysticism, it appears to us evident that the process leading toward Mystical Culmination is far richer in the case of the psychedelic subject than is the *via negativa* or path of obliteration of the traditional mystic. This is an area in which our conclusions have not yet crystallized and to the consideration of which we plan to give much further attention. However, we do feel it possible to suggest that the disparate processes involved in these two mysticisms may do much to explain the withdrawal from life of many of the traditional mystics as compared to the psychedelic mystic's oft-observed tendency to move towards a fullness of experience.

In the case of our six subjects who experienced the introvertive mystical state, the only significant change in post-session behavior observed by either us or the subject was a change toward increasing concern with and appreciation of the particulars of existence. For if one were to note any single deficiency characteristic of all of these subjects, it would be the somewhat abstracted attitude they had acquired as a result of their years of preparational devotions. The beneficial effect of the psychedelic mystical experience, then, was to take the subject through a process of experiencing Essence in such a way that it illuminated all of existence, making him more interested in and responsive to the phenomena of existence than he had been before. Thus, instead of retreating from the phenomenal world, as often occurs with the traditional mystic, the psychedelic subject was inspired by the process of his experience to a kind of flight *towards* reality.[32]

Epilogue

To comment first of all on the preceding chapter, it should be clearly understood that we make no judgment as to whether confrontation or union with a literal God has occurred in the experiences described. Such a determination could have no foundation other than our own wishes and personal beliefs. No more could we make such a judgment were we present with a Saint Theresa in her cell or a Saint Francis of Assisi in the chapel. Only within the accepted limitations of our phenomenological approach do we say that some of these experiences are "authentic."

But if we cannot say of the psychedelic journey that God certainly is waiting to welcome each voyager, still it should be clear that this experience holds out the promise of rewards of incalculable value. Can there be any justified doubt, for example, that we have been describing regions of mind and states of consciousness hitherto inaccessible or accessible only very rarely and under conditions hardly favorable to careful study? We think there can be no such doubt and that we have done what we said at the outset we would do—"make credible our belief that the psychedelic drugs afford the best access yet to the contents and processes of the human mind."

Do these drugs then promise discoveries about mind as important and far-reaching in their ultimate effects as have been the revolutionary findings of this century concerning the physical universe? At the very least, the promise is so great that every effort should be made to determine whether, with the new psycho-chemicals, we now have the means of exploring and charting the whole or large segments of the human psyche, or a tool of more limited application. That the right kind of research will, in any case, yield rewards of very great value seems to us absolutely certain.

The question thus arises: Shall this potential slip from our grasp, or its realization be for long delayed, because of unwarranted restrictions imposed on the basis of excessive caution or for reasons even less worthy? Or shall we work out a practical program of research with essential safeguards provided, but without the crippling limitation of control by a single profession whose members necessarily are ignorant in many of the areas where psychedelic work could be most fruitful? Overcoming the psychedelic drug status quo with its unrealistic prohibitions and misunderstandings will be very difficult; but surely the effort should be made.

As regards our own work, it has been pioneering and therefore is crude and tentative, as such work has to be. Had legal restrictions not blocked its continuance, refinement and perhaps some additional and altered conclusions would have been possible. As it is, we must present only partial findings—with the hope that others will be able to use our work as a foundation upon which to build.

Nonetheless, we have thought a book warranted at this time. For one thing, there has not existed up to now a single realistic work detailing an approach to guiding drug sessions or providing any theoretical basis for psychedelic work that is *grounded in the psychedelic experience itself*. These we have sought to provide, and now it remains for others to test our approach and attempt to repeat our results in their own work. We look forward to learning the outcome of any and all such efforts.

We want to mention, too, that we hope we have established the very great importance and challenge of the eidetic images and the need to study them exhaustively both within the context of the psychedelic drug-state and outside it. Most curiously, the importance of these images has been all but overlooked by most workers, and the symbolic dramas have been ignored or barely mentioned by writers with whose work we are familiar. If these images and dramas still are but little understood, at least we now have a much better understanding of their potential value for the psychedelic subject.

The revolution in the study of mind is at hand. *The Varieties of*

Psychedelic Experience may suggest that that revolution can effect an *evolution* of mind also. For we doubt that extensive work in this area can fail to result in eventually pushing human consciousness beyond its present limitations and on towards capacities not yet realized and perhaps undreamed of.

Notes

Chapter One

1. A breakdown of the 206 sessions guided or observed by the authors shows the number of subjects taking the various drugs to be as follows: LSD, 112; Peyote, 85; Mescaline, 4; DMT, 3; and Psilocybin, 2. In this book we deal almost exclusively with LSD and peyote experiences.

2. Psychedelic subjects repeatedly have said that they regard their drug experience or some aspect of it as their "richest" or "most important" experience, etc. This occurs not just in our work, but also in the work of a great many other researchers.

Chapter Two

1. For extended discussions see Masters, R.E.L., *Eros and Evil: The Sexual Psychopathology of Witchcraft.* Julian Press, New York, 1962; also, by the same author, *Forbidden Sexual Behavior and Morality.* Julian Press, New York, 1962.

2. In some of the older literature: *Anhalonium lewinii.*

3. The literature of peyotism among the American Indians is substantial. The most important volume is Weston La Barre's *The Peyote Cult,* reissued in an updated edition in 1964 by the Shoe String Press of Hamden, Connecticut. The reader may also profitably consult J.S. Slotkin's *The Peyote Religion,* Free Press of Glencoe, Illinois, 1956. No one attempting a study of peyote should neglect, at the very beginning, to avail himself of La Barre's outstanding bibliographies.

4. Osmond, H., "Peyote Night," in *Tomorrow.* Spring, 1961, p. 113.

5. That peyote ought not to be considered along with such narcotic drugs as heroin and morphine was clearly set forth in an admirable decision at Flagstaff, Arizona, in July of 1960. At that time, the Hon. Yale McFate, considering action against a Navaho woman, ruled that "Peyote is not a narcotic. It is not habit-forming. . . . The use of Peyote is essential to the existence of the peyote religion. Without it, the practice of the religion would be effectively prevented. . . . It is significant that many states which formerly outlawed the use of peyote have abolished or amended their laws to permit its use for religious purposes. It is also significant that the Federal Government has in nowise prevented the use of peyote by Indians or others." However, in 1964, the California Fourth District Court of Appeals ruled against the use of peyote in that state and found that ". . . the use of peyote in Indian religious ceremonies constitutes enough of a threat to public safety to make the act illegal without violating constitutional rights of religious freedom." The wording of parts of this ruling made it clear that the court was more concerned with keeping peyote away from "Beatniks" than it was with barring peyote use by Indians. This brings to mind famed botanist Richard Schultes' axiom that when problems arise in connection with drug use, they tend to "arise after the narcotics have passed from ceremonial to purely hedonic or recreational use." Whether this fear of "hedonic" (and other nonreligious) use is warranted in the case of peyote is a question this book may help to answer.

6. Lewin, L., *Phantastica, Narcotic and Stimulating Drugs*. E.P. Dutton & Co., New York, 1964, p. xvi.

7. Mitchell, S. Weir, "The effects of Anhalonium Lewinii (the mescal button)," *British Medical Journal*. 1896, 2: 1625.

8. Ellis, H., "Mescal: A New Artificial Paradise," *The Contemporary Review*. January, 1898. Also in *Annual Report of the Smithsonian Institution*, 1898, pp. 537-548.

9. Cohen, S., *The Beyond Within: The LSD Story*. Atheneum, New York, 1964, p. 231.

10. See, for instance, Fisher, G., "Some Comments Concerning Dosage Levels of Psychedelic Compounds for Psychotherapeutic Experiences," *Psychedelic Review*. Vol. 1, No. 2, 1963. However, we consider Fisher's recommended dosages to be on the high side and call especial attention to his warning that extremely drug-sensitive persons always should be given lesser amounts of a psychedelic drug.

11. A "good" example of this is the article, "They Split My Personality," by Harry Asher, which appeared in *Saturday Review*, June 1, 1963. Asher's unfortunate LSD experience, and its still more unfortunate aftermath, doubtless makes fairly entertaining reading; but it cannot do other than create a misleading and damaging impression of the LSD experience as it unfolds in the vast majority of cases.

12. Cf. Hyde, R.W., "Psychological and Social Determinants of Drug Action," in Sarwer-Foner, G.J., *The Dynamics of Psychiatric Drug Therapy*. Charles C. Thomas, Springfield, Illinois, 1960, p. 297, as regards the importance of the "situational determinants." Reporting on sessions in which the subjects (dose usually 1 microgram per kilogram of body weight) were students, nurses, attendants, and physicians, he found that impersonal, hostile, and investigative attitudes on the part of others led to devaluative distortions and hostile responses in the subjects. Flexibility, familiarity, acceptance, and presence of others with common culture ameliorated the LSD reaction, while rigidity, unfamiliarity, nonacceptance, and absence of others with a common culture potentiate the (psychotic) reaction.

13. Turner, W., Almudevar, M., and Merlis, S., "Chemotherapeutic Trials in Psychosis," *American Journal of Psychiatry*, 116: 261, 1959, abstract in

Delysid (LSD-25), Annotated Bibliography, Addendum #2, Sandoz Pharmaceuticals, p. 226.

14. See, for example, Sandison, R., "Discussion Fourth Symposium: Comparison of Drug-Induced and Endogenous Psychoses in Man," in Bradley, P., Deniker, P., and Radouco-Thomas, C., Neuro-Psychopharmacology. Elsevier, Amsterdam, 1959, p. 176. Abstract in Delysid, Addendum #4, p. 330.

15. Smith, C., "A New Adjunct to the Treatment of Alcoholism," Quarterly Journal of Studies on Alcohol, 19: 406-417, 1958; Chwelos, N., Blewett, D., Smith, C., and Hoffer, A., "Use of d-lysergic acid diethylamide in the Treatment of Alcoholism," Ibid., 20: 577-590, 1959; MacLean, J., MacDonald, D., Byrne, U., and Hubbard, A., "The Use of LSD-25 in the Treatment of Alcoholism and Other Psychiatric Problems," Ibid., 22: 34-45, 1961; and Jensen, S., "A Treatment Program for Alcoholics in a Mental Hospital," Ibid., 23: 315-320, 1962. In a subsequent report published in the same journal (24: 443, 1963), Jensen reported that taking LSD is a "transcendental" experience for many alcoholics, producing a subsequent intensification of religious feeling.

16. "Alcoholics Aided in Mind Drug Test," New York Times, May 11, 1965. This same article reports on recent Canadian work and quotes Dr. A. Hoffer, director of psychiatric research at University Hospital, Saskatoon, as saying that out of 600 alcoholic subjects treated with psychedelic drugs, a third have achieved complete abstinence and a quarter have showed "marked improvement."

17. These findings have been much criticized on a variety of grounds including lack of a control group. Unfortunately, more effort seems to have been put into attacking Leary than into trying to duplicate his results.

18. Arendsen-Hein, G., "LSD Therapy: Criminal Psychopaths," in Crocket, R., Sandison, R., and Walk, A. (Eds.), Hallucinogenic Drugs and Their Psy-

chotherapeutic Use. Charles C. Thomas, Springfield, Illinois, 1963, p. 102.

19. "A Simple Tool For Psychiatry," San Francisco Chronicle, June 7, 1965, p. 7. This interview with a Czech psychiatrist, Dr. Stanislav Grof, of the Psychiatric Research Institute of Prague, suggests that Iron Curtain countries are engaging in LSD work quite different from our own and meriting thorough study and investigation.

20. "Euphoria Induced to Ease Pain," Medical World News, August 30, 1963.

21. Kast, E., "Pain and LSD-25: A Theory of Attenuation of Anticipation," in Solomon, D. (Ed.), LSD: The Consciousness-Expanding Drug. G.P. Putnam's Sons, New York, 1964, pp. 241-256.

22. As recently as 1961 a Lancet editorial could declare that "Much more knowledge of good (and ill) effect is needed before LSD can be introduced into the mental welfare curriculum. It remains a talking point whether drug psychosis has most in common with schizophrenia, affective disorder, toxic delirious state, or extended temporal lobe aura, and it is even more doubtful how far it is therapeutically effective." (Lancet 1: 445, 1961.)

23. See, for example, Cohen, S., "Lysergic Acid Diethylamide: Side Effects and Complications," Journal of Nervous and Mental Disorders, 130: 30, 1960. Cohen's report is based on 5,000 LSD and mescaline subjects who received the drugs 25,000 times (LSD dosages 25 to 1,500 micrograms). Among experimental subjects there were no suicide attempts and psychotic reactions lasting longer than forty-eight hours were met with in only 0.8/1,000 of the cases. In patients undergoing therapy the rates were attempted suicide: 1.2/1,000; completed suicide: 0.4/1,000; psychotic reaction over forty-eight hours: 1.8/1,000. Cohen additionally found in this study that exposure to LSD produced no serious prolonged physical side effects. He found LSD to be contraindicated in

the cases of schizoid personalities, epileptics, obsessive compulsives, seriously depressed patients, and persons with serious physical diseases, such as liver damage.

During the course of our own research, no subject ever experienced a post-session psychotic reaction, much less attempted or completed suicide.
24. Cohen, S., *The Beyond Within*, p. 36.
25. Cf. "How Drugs Act on Brain," *MD*, March, 1965, p. 114. (Abstract of a paper by Prof. P. Bradley, Department of Experimental Neuropharmacology, Birmingham University, England.) A thorough discussion of chemical and biochemical aspects of LSD pharmacology is that of Metzner, Ralph, "The Pharmacology of Psychedelic Drugs," *Psychedelic Review*,

June, 1963. An extensive bibliography is appended.
26. If psychotherapy-in-general may be so described.
27. Blum, R., & Associates, *Utopiates: The Use and Users of LSD 25*, Atherton, New York, 1964, pp. 6, 7.
28. This type of reaction to a drug-state "psychosis" is one we have encountered several times. After describing in hair-raising detail the most harrowing sort of experience, the person will go on to say that it was valuable, and claims of consequent enhancement of self-esteem and specific therapeutic benefits may be made. We have never heard a recovered schizophrenic give a similar estimate of the "value" of his psychosis —perhaps another point of differentiation between (some) drug-induced and otherwise originating psychoses.

Chapter Three

1. This latter type of (robot or mechanical man) experience has occurred in sessions conducted by one guide (R.M.), but not in sessions conducted

by the other guide. It appears to be related to this guide's more "materialistic" orientation.

Chapter Four

1. For relevant discussions of the psychology and principles of caricature, see the section on "The Comic" in Ernst Kris, *Psychoanalytic Explorations in Art*, George Allen & Unwin, London, 1953.
2. Same subject previously identified in this chapter as S-4.
3. We might note here that even among professionals in the fields of aesthetics and psychology "empathy" is a rather vague and ill-defined term when its meaning is not drastically limited to such behavior as adopting postures imitative of art works. The drug subjects, like the professionals, find "empathy" a conveniently elastic category.
4. McGovern, W.M., *Jungle Paths and Inca Ruins*, Grosset & Dunlap, 1927, p. 263.
5. Wilkins, H.T., *Devil Trees and Plants of Africa, Asia and South America*,

Haldeman-Julius, Girard, Kansas, 1948, p. 22.
6. "Editor's Essay," *MD*, June, 1965, p. 11.
7. Compare, for example, Duncan Blewett, "Psychedelic Drugs in Parapsychological Research," *International Journal of Parapsychology*, Vol. 5, No. 1, p. 65:

"In order to serve this computer function, the cortex must also serve as a sorting or selective filtering mechanism, such that one idea or quantum of information at a time is called to awareness. This aspect of cortical behavior has been widely discussed. This inhibiting or shutting-out was discussed by Bergson and is cited, for example, by Smythies, who states: 'Usually, ideas of mind-brain relation are thought of wholly in terms of excitation. Brain events excite certain mental events in the mind. However, it is also possible that some brain events normally actively inhibit the spontaneous activity of the mind. When this inhibition is, in turn, suppressed by the specific action of the psychedelic drugs, then the spontaneous activity of the human psyche becomes released or revealed. . . .' "

This theory, and its variations, has been used to explain not just ESP phenomena, but a large part of the entire psychedelic experience.

8. The child's search for the cookie jar was apprehended by the subject as a "vivid mental impression"—she "saw" not eidetic images, but "with the mind's eye."

9. Puharich, Andrija, *Beyond Telepathy*. Doubleday, New York, 1962.

10. We are speaking here mainly of conscious, nondrug-state concern. In the psychedelic sessions the subject very often evidences a concern for his cosmic significance and relationship to God that is far in excess of the interest he displays at other times. Even so, for a majority of subjects, the relationships with other persons are probably of still greater importance.

Chapter Five

1. Another six may have reached this level, and these six did achieve what we regard as authentic mystical experiences, but without the "transformation," or experiencing of drastic and positive change. We will deal with these six "special cases" in our section on mysticism and explain why we separate them from the other eleven. We would add here, too, that the *integral* level has been reached by ten percent of the last sixty subjects, suggesting that as the guiding methodology was refined the percentages tended to increase.

Chapter Six

1. Various other writers have made this distinction between "simple" and "complex" images or, as some misleadingly call them, "hallucinations." For example, Balestrieri, A., "Hallucinatory Mechanisms and the Content of Drug Induced Hallucinations," in Bradley, P., Flügel, F., and Hoch, P., *Neuro-Psychopharmacology*, Vol. 3, Elsevier, Amsterdam, 1964, pp. 388-390. Balestrieri mentions as simple "hallucinations" images and other phenomena including "geometries, colours, sounds without significance, 'stars,' 'lights,' changes in shape, in number, in localization, and so on." His complex "hallucinations" include "images of persons and things, autoscopies, landscapes, etc." He writes (p. 389) that "We believe that rough variances in sensory systems or an interference with the nervous mechanisms indicated by Klüver are more apt to cause elementary or simple hallucinations, at least at first. However, more complex phenomena could, at least in some cases, derive from the activation of images already recorded and retained in the brain." Balestrieri reports simple "hallucinations" in about ninety percent of his subjects. In eighty percent of the cases these were the only ones to appear or else preceded the appearance of the complex "hallucinations." The complex "hallucinations" occurred with twenty percent of the subjects. Without preceding simple "hallucinations," they occurred with only ten and a half percent; and the complex "hallucinations" never preceded the simple ones. It should be noted that his subjects are described as "psychoneurotics or affected by neurological diseases." In our opinion, intelligence and "creativity" may be important factors in determining the occurrence and incidence of complex images. Thus, the very high frequency (almost all) of complex

images among our own subjects who were almost all of superior intelligence and many of whom were engaged in some kind of creative work or displayed considerable imagination.

2. In all of our cases drugs were given orally. Administration by injection seems warranted, if it ever is warranted at all, only for medical purposes.

3. The effects of DMT, in many ways similar to those of LSD, last for only about thirty minutes, as compared to the eight to twelve hours of the typical LSD and peyote intoxications. Also, the injected DMT takes effect almost instantly as compared to the several minutes typically required by the injected LSD.

4. In these cases the reader may wonder

why the subject does not simply open his eyes to escape the horror of the image? Some do, as this subject does, eventually; but, for a while at least, the subject is fascinated by the image and it does not occur to him that he might escape in such a way. In any case, opening the eyes is no guarantee of escape from the anxiety, which then may be projected onto the environment. There would seem to be no way to predict whether, in a particular instance, it would be better to stay with the images or to "change the scene" and risk something even worse.

5. De Beauvoir, Simone, *The Prime of Life*. The World Publishing Company, New York, 1962, pp. 168-170.

Chapter Seven

1. It should be noted that the subject retained this repulsive self-image at the time of his session. The self-image is not in accord with the facts, since the subject has an intelligent, not at all

unattractive appearance.

2. Heard, Gerald, *Explorations*, Vol. 2, "Part Three: Rebirth." World Pacific Records, Hollywood, 1961.

Chapter Eight

1. Huxley, A., "Mescaline and the 'Other World,'" in Cholden, L. (Ed.), *Lysergic Acid Diethylamide and Mescaline in Experimental Psychiatry*. Grune & Stratton, New York, 1956, pp. 48-49.

2. After his session, S steadfastly claimed to be conscious of no information of the sort contained in his account. He agreed, however, that it was "quite possible" that he might have subliminally "picked up" this information through casual reading of a weekly magazine to which he and his family had been regular subscribers since his childhood; but if so, he was not aware of it.

3. It is a frequent occurrence for subjects to experience symbolic or literal materials relating to being in the womb. Thus subjects have reported being locked up in some kind of small confine, being buried in the depths of the earth or swallowed by a monster, etc.

Through some of these symbols the subject experiences a symbolic death with regression to an embryonic state then followed by the experience of being reborn.

4. This proposal to subjects that they consider symbols of religious significance was made in only a few cases and does not substantially affect the statistical incidence of the religious and religious-type experiences as they have occurred in the totality of our cases. Also, the religious symbols were presented only to strongly religious individuals—i.e., persons who would, in any case, almost certainly have introduced religious elements into their drug experience.

5. That is, anachronistic. This bringing together in the same spatial context persons and objects from different temporal ones, is a fairly common experience and sometimes discloses hitherto

unrecognized parallels between individuals, events, ideas, etc.

6. The Prometheus-Faust myth receives extended exemplification in the case of S-3 in the following chapter on religious and mystical experience. That case involves also some of the other mythic motifs.

7. For an interesting and relevant discussion of the place of this motif in patterns relating both to mythology and the unconscious, see Carl Jung's essay, "The Psychology of the Child-Archetype," in Jung, C.G., and Kerenyi, C., *Essays on a Science of Mythology: The Myths of the Divine Child and the Divine Maiden.* Harper Torchbooks, New York, 1963, pp. 70-100.

8. For a further exploration of the meaning and source of the motifs of this subject's experience the reader is referred to Weston, Jessie, *From Ritual to Romance.* Doubleday Anchor Books, Garden City, New York, 1957.

9. Jung, C.G., *op. cit.*, p. 85.

10. Zimmer, H., *The King and the Corpse.* Pantheon Books, Bollingen Series XI, New York, 1948, p. 193.

11. That such props may indicate regression to a childish state is obvious—and one of the cases to follow will illustrate the fact. However, this element is not always present, or certainly is not a factor of major significance in some of the cases we have observed.

12. There would seem to be only very rarely any question of the individual experiencing the *symbolic dramas* because he is not able to approach his conflicts directly and insightfully (as suggested by Betty Eisner, "Observations on Possible Order Within the Unconscious," in Bradley, P., Deniker, P., and Radouco-Thomas, C., *Neuro-Psychopharmacology.* Elsevier, Amsterdam, 1959, p. 441). Rarely, this may be true and then the symbolic drama may provide a means of escaping direct confrontation with the literal materials so that the resolution of problems may occur in a form that does not provoke any strong resistance. (Or so we speculate on the basis of our non-therapeutic experience with experimental subjects.) But much more often, we think, the symbolic drama will require as a constituent prerequisite the working through of the psychodynamic materials on the preceding level; just as the following experience of the integral level usually requires as a constituent prerequisite certain experiences on the symbolic level.

Chapter Nine

1. See, for example, Huxley, Aldous, *The Doors of Perception* and *Heaven and Hell.* Harper & Row, New York, 1963; Heard, Gerald, *The Five Ages of Man.* Julian Press, New York, 1964; Watts, Alan, *The Joyous Cosmology.* Pantheon Books, New York, 1962; and Zaehner, R., *Mysticism, Sacred and Profane,* Oxford University Press, New York, 1961.

At the present writing most of this controversy has not yet erupted into print; but the authors are amazed at the easy acquiescence of seminarians and theologians to the claims of religious and mystic efficacy made for the psychedelic drugs.

2. For a discussion of the physiology of fasting and the psychological changes it produces, see Keys, Ansel, *The Biology of Human Starvation.* University of Minnesota Press, 1950.

3. Huxley owes this phrase to the theory of Henri Bergson that the brain, sense organs, and central nervous system function essentially as organs of selection and elimination. This eliminative process, referred to before, helps protect us from being overwhelmed and disoriented by the vast quantities of useless and irrelevant knowledge that would be ours were we able to perceive the multiplicity of phenomena within our sensory and cognitive field. By screening out the multiplicity and leaving only those perceptions with prag-

matic potential to survival, our awareness is organically inhibited and we
perceive only a fraction of our world.
As Huxley has put it: "Mind at large
is funneled through the reducing valve
of the brain and the nervous system"
and what survives the journey through
the funnel is only "a measly trickle of
the kind of consciousness which will
help us to stay alive on the surface of
this planet." Huxley, *op. cit.*, p. 23.

4. De Felice, Philippe, *Poisons Sacrés,
Ivresses Divines.* Editions Albin, Paris,
1936, p. 363.
5. An interesting reconsideration of these
ideas is to be found in Mary Barnard's
"The God in the Flowerpot," *The
American Scholar,* Autumn, 1963, pp.
578-586: "What . . . was more likely
to happen first," she asks, "the spontaneously generated idea of an afterlife
in which the disembodied soul, liberated from the restrictions of time and
space, experiences eternal bliss, or the
accidental discovery of hallucinogenic
plants that give a sense of euphoria,
dislocate the center of consciousness,
and distort time and space, make
them balloon outward in greatly expanded vistas? . . . the (latter) experience might have had . . . an almost
explosive effect on the largely dormant
minds of men, causing them to think
of things they had never thought of
before. This, if you like, is direct revelation." Miss Barnard goes on to suggest
that "fifty theo-botanists working for
fifty years would make the current
theories concerning the origins of much
mythology and theology as out-of-date
as the pre-Copernican astronomy."
6. Wasson, R.G., "The Hallucinogenic
Fungi of Mexico: An Inquiry into the
Origins of the Religious Idea Among
Primitive Peoples," *Botanical Museum
leaflets Harvard University,* Vol. 19,
No. 7, Cambridge, Massachusetts, Feb.
17, 1961, pp. 156-157.
7. Wasson, R.G., and Wasson, V.,
Mushrooms, Russia and History, Pantheon Books, New York, 1957.
8. Aristides writes in part: "Eleusis is a
shrine common to the whole earth,
and of all the divine things that exist
among men, it is both the most awesome and the most luminous. At what
place in the world have more miraculous tidings been sung, where have the
dromena called forth greater emotion,
*where has there been greater rivalry
between seeing and hearing?"* Quoted
in Otto, W.F., "The Meaning of the
Eleusinian Mysteries," in *The Mysteries: Papers from the Eranos Year-
books,* Joseph Campbell (Ed.), Pantheon Books, Bollingen Series XXX, 2,
New York, 1955, p. 20.
9. Wasson, R.G., "The Hallucinogenic
Fungi of Mexico," pp. 149-150. The
Porphyrius reference is taken from
Giambattista della Porta, *Villa,* Frank-
fort, 1592, p. 764.
10. Quoted in Harman, W.W., "The
Issue of the Consciousness-Expanding
Drugs," *Main Currents in Modern
Thought,* Vol. 20, No. 1, Sept.-Oct.
1963, p. 6.
11. It should also be noted, however,
that Huxley was the first to caution
moderation with regard to the expectation of the mystical efficacy of the psychedelic drugs. "I am not so foolish,"
he wrote, "as to equate what happens
under the influence of mescalin or of
any other drug, prepared or in the future preparable, with the realization of
the end and ultimate purpose of human life: Enlightenment, the Beatific
Vision. All I am suggesting is that the
mescalin experience is what the Catholic theologians call 'a gratuitous grace,'
not necessary to salvation but potentially helpful and to be accepted thank-
fully, if made available. To be shaken
out of the ruts of ordinary perception,
to be shown for a few timeless hours
the outer and the inner world, not as
they appear to an animal obsessed with
survival or to a human being obsessed
with words and notions, but as they are
apprehended, directly and uncondition-
ally, by Mind at Large—this is an
experience of inestimable value to
everyone and especially to the intellectual." Huxley, *op. cit.*, p. 73.
12. Stace, W.T., *Mysticism and Philosophy,* J.B. Lippincott Co., Philadelphia
and New York, 1960.

13. Pahnke, Walter N., *Drugs and Mysticism: An Analysis of the Relationship between Psychedelic Drugs and the Mystical Consciousness.* A thesis presented to the Committee on Higher Degrees in History and Philosophy of Religion, Harvard University, June, 1963. This thesis is available at the Harvard University Library, Cambridge, Massachusetts, although restricted for five years. Before this time persons may write the author at 277 West 14 Place, Chicago Heights, Illinois, for permission to obtain a microfilm of the thesis.

14. Leary, T., "The Religious Experience: Its Production and Interpretation," *Psychedelic Review*, Vol. 1, No. 3 (1964), p. 325.

15. McGlothlin, W.H., *Long-Lasting Effects of LSD on Certain Attitudes in Normals.* Printed for private distribution by the RAND Corporation.

16. Ditman, K.S., Hayman, M., and Whittlesay, J.R.B., "Nature and Frequency of Claims Following LSD," *Journal of Nervous and Mental Disease*, Vol. 134 (1962), pp. 336-352. And:
Savage, C., Harman, W.W., Fadiman, J., and Savage, E., "A Follow-up Note on the Psychedelic Experience." Paper delivered at a meeting of the American Psychiatric Association, St. Louis, Missouri, May, 1963.

17. Slotkin, J., *The Peyote Religion.* Free Press, Glencoe, Illinois, 1956.

18. Smith, Huston, "Do Drugs Have Religious Import?" *The Journal of Philosophy*, Vol. LXI, No. 18, Sept. 17, 1964. This article has been reprinted in Solomon, D. (Ed.), *LSD: The Consciousness-Expanding Drug*, G.P. Putnam's Sons, New York, 1964, and the above quotation may be found on p. 159 of that volume. In the same article Dr. Smith suggests that Zaehner's disaffection with the drug may be due in part to the fact that his own mescaline experience was by his own admission "utterly trivial." Also, Zaehner is a convert to Roman Catholicism and thus may feel bound to uphold the Church's official position that mystical experience is a gift of grace and as such can never come under man's control.

19. On the other hand, and as we noted at the outset, it is possible to go to the opposite extreme. Then, only pathology is perceived and, through reduction and misunderstanding, authentic mystical experience becomes nothing more than depersonalization, etc.

20. James, William, *The Varieties of Religious Experience*, Modern Library, New York, 1902, pp. 378-379.

21. This notion of a kind of symbolic animal hierarchy related to stages of human development has come up with several of the psychedelic drug subjects. The case of S-7 in our chapter on the body image offers, as will become clear, some especially striking correspondences to the present case.

22. Dosages on each occasion was 250 micrograms LSD.

23. This incident of "sitting down before the Majesty of God" carried with it no real sense of confronting God. Later, S was not certain that "God was there at all. Perhaps this was only a place where meetings with God were supposed to be held."

24. Stace, W.T., *Mysticism and Philosophy*, pp. 110-111.

25. Stace, *ibid.*, p. 79.

26. William Blake, "The Marriage of Heaven and Hell," xxii.

27. William Wordsworth, "Tintern Abbey."

Compare with this the similar sentiments in Robert Browning when he has the young David sing:
"I but open my eyes,—and perfection, no more and no less,
In the kind I imagined full-fronts me, and God is seen God
In the star, in the stone, in the flesh, in the soul and the clod."
("Saul," xvii.)

28. Underhill, E., *Mysticism*, Meridian Books, New York, 1955, pp. 255-256.
In the same work, Evelyn Underhill records a remarkable instance of cosmological mysticism to be found in the *Journal* of George Fox. Here, as in Boehme's case, there is the insistence

on having been the recipient of a revelation concerning the nature of objective reality:

"Now I was come up in spirit through the flaming sword into the Paradise of God. All things were new: and all the creation gave another smell unto me than before, beyond what words can utter. . . . The creation was opened to me; and it was showed me how all things had their names given them, according to their nature and virtue. And I was at a stand in my mind whether I should practice physic for the good of mankind, seeing the nature and virtue of the creatures were so opened to me by the Lord . . . Great things did the Lord lead me unto, and wonderful depths were opened unto me beyond what can by words be declared; but as people come into subjection to the Spirit of God, and grow up in the image and power of the Almighty, they may receive the word of wisdom that opens all things, and come to know the

hidden unity and the Eternal Being." (George Fox, *Journal*, Vol. 1, cap. ii; quoted on pp. 257-258 of the Underhill volume.)

29. Leary, T., "The Religious Experience: Its Production and Interpretation," *Psychedelic Review*, Vol. 1, No. 3, 1964, pp. 324-346.

30. In this case, the fact that S had been for many years a dedicated student of Eastern disciplines explains certain epiphenomena—especially, the initiation in which she received the "third eye" as a mark of her enlightenment— which may seem puzzling to the reader not too well acquainted with this field.

31. Quoted by Huston Smith, *op. cit.*, p. 159.

32. Some portions of this and the preceding chapter first appeared in Jean Houston's article, "Psycho-Chemistry and the Religious Consciousness." *International Philosophical Quarterly*, Vol. V, No. 3, September, 1965, Pp. 397-413.